The Enlightened Eater

Rosie Schwartz

The Enlightened Eater

Macmillan Canada
Toronto

Canadian Cataloguing in Publication Data
Schwartz, Rosie
    The enlightened eater

4th ed.
First ed. by Marion Kane and Rosie Schwartz. Includes index.
ISBN 0-7715-9050-4

1. Cookery. 2. Diet. 3. Nutrition. I. Title.

TX355.K35 1994   641.1   C94-930582-0

Design: Ivan Holmes
Cover: Gillian Tsintziras/The Brookview Group

Macmillan Canada wishes to thank the Canada Council and the Ontario Ministry of Culture and Communications for supporting its publishing program.

Macmillan Canada
A Division of Canada Publishing Corporation
Toronto, Canada

   2 3 4 5 — 98 97 96 95

Printed in Canada

To my husband, Earl, who besides being the best taster has been invaluable in his role as an editor as well as medical consultant; to my daughters, Alyssa for her willingness to try new dishes, and Farrah, who is a joy to watch in the kitchen.

Contents

Acknowledgments

Many thanks to Janet Cornish for her help in testing the recipes of the first edition; and to Mary Fabiano and Marg Howard for their assistance in the recipe testing.

I would also like to thank my parents, Julius and Elsa Fuss, for their support, with a special thanks to my mother for her endless help in coming up with recipe ideas.

Through the Nutrition Maze

Nutrition continues to be one of the hottest topics around as more and more evidence surfaces about how our food choices affect our well-being. There's no question that this trend will continue right through the 1990s. But with this new awareness of food and nutrition has come some not so welcome attitudes. Eating right has almost become a moral issue. Those who opt for less wholesome fare are sometimes looked down upon for "loose behaviour."

Others live their lives in fear of food. Eating has become an exercise in avoidance. Every media report panning a food item is taken to heart, and purveyors of supplements then coax these people into a diet of capsules. Food can no longer be enjoyed.

It's time to get back to the pleasures of eating.

On the other hand, we can't ignore that heart disease, cancer and osteoporosis are but a few of society's ailments that have been linked to what's on our plates.

We're living in a time of increasing travel abroad and enjoying greater ethnic diversity in our cities. As a result, we're exposed to a cornucopia of different foods in our own neighbourhoods. All of this adds up to a lot of confusion over what's in our foods as well as what we should be eating.

We're also inundated with information on the subject of weight loss. Every week it seems we hear about a new "magic" diet. Someone at a party swears that she has lost ten pounds in two weeks by eating nothing but fruit for breakfast. A celebrity on a TV talk show gushes about his instant formula for shedding pounds. And we fall prey to these diets, in spite of the "anti-diet" messages we hear. "This will be the last crash diet." Today more than half the North American population thinks it's overweight, so little wonder that fad diets continue to be the scam of the decade.

Instead, we should try to maintain a healthy body weight and at the same time teach our children to accept the different shapes and sizes of those who make up our society. Maybe then we'll begin to see a decline in the alarming incidence of eating disorders.

The Enlightened Eater addresses nutrition for the life cycle from infancy through the golden years. Topics such as nutrition for singles, vegetarianism, caffeine, alcohol, and the role that exercise plays in nutrition are included.

Eating right rather than *not eating* is my focus for successful weight loss and a more natural weight-management plan.

In my private practice I find that many people are very much aware of what's current on the nutrition scene but aren't able to make the necessary changes. My role is to help bridge the gap between what they know they should be eating and what they actually are eating. I hope that *The Enlightened Eater* will help readers bridge that gap too.

Above all else, when we're trying to be well-nourished the food must taste good. It's got to be even better than good if we're trying to change our daily food habits by eating lighter when eating alone, feeding a family, or entertaining friends. This new way of eating has to compete with the food of days gone by when the sky was the limit and you could just throw on lots of butter or salt to "improve" the taste of a dish.

The Enlightened Eater contains recipes which will show you that healthful eating can be a most pleasurable experience. I hope you will enjoy the recipes in *The Enlightened Eater* and that they'll help you learn to adapt old favourites to a new style of eating.

Accompanying the recipes are nutrient values per individual serving. When recipes make variable servings, the nutrient values apply to the smaller serving. For example, if a recipe makes twelve to fifteen muffins, the nutrient values apply to one muffin out of a batch of fifteen.

The appendixes are tables of nutrient contents of various foods. These will be helpful to those of you who want more specific nutritional information about your food. For example, if you want to increase the amount of fibre in your diet, you can skim down the fibre column in Appendix A to find a high-fibre food you like to eat. Another use of the nutrient tables can be to determine one day's intake of a particular vitamin, mineral, or other nutrient.

Finally, keep in mind that although the information in this book may help enlighten you on the subject of food and nutrition, you must adapt your eating habits to your own likes, dislikes, and lifestyle. Saying that you'll eat better when you start eating at home isn't going to work if you eat most of your meals in restaurants.

Remember, even though food and nutrition play a vital role in health and well-being, eating is one of life's great pleasures. Let's not misuse our knowledge of nutrition and turn the art of eating into a science. Eat and enjoy!

The
Enlightened
Eater

1   Food Group Dynamics

Our bodies need more than 50 nutrients every day to achieve optimal health. These nutrients are carbohydrate, fat, protein, vitamins, minerals, fibre, and water. Optimal health means that all body functions, which run the gamut from building and maintaining cells to regulating bodily processes and supplying energy, are working efficiently.

As for the amounts in which these nutrients should be consumed, studies have come up with recommended levels of intake to maintain the health of an already healthy individual. In Canada these recommendations are called *Recommended Nutrient Intakes* (RNI). In the United States they have the title *Recommended Dietary Allowances* (RDA). However, figures showing these recommended intakes are of little help unless nutrient requirements are translated into actual foods. In Canada, the *Canada's Food Guide For Healthy Eating* was developed to do just this. This framework groups together those foods that have similar nutrients. Because these nutrients are similar, not identical, it is important to remember that a great variety of foods must be eaten to achieve top-notch nutrient balance.

No one food group can provide all the necessary nutrients. Nor are there any redundant food groups. A person who misses out on one food group on a regular basis is likely to suffer from nutritional deficiencies. Someone who is forced to do so because of allergies, for example, must make special adjustments to his or her diet.

The key is balance. And a balanced meal pattern for the average person means eating foods from all the food groups. Because the science of nutrition is currently attracting more and more attention, research into it is growing. And more connections between various nutrients and health are being discovered. One must therefore keep in mind that nutritional recommendations are not written in stone and may be revised as more information is assessed.

When you are choosing from the four basic food groups (meat and alternatives, grains, vegetables and fruits, and dairy products), it is important to keep other factors in mind too—in particular, how much fat and fibre go hand in hand with other nutrients. After all, there's a big nutritional difference between a baked potato consumer with its fibre-laden skin and a plate of oily french fries!

The Enlightened Eater's Food Guide on pages 4 and 5 adds an extra dimension to the food group framework because it shows the four food groups *and* breaks down foods in each group by their nutritional quality. The "Cream of the Crop" are the best overall food choices because they take into account fat, fibre, sugar, and salt. "Go for It" includes good choices that do not, however, get a top-notch rating. "Proceed with Caution" includes foods that are lower on the nutritional scale or foods that may be loaded with nutrition but have drawbacks. Examples are eggs and liver, which contain high levels of cholesterol along with valuable protein, vitamins, and minerals. "Food Group Flunkies" may or may not contain nutrients, but their drawbacks outweigh their virtues. It's a good idea not to eat such foods on a regular basis.

Two things are crucial to remember: first, when it comes to eating well, variety truly is the spice of life; and second, an individual's stage in the life cycle can affect the amounts of food eaten from each food group. For example, a growing adolescent or menopausal woman needs to dip more heavily into the dairy food group than does a 25-year-old man.

Energy-Yielding Nutrients
The nutrients required by our bodies can be divided into two main categories: those that yield energy (calories) and those that do not. Nutrients that yield energy are carbohydrate, protein, and fat. Alcohol is the only substance that contains calories but no nutrients.

Calorie

A calorie is the amount of energy or heat required to raise one litre of water one degree. When foods are burned up by the body, they give off energy or heat, which can be measured in calories. Protein and carbohydrate both contain four calories per gram. Fat harbours nine calories per gram and alcohol seven. A balanced diet should be made up of at least 55 percent of total calories from carbohydrate, 15 percent of total calories from protein, and no more than 30 percent of total calories from fat.

Carbohydrate

Carbohydrate consists either of simple sugars or of starch broken down by the body to yield energy.

Natural sugars are sugars that exist naturally in food. For example, lactose is the sugar in milk. Fructose is the sugar in fruits and vegetables, and sucrose is the sugar found in refined table sugar. Sugars, which can be identified by their *ose* ending, also include dextrose, maltose, and glucose, among others.

Refined sugars contribute calories without any redeeming nutrients and are often referred to as "empty calorie" foods. Our society's excessive sugar consumption goes hand in hand with eating too much fat and not enough nutrient-rich foods. Hence a large number of people are overweight.

A spoonful of sugar may make the medicine go down, and it often comes from obvious sources. But sugar does not always come on spoons, and it is particularly prevalent in many processed foods. Refined sugars sometimes appear on package labels simply as sugar (white or brown), but they can also show up in a number of disguises: as honey, glucose, fructose, corn syrup, dextrose, and liquid invert sugar. Because ingredients are listed in descending order of quantity, the closer sugar is to the beginning of the list, the higher the sugar content of the food. Even if sugar is not the first ingredient, it may be the dominant one when the various versions listed are combined.

Long chains of simple sugars are called *complex carbohydrates*. In humans complex carbohydrates are stored as glycogen. In plants they are stored as starch. When starch is broken down by the body, it becomes simple sugars that end up in the blood as blood sugar, or *glucose*. Glucose is essential to fuel our brain and muscles. If we consume too much carbohydrate, the excess glucose is removed from the bloodstream and stored in small amounts in the liver and muscles as glycogen. Once these glycogen stores are filled, excess carbohydrate is turned into fat and stored for future energy.

Protein
Protein is essential to build and repair body tissues, and this is its primary function. It can also provide energy in the absence of adequate carbohydrate. However, this is not the best use of protein because many of its benefits are not taken advantage of.

Fat
Fat can be used for energy when carbohydrate is not available. However, it produces more than twice as much energy (calories) as carbohydrate and can have other negative nutritional effects too.

THE ENLIGHTENED EATER'S FOOD GUIDE

Recommended servings are per day.	MILK PRODUCTS Children up to 11 years: 2–3 servings Adolescents: 3–4 servings Pregnant, nursing, and post- menopausal women: 3–4 servings Adults: 2 servings	GRAIN PRODUCTS 6 or more servings

Cream of the Crop	1 cup/250 mL skim milk
	4 tbsp./20 mL skim-milk powder
	$\frac{3}{4}$ cup/175 mL skim-milk yogurt
	$1\frac{1}{2}$ oz./45 g skim-milk cheese
	$\frac{1}{2}$ cup/125 mL evaporated
	  skim milk
		1 slice whole-grain bread
		$\frac{1}{2}$ cup/125 mL whole-grain
		  cereal
		Snack foods like air-popped,
		  unsalted popcorn, $1\frac{1}{2}$ cups/
		  375 mL

Go for It	1 cup/250 mL 2% milk
	$\frac{3}{4}$ cup/175 mL 2% yogurt
	$1\frac{1}{2}$ oz./45 g part-skim cheese
	  (less than 15% B.F.)
	Fruit-flavoured skim-milk yogurt
	$\frac{1}{2}$ cup/125 mL evaporated
	  2% milk
		Refined, enriched breads and
		  cereals
		Whole-grain baked goods like
		  muffins
		Homemade granolas

Proceed with Caution	1 cup/250 mL whole milk $\frac{3}{4}$ cup/175 mL whole-milk yogurt $1\frac{1}{2}$ oz./45 g whole-milk cheese Fruit-flavoured yogurt Low-fat chocolate milk	Enriched, sugared cereals Buttered popcorn Commercial granolas High-fat crackers

Food Group Flunkies	Whipping cream
	Cream cheese
	Sour cream
	Ice cream
	Sweetened condensed milk
	Butter
	High-fat processed cheese
	  spreads
		Commercial granola bars
		Cakes, pies, pastries
		Croissants
		Doughnuts
		High-fat snack foods like
		  commercial tortilla chips,
		  cheese puffs, etc.

MEAT AND ALTERNATIVES
2 regular or 3 smaller servings

VEGETABLES AND FRUITS
5 or more servings
Choose at least 2 vegetables.
Include orange and dark
green vegetables and
orange fruit.

2–3 oz./60–85 g lean fish, fresh, frozen, or canned in water and unsalted

$\frac{1}{2}$ cup/125 mL cottage cheese

1 cup/250 mL dried legumes (peas, beans), when complemented

Fresh fruits and vegetables, properly stored, $\frac{1}{2}$ cup/125 mL or 1 medium

Frozen vegetables, no sauce

Canned vegetables, no salt added

2–3 oz./60–85 g lean meat, chicken, turkey, fatty fish, or shellfish, fresh, frozen, or canned in oil and salt, rinsed

Canned fish in broth or oil and salt, rinsed

2 oz./60 g skim-milk cheese

$\frac{1}{2}$ cup/125 mL unsweetened fruit juice

$\frac{1}{2}$ cup/125 mL canned fruit in its juice

Canned vegetables, salt added

$\frac{1}{2}$ cup/125 mL nuts or seeds

4 tbsp./20 mL peanut butter

2 eggs

2 oz./60 g liver

2 oz./60 g duck or goose

2 oz./60 g untrimmed meat or lean processed meat

2 oz./60 g battered or fried fish or chicken

2 oz./60 g whole-milk cheese

2 oz./60 g pickled or smoked meat

$\frac{1}{2}$ cup/125 mL sweetened fruit juice

$\frac{1}{2}$ cup/125 mL canned fruit in sugar syrup

Frozen vegetables in sauce

Hot dogs

Salty, high-fat processed meats

Side bacon or bacon bits, regular or simulated

Fruit drinks

Gelatin desserts

Fruit pies

Potato chips, regular french fries, onion rings

Fruit-flavoured yogurt

On the positive side, fat contains linoleic acid—our one essential fatty acid because it cannot be manufactured by our bodies. Fat also aids in the absorption of fat-soluble vitamins and acts as insulation as well as a sort of cushion for the body.

Vital Vitamins

Vitamins are organic (living) compounds that the body needs, in small amounts, to promote growth and maintain life. Minerals, which the body also needs in small amounts, are inorganic (non-living) and are thus classified separately from vitamins.

The key to any discussion of vitamins is the phrase *in small amounts*, because this is how they exist in food. Vitamins consumed in larger amounts, such as in the treatment of illness, are another matter; they should be considered drugs or therapeutic agents rather than food. Vitamins should be consumed not indiscriminately, but with the same caution as medication.

Regular, consistent intake of both vitamins and minerals is, however, very important. Although a lack of either may not cause a deficiency immediately (it could take a long time, sometimes years, to manifest itself), a deficiency could remain at a subclinical, barely discernible level and be detrimental to a person's health. Regular, day-to-day intake of vitamins and minerals is crucial; small lapses can easily add up.

There are two main categories of vitamins: water-soluble and fat-soluble.

Water-Soluble Vitamins

Because they are soluble in water, these vitamins can easily be lost by leaching into cooking water during food preparation. (This is discussed in detail in Chapter 5.) Water-soluble vitamins consist of the B vitamins and vitamin C.

Thiamin
(Vitamin B1)

Sources of thiamin are whole-grain and enriched cereals, meats like pork, beef, and lamb, nuts, and legumes.
Thiamin helps the body use carbohydrates as energy. It also promotes normal appetite and contributes to the functioning of the body's nervous system. The greater the carbohydrate intake, the greater the need for thiamin. The same is true for alcohol: the more it is consumed, the greater the recommended requirement for thiamin.

Riboflavin

The best source of riboflavin is milk and its by-products.

Other sources include green vegetables, fish, eggs, liver, meat, and enriched breads and cereals. Riboflavin is sensitive to light, so storing milk in a clear container results in some loss of this nutrient.

Riboflavin is needed to convert protein, fat, and carbohydrate into energy. It also does wonders for the skin, eyes, and nervous system.

Niacin

Niacin comes from liver, meat, fish, poultry, peanuts, and enriched cereals. It helps the body get energy from carbohydrates, protein, and fat. It also helps keep the nervous system and digestive tract healthy.

Some physicians are prescribing niacin in large doses in the fight against heart disease. The amounts prescribed can really be considered a drug, however, because of the possible side effects: severe body flushing, dry skin, intestinal disorders and, sometimes, abnormal liver function. Because of these possible side effects, niacin as a treatment for lowering blood cholesterol should be used only under the supervision of a physician.

Pyridoxine
(Vitamin B6)

Liver, beef, lamb, pork, salmon, whole-grain cereals, lima beans, cabbage, potatoes, spinach, and grapes are prime sources of pyridoxine.

Pyridoxine is necessary for the metabolism of protein and helps the nervous system function normally. As well, women who take oral contraceptives should eat plenty of pyridoxine-rich foods, because it is thought that the pill increases one's need for this vitamin. The verdict is not yet in on whether vitamin B6 is an effective treatment for Pre-Menstrual Syndrome (PMS), but the side effects of taking too much have been documented. Even 50 mg a day over a long period of time can cause sensory nerve changes that decrease a person's sensitivity to hot and cold. Once the person stops taking the vitamin, these symptoms disappear. However, very large doses may result in permanent nerve damage.

Pantothenic Acid

Almost all foods contain pantothenic acid, but especially good sources are whole-grain cereals and organ meats. Pantothenic acid is required for the metabolism of protein, fat, and carbohydrate. It also plays an important role in the manufacture of hemoglobin, steroid hormones, cholesterol, and fatty acids.

Biotin

Among the foods high in biotin are egg yolks, milk, and organ meats. Nuts, cereals, and legumes are other sources. Biotin is necessary for the release of energy from carbohydrates as well as for the metabolism of fat and protein.

Folacin
(Folic Acid)

Folacin comes from dark green, leafy vegetables like spinach and also from liver and kidneys. As with the other B vitamins, this vitamin can easily be lost during food preparation.

Folacin is needed to keep red blood cells healthy, to prevent macrocytic anemia and in the manufacture of genes. Lack of it may play a role in the development of certain birth defects called neural tube defects. Supplementing the diets of women likely to give birth to infants with these defects has been shown to decrease the risk. Pregnant women need a folacin-rich diet, too.

Vitamin B12

Liver and kidneys are especially rich in vitamin B12. It is also found in meat, fish, eggs, milk, and milk products. The only natural sources of B12 are animal ones. Some foods, such as soy milk, are fortified with it.

Vitamin B12 is of prime importance in the synthesis of hemoglobin and maintenance of healthy red blood cells. A lack can result in pernicious anemia. It is also important for the nervous and digestive systems.

Ascorbic Acid
(Vitamin C)

Good sources of vitamin C are fruit and vegetables such as citrus fruits, broccoli, cabbage, tomatoes, peppers, cantaloupe, and strawberries.

Vitamin C is important for the manufacture of collagen, which acts as a cementing agent, binding cells together. It also helps to heal wounds, absorb iron, and maintain healthy teeth and gums. Vitamin C–rich foods may play a role in preventing certain cancers.

Vitamin C has been touted as a cure-all for a number of ailments, in particular the common cold. Doses advocated in such cases are sometimes more than 100 times the recommended amount. Studies have not conclusively proved the benefits of such megadoses of vitamin C. It doesn't appear to prevent colds, though large doses may decrease the severity of the symptoms. In some people, these megadoses may result in nausea and diarrhea or nosebleeds. Cigarette smoking has been shown to increase the need for vitamin C, so smokers might do well to boost their consumption of vitamin C-rich foods.

Fat-Soluble Vitamins
These vitamins are soluble in fat and, in most cases, when consumed in excess, are stored in the body.

Vitamin A Good sources of vitamin A are liver, kidneys, eggs, milk, yellow and dark green leafy vegetables, and fruit.

One of the main benefits of vitamin A is taught by the old adage that carrots help you see in the dark. Because this vitamin aids in the formation of "visual purple" (rhodopsin), it is necessary for night vision. It is also important for keeping the skin and the body's inner linings healthy, helping the body resist infection, promoting growth, and maintaining teeth, hair, bones, and glands.

However, taking large doses of vitamin A supplements can be dangerous. The symptoms of vitamin A toxicity include fatigue, headaches, loss of hair and nails, vomiting, skin changes, and enlargement of the liver. Beta-carotene, also known as provitamin A is a yellowish-orange pigment found in fruits and vegetables and appears to play a role in decreasing the risk of heart disease and certain cancers. (See Radical Behaviour, page 127.) Beta-carotene supplements do not have the same toxic effects as their relative, vitamin A.

Vitamin D The main source of vitamin D is milk that has been fortified with it. Vitamin D does not occur naturally in plant foods but is found in certain fish, such as salmon. It also exists in limited amounts in eggs and meat.

Vitamin D is produced by the body when sunlight irradiates a compound called 7-dehydrocholesterol, which is present in the skin. (This is one example of how the body needs a certain amount of cholesterol.) Vitamin D requirements can be met by food alone, by sunlight alone, or by a combination of the two.

Vitamin D is important for the body's absorption of calcium and phosphorus, two minerals needed to keep bones and teeth healthy. It also helps regulate certain substances in the blood.

Because this vitamin is fat-soluble, excess amounts are stored in the body. Toxic doses can cause loss of appetite, vomiting, and weight loss. They can also cause high levels of calcium in the blood, which can in turn produce calcium deposits in such tissues as the lungs and kidneys. Overdoses of vitamin D over long periods of time can even result in death. Foods are therefore fortified with care. Individuals must also be careful when taking vitamin D supplements such as fish liver oils. However, a person whose diet is low in calcium, who does not drink milk, and who has little exposure to sunlight should ensure that he or she has some dietary source of vitamin D.

Vitamin E is found in polyunsaturated fats such as poyunsaturated oils and margarines, leafy green vegetables, and some nuts and seeds like almonds and sunflower seeds. It is present to a lesser extent in whole grains, meat, and eggs. It is added to some foods as a preservative to prolong shelf life.

Contrary to popular belief, vitamin E has no magic powers that will do wonders for your sex life! One beneficial property it does possess, though, is that it takes up oxygen (is oxidized) before other compounds in the body. This is particularly beneficial for preventing the oxidization—the destruction—of vitamins A and C. The same process occurs with polyunsaturated fats, a fact that explains why vitamin E is used to prevent them from going rancid. This vitamin also helps keep the body's cell membranes intact. Research is pointing towards a protective effect of vitamin E against heart disease and certain cancers. (See Radical Behaviour, page 127.)

More research is needed before safe doses of supplementation can be determined.

Vitamin K   Vitamin K comes from soybean oil, liver, and dark green leafy vegetables. It plays an important role in blood coagulation. Without it, blood cannot clot, and uncontrolled bleeding can result.

Mineral Matters
Minerals are inorganic compounds found in all foods, whether of animal or plant origin. They come from the earth and are passed on through living things by foods and water.

Minerals exist in varying amounts from soil to soil. If certain minerals have become depleted in the soil of a particular area, crops grown in it will be deficient in those minerals. As well as minerals that act as nutrients, there are those—arsenic, lead, and mercury—that should be avoided because of their toxicity.

Minerals fall into two categories depending on the amounts stored in our bodies. *Macronutrient minerals* found in larger amounts are calcium, phosphorus, sodium, chlorine, potassium, magnesium, and sulphur. *Micronutrient*, or *trace, minerals*, although stored in extremely small amounts, are just as vital to good health. These are iron, fluorine, iodine, molybdenum, chromium, cobalt, copper, zinc, selenium, and manganese.

Calcium   Calcium has lately been the subject of much discussion in nutrition circles. It is stored by the body to be used as needed and is required for several functions. It is necessary for digestion and aids in blood clotting. Current research is also investigating a lack of calcium in the diet as a possible role in the development of hypertension. In addition, calcium is a crucial component in nerve-impulse transmission and muscle contraction, the latter of which is particularly important for the normal contraction and relaxation of the heart muscle. If necessary, the body will dip into its calcium storage spots, namely bones and teeth, to enable the heart to function normally.

One buzzword we hear these days is the disease caused by the lack of calcium—*osteoporosis*. The bones of a tiny infant are softer than the bones of an adult. As the child matures, calcium, along with other minerals like phosphorus, is deposited in the bone tissue and builds strong, hard bones. As the body needs calcium for other purposes, it takes it from the bones. This process is called *calcium exchange*. If our diet is rich in calcium, this mineral is constantly replaced, and so the process continues. However, if our diet is lacking in calcium, osteoporosis can result.

Osteoporosis causes the bones to become brittle and porous. This means that they can easily break or fracture. A person who has osteoporosis often has a "dowager's hump," or curvature of the spine, and problems with his or her teeth caused by a deterioration in the jawbones. An afflicted person becomes so fragile that he or she can fracture a bone from merely a sneeze or a hug. Particularly unfortunate is the fact that once osteoporosis has developed, the bones cannot be strengthened. Although treatments are being studied that could stop the disease from progressing, the only way we can currently deal with it is by prevention.

Osteoporosis strikes one in four women in varying degrees but can also affect men. Other factors associated with it are heredity, fair skin, lack of sex hormones in women, lack of weight-bearing exercise, and diet. Although we cannot control our skin colour, we can regulate the amount of exercise we do and what we eat. Inadequate calcium is a known cause of osteoporosis; caffeine, cigarette smoke, and alcohol are considered possible causes. Pre- and post-menopausal women are thought to need 1,200 to 1,500 mg of calcium a day, compared to the 800-mg daily requirement of average adult women.

CALCIUM CONTENT OF VARIOUS FOODS

Food	Amount	Calcium Content (mg) (approximate)
Milk, low fat or whole	1 cup/250 mL	314
Skim milk powder, dry	$\frac{1}{4}$ cup/50 mL	375
Yogurt, plain	$\frac{3}{4}$ cup/175 mL	319
Yogurt, fruit-flavoured	$\frac{3}{4}$ cup/175 mL	296
Cheese, hard, natural	$1\frac{1}{2}$ oz./45 g	325
Cheese, processed	1 1-oz./30-g slice	277
Cottage cheese	1 cup/250 mL	164
Ice cream	$\frac{1}{2}$ cup/125 mL	80
Sardines, canned	$3\frac{1}{2}$ oz./100 g	437
Salmon, canned with bones	3 oz./90 g	250
Tofu, made with calcium	$\frac{1}{2}$ cup/125 mL	150
Beans (kidney, lima, chickpeas), cooked	1 cup/250 mL	74
Soybeans, cooked	1 cup/250 mL	139
Almonds	2 tbsp./25 mL	50
Broccoli	$\frac{1}{2}$ cup/125 mL	45
Greens, mustard and beet	$\frac{1}{2}$ cup/125 mL	86
Rhubarb, cooked	$\frac{1}{2}$ cup/125 mL	184
Orange	1 medium	52
Molasses, blackstrap	1 tbsp./15 mL	144

Calcium is as crucial for the development and maintenance of strong teeth as it is for those of bones, but there is less calcium exchange between teeth and the rest of the body than is the case with bones. It is therefore vital that children consume enough calcium when their teeth are forming; otherwise, their teeth will become soft, with all the problems that ensue. Conversely, children who get plenty of calcium have a good chance of developing strong, healthy teeth that are resistant to decay.

A calcium-rich diet may have other perks for women. A six-month study of 78 women in New York found that those who supplemented their diets with calcium had fewer symptoms of Premenstral Syndrome.

The mineral may also have an effect in lowering blood pressure. A recent study at the University of Montreal showed that people with a low intake of dietary calcium may be more at risk of developing hypertension. The effects of diet in terms of sodium, calcium, and alcohol intake were examined, and some of the findings were not unexpected. Sodium and alcohol were found to contribute to the elevation of blood pressure; but in those who also consumed large amounts of dietary calcium, sodium was found to have no effect on blood pressure. Calcium seemed to have a protective effect on those consuming alcohol, as well.

Absorption is another important factor to consider when discussing calcium. Both vitamin D- and lactose-containing foods such as milk enhance calcium absorption. So does lactose-hydrolyzed milk; thus, people with lactose intolerance need not miss out. It used to be thought that if the body's intake of phosphorus was higher than that of calcium, calcium absorption would be reduced, but recent studies have proved this invalid. However, an adequate phosphorus intake ensures good calcium absorption.

A severe excess of protein in the diet can hinder calcium absorption. So can such compounds as phytic and oxalic acid, which bind some of the calcium in food, making it unavailable for absorption. Phytic acid is found mainly in cereals but also in some other foods including nuts; oxalic acid occurs mainly in vegetables like spinach, beets, and rhubarb. These foods are all high in fibre, and because we are being encouraged to boost our fibre intake, it is particularly important that our diets are also rich in calcium.

Smoking also appears to have a negative influence

on the body's calcium balance, as does a lack of exercise. People who are inactive or bedridden have a negative calcium balance, which means that their bodies are taking calcium from their bones for other needs. Research is currently investigating the effects of regular, weight-bearing exercise on the body's use of calcium. Aluminum-containing antacids taken for gastric discomfort can also negatively affect calcium absorption, something that is especially important for the elderly to consider, for they are often on long-term antacid therapy.

This discussion points to a pretty positive picture of one food as the ideal source of calcium—namely, milk.

Milk contains vitamin D, lactose, and phosphorus without the binding effects of the phytic and oxalic acids in plant foods. This makes milk the best choice for people who tolerate it. Other sources of calcium, however, such as sardines and salmon with their bones (conveniently precooked in the can), should not be ignored, because they can contribute appreciable amounts of calcium as well as variety to the diet.

With all the concern over what a lack of calcium in the diet can do, many people are turning to supplements. This is not advisable without consulting a physician about possible side effects, such as the formation of kidney stones.

Phosphorus
Sources of phosphorus are plentiful: dairy products, meats, fish, eggs, and peanuts.

The body uses phosphorus in the form of *phosphate*, which is required for the formation of teeth and bones. Like calcium, phosphorus also plays a role in energy release, protein synthesis, and fat transport, as well as being a component in the body's manufacture of genes. We also need phosphorus in our diets to ensure calcium absorption.

Protein foods yield a high amount of phosphates. Carbonated drinks contain considerable amounts of phosphates, but they are a kind that do not help with calcium absorption.

Iron
Iron is necessary for the production of hemoglobin—that part of the red blood cells that carries oxygen throughout the body. When the body lacks iron, there is not enough oxygen in the blood. This causes fatigue and explains why being tired is one symptom of an iron deficiency. Iron is also important for other bodily functions, such as the transformation of provitamin A to vitamin A.

IRON CONTENT OF VARIOUS FOODS

Food	Amount	Iron Content (mg)
Pork liver	3 oz./85 g	15
Beef kidney	3 oz./85 g	6
Beef liver	3 oz./85 g	8
Cream of wheat, enriched, cooked	$\frac{1}{2}$ cup/125 mL	8
Prune juice	$\frac{1}{2}$ cup/125 mL	2
Cereals, whole-grain, enriched	$\frac{3}{4}$ cup/175 mL	4
Beef, ham, pork, veal	3 oz./85 g	2
Blackstrap molasses	1 tbsp./15 mL	3
Legumes, cooked	$\frac{1}{2}$ cup/125 mL	2–3
Spinach	$\frac{1}{2}$ cup/125 mL	4
Sunflower seeds	$\frac{1}{4}$ cup/50 mL	3
Almonds	$\frac{1}{4}$ cup/50 mL	2
Wheat germ	1 tbsp./15 mL	1
Apricots	3	2
Bran muffin	1	2
Rice, brown or white	1 cup/250 mL	2
Broccoli	1 stalk	1
Chicken, turkey	3 oz./85 g	1
Egg	1 large	1
Dates, raisins, prunes	$\frac{1}{4}$ cup/50 mL	1
Tomato juice	$\frac{1}{2}$ cup/125 mL	1

Food sources of iron fall into two groups: heme and non-heme. Heme iron comes from meat; non-heme iron comes from non-meat sources. The body absorbs heme iron more easily than non-heme iron, which, it has been found, is more easily absorbed when consumed with vitamin C. This means that eating an orange with your iron-enriched cereal at breakfast will boost your body's absorption of iron.

People likely to suffer from an iron deficiency include teenagers, menstruating women (particularly teenagers), pregnant women, preschool children, and some athletes (see Chapter 9).

Sodium

Sodium winds up in our food via two routes. It can occur naturally or be added during processing or preparation of food. Milk and cheeses are natural sources of sodium, while salted snack foods or condiments acquire it during processing. In fact, processed foods account for about one-third the sodium we eat.

Sodium has several functions in the body. It maintains the *acid-base balance* (the balance of acid and alkaline), sends nerve impulses, and aids muscle contraction. It also helps maintain the balance of fluids inside and outside the body's cells. Sodium is found mainly in the outside fluids of cells and functions with potassium, which is found mainly in the cells' inside fluids. Sodium is a necessary part of our diet, but not often in the excessive amounts consumed by many North Americans.

The body rids itself of excess sodium through the kidneys and perspiration. People who perspire heavily during strenuous work or exercise could have a greater-than-average need for sodium. Research is continually in progress to discover the long-term effects of high sodium intake and the relationship between it and diseases like hypertension. In Western nations, blood pressure rises along with age, but this pattern is not seen in countries where salt consumption is low. As well, studies have shown that mild hypertension can be controlled by reducing the amount of salt we eat. Researchers recently reported in the *British Medical Journal*, after reviewing a whopping 78 studies which involved more than 47,000 people, that it's time to shake our salt habit.

They faulted studies that showed no link between high blood pressure and salt intake for being too short in duration. Each of the studies that found no connection lasted less than five weeks—too short a period to show any link.

SODIUM CONTENT OF VARIOUS FOODS

Food	Amount	Sodium Content (mg)
Beef, cooked	$3\frac{1}{2}$ oz./100 g	71
Corned beef	$3\frac{1}{2}$ oz./100 g	1,134
Frankfurter, beef	1	414
Chicken, roasted	$3\frac{1}{2}$ oz./100 g	65
Chicken, canned	$3\frac{1}{2}$ oz./100 g	438
Salmon, fresh, cooked	$3\frac{1}{2}$ oz./100 g	127
Salmon, canned	$3\frac{1}{2}$ oz./100 g	522
Fish, batter-dipped, frozen	$3\frac{1}{2}$ oz./100 g	411
Pork and beans in tomato sauce	$\frac{1}{2}$ cup/125 mL	450
Broccoli, frozen	$\frac{1}{2}$ cup/125 mL	14
Broccoli, frozen with cheese sauce	$\frac{1}{2}$ cup/125 mL	479
Cottage cheese, creamed	$\frac{1}{2}$ cup/125 mL	485
Cheddar cheese	1 oz./85 g	186
Cheddar cheese, processed	1 oz./85 g	430
Milk	1 cup/250 mL	296
Chicken noodle soup, dehydrated, reconstituted	1 cup/250 mL	1,280
Chicken noodle soup, canned	1 cup/250 mL	1,100

Sodium Content of Various Foods (continued)

Food	Amount	Sodium Content (mg)
Puffed wheat	1 cup/250 mL	Less than 1
Corn flake–type cereal	1 cup/250 mL	230
Popcorn, unsalted	1 cup/250 mL	Less than 1
Potato chips, plain	1 oz./30 g	213
Potato chips, BBQ flavour	1 oz./30 g	317
Bouillon cube	1	1,440
Ketchup	1 tbsp./15 mL	177
Mustard	1 tbsp./15 mL	200
Soya sauce	1 tbsp./15 mL	1,030
Steak sauce	1 tbsp./15 mL	149
Teriyaki sauce, bottled	1 tbsp./15 mL	700
Pickle, kosher	1	581
Pickle relish	1 oz./30 g	375
Olives, green	2 medium	192
Soda, diet	12 oz./375 g	70
Mineral water (Perrier)	8 oz./250 g	5

Salt contains about 40 percent sodium by weight and is used widely in the preservation, processing, and preparation of foods. Recommended levels of sodium intake appear to be 1.1 to 3 grams per day, but our average daily intake is about 4 to 6 grams. Not everyone is predisposed to a salt sensitivity. However, because of the great incidence of high blood pressure and stroke along with a lack of testing to determine who is sensitive, it seems that moderation should be the order of the day.

Because about one-third of our sodium intake comes from the salt that we add to food, we can, by slowly reducing the amount of salt we pour from the shaker, lower our consumption. Salt is an acquired taste and we can gradually modify our intake. After a while, food seasoned with the old heavy hand will taste too salty.

Potassium

Bananas and oranges are well known as good sources of potassium. It is also present in varying quantities in dried fruit, kiwi fruit, tomatoes, potatoes, and some others.

Potassium works with sodium to maintain the body's balance of fluids. Too high a sodium intake can upset the balance and result in a need for more potassium. An eating plan chock-full of potassium-rich foods may have the same effect on blood pressure regulation as lowering the sodium content of the diet. Diuretics, severe diarrhea, and vomiting can cause potassium loss. Potassium is also necessary to maintain the acid-base balance in the body, transmit nerve impulses, and release energy from carbohydrate, protein, and fat.

Chloride

Table salt, sodium chloride, provides enough chloride for the body. Meat, milk, and eggs are other chloride sources. Chloride maintains the body's acid-base balance. It is an important part of hydrochloric acid, found in the stomach, which is needed for the early stages of digestion.

Fluoride

Fluoridated water is our main source of fluoride and is monitored to keep amounts safe. A person who relies heavily on bottled water as an alternative to tap water should therefore consider some kind of supplement. This mineral can also be found in sardines with their bones.

Fluoride helps build strong bones and teeth. A lack of it not only causes weak teeth but can also contribute to osteoporosis. Too much causes mottled teeth.

Magnesium

Magnesium is found in whole-grain breads and cereals, green leafy vegetables, nuts, beans, and milk. It is needed to release energy from carbohydrates, synthesize protein, stimulate nerve and muscle action, and retain calcium in tooth enamel. Its status is not affected, however, by increasing calcium in the diet, as claimed by some food faddists. There is therefore no reason to take magnesium supplements simply because you are taking calcium supplements.

Manganese

Manganese occurs in nuts and whole-grain cereals and is required for normal bone development. Toxic amounts of this mineral can result in reduced iron absorption and anemia.

Iodine

Sources of iodine are saltwater fish, shellfish, and iodized salt. Iodine is a crucial component of the hormone thyroxin, which regulates the thyroid gland. This gland plays an important role in controlling the body's basal metabolic rate. A lack of adequate iodine results in goitre (enlargement of the thyroid). Strangely enough, too much iodine can have a similar effect.

Iodine exists only at low levels in most foods, so it is added to table salt to compensate for this.

Selenium

Selenium is obtained from cereals and fish and acts as an anti-oxidant much like vitamin E. Vitamin E seems to protect selenium by binding with oxygen before the selenium and oxygen can combine. Too large a dose of selenium supplements can be toxic, causing hair loss as well as changes in teeth and nails.

Research is going on into the possible role of selenium in cancer prevention. It is thought that a low selenium intake might be linked to cancers of the esophagus, stomach, and rectum. Because of the dangers of ingesting too much selenium, more human studies are needed to determine safe levels of supplementation. The wisest way to obtain this mineral is be eating foods rich in it.

Zinc

Meat, eggs, liver, and shellfish are good sources of zinc. It is also contained in whole grains and milk. Zinc is important for its role in the body's metabolism of protein and carbohydrate and for insulin production. Dwarfism has been documented as one possible result of a zinc deficiency. Overdoing it on zinc supplements may disturb the balance of other constituents of the body. An excess of zinc can, for example, throw off the body's copper balance and also affect HDL cholesterol levels (see page 23).

2   Go for Fibre—Forgo Fat

If anything is for sure in this entire, often confusing debate about nutrition, it is that the North American diet is long on fat and short on fibre. And what seems increasingly clear is that there is a link between this and the continent's two major diseases—heart disease and cancer.

In 1990, Health and Welfare Canada came out with their recommendations for a diet to promote health and prevent disease:

• Enjoy a _variety_ of foods.

• Emphasize cereals, breads, other grain products, vegetables, and fruits.

• Choose lower-fat dairy products, leaner meats, and foods prepared with little or no fat.

• Achieve and maintain a healthy body weight by enjoying regular physical activity and healthy eating.

• Limit salt, alcohol, and caffeine.

The Canadian Cancer Society has stated that 35 percent of all cancers can be linked to diet, and the main culprit seems to be fat. In addition, dietary fats, and cholesterol in particular, are major contributors to heart disease.

Lessons from Jack Sprat
The evidence is steadily growing to connect a diet high in fats with certain cancers. At the top of the list are cancers of the colon and rectum, followed by cancers of the breast, endometrium, and the ovaries in women, and prostate cancer in men. Some foods actually contain _carcinogens_ (cancer-causing agents), while others harbour substances that promote their production. There is a great deal of research currently underway and much debate about which foods can cause cancer. Some of these will be discussed in Chapter 3.

Heart of the Matter
On the North American continent, where the burger with fries still reigns supreme and where we have one of the

highest standards of living in the world, we can lay claim to another less welcome record—one of the highest rates of heart disease, a bigger cause of death than all the others combined. And high blood cholesterol, kissing cousin to dietary fat, is now known to be a major cause.

What is the cholesterol–heart disease connection?

Atherosclerosis, also known as hardening of the arteries, is a major form of heart disease. It is caused by a buildup of cholesterol deposits—a process that can begin during childhood—on the artery walls. These arteries eventually lose their elasticity and become narrow, sometimes even blocked.

In spite of ongoing research, the exact cause of atherosclerosis is not known, but heart disease has been linked to seven major factors: heredity, lack of exercise, diabetes, obesity, high blood pressure, smoking, and high levels of cholesterol in the blood. Several of these are related to diet and are therefore within our control. In 1985, the National Institute of Health in the United States recommended that we North Americans lower our cholesterol levels. And when the Canadian Consensus Conference on Cholesterol also recommends that we lower what we previously considered as acceptable blood cholesterol levels, as it did in March 1988, it's time to sit up and take a good look at what's on our plates.

The North America–wide Lipid Research Clinics conducted a ten-year study on the prevention of heart disease, the results of which were published in 1984. Although it was already known that high blood cholesterol was a factor in the development of heart disease, no definite connection had been made between lowering blood cholesterol and preventing heart disease. The Lipid Research Clinics study concluded that a 1 percent reduction in cholesterol resulted in a 2 percent lower risk of coronary disease; this gives a 10 to 20 percent cholesterol–heart disease prevention ratio.

Criticisms of this study point to the use of drugs in conjunction with a cholesterol-reduced diet and to the fact that people used in the study, who had high cholesterol levels, were not typical. It would be extremely difficult, however, to conduct a long-term study such as this without using drugs (those with high cholesterol would be at risk), and the principles advocated in the study are in keeping with other disease-prevention strategies. Still, research has now shown that lowering blood cholesterol can actually reverse the buildup of fatty deposits that have already accumulated in the arteries.

Cholesterol—Heroes and Villains

Cholesterol is a waxy, fat-like substance that occurs naturally in the blood of all animals, including humans. It is required, but only in the right amounts, to help produce hormones, make the brain function properly, and maintain the body's nerve structure. Problems begin when cholesterol occurs in excess—and this means that the North American diet that's heavy on burgers and fries but light on fresh fruit and veg could well do with a cholesterol-reducing overhaul!

Too high a cholesterol level is often hereditary. But eating too many fat- and cholesterol-laden foods is certainly not good for anyone. Saturated fats, such as those contained in butter, can work a little cholesterol trickery by increasing the body's cholesterol production, sometimes to an unhealthy degree.

Because of the medical risks of high blood cholesterol, it is advisable for everyone to have their blood cholesterol level checked periodically. Individuals with an unhealthy high cholesterol count can then determine what dietary changes to make.

An emerging fact about cholesterol compounds is that there are two kinds—the bad and the good.

Most of us have heard plenty about the bad kind, known as LDL (*low-density lipoprotein*) or VLDL (*very low-density lipoprotein*) cholesterol. (And when we use the word *cholesterol* by itself, this is the kind we mean.) But many of us have never heard of the good kind of cholesterol, called HDL (*high-density lipoprotein*). HDL has the amazing property, so it seems, of removing cholesterol from the artery walls. The higher a person's HDL, therefore, the better. While regular exercise can increase one's HDL, smoking and stress both reduce it. (Taking large doses of zinc may block the beneficial effect of exercise on the HDL levels. A University of Wyoming study of two groups looked at the effect of zinc supplementation on HDL cholesterol levels. It found that the group taking oral zinc daily had lower HDL levels than the group that did not take any oral zinc.) Diet, body weight, and heredity, on the other hand, are the main factors controlling LDL.

The bottom line is that we must find ways to eat, to cook, and to organize our lives that promote the production of HDL cholesterol and diminish our levels of LDL cholesterol.

The fat in foods and the fat in our bodies are made up of substances called *triglycerides*. Triglycerides are the form in which our bodies store fat to be used for extra

CHOLESTEROL CONTENT OF VARIOUS FOODS

Food	Amount	Cholesterol Content (mg)
Egg yolk	1 large	215
Liver, beef	3 oz./85 g	375
Kidneys, beef	3 oz./85 g	328
Sweetbreads, beef	3 oz./85 g	400
Brains	3 oz./85 g	1,785
Beef, lean	3 oz./85 g	73
Lamb, lean	3 oz./85 g	83
Pork, lean	3 oz./85 g	82
Veal, lean	3 oz./85 g	87
Poultry, skin removed	3 oz./85 g	80
Fish, lean	3 oz./85 g	60
Fish, fatty	3 oz./85 g	50
Clams	8 large	48
Crab	3 oz./85 g	70
Lobster	3 oz./85 g	72
Oysters	3 oz./85 g	43
Scallops	3 oz./85 g	45
Shrimp	10 large	110
Butter	1 tbsp./15 mL	31
Lard	1 tbsp./15 mL	12
Bacon, crisp	3 slices	15

The Enlightened Eater

Milk, whole	1 cup/250 mL	35
Milk, 2%	1 cup/250 mL	19
Milk, skim	1 cup/250 mL	5
Cheese, whole milk	1 oz./30 g	25–35
Cheese, part skim	1 oz./30 g	18
Cottage cheese, creamed	1 cup/250 mL	33
Cottage cheese, 2%	1 cup/250 mL	20
Ice cream	1 cup/250 mL	90

energy or to insulate our bodies and protect our vital organs.

Triglycerides, which circulate throughout the body in the bloodstream, seem to act somewhat like cholesterol when they occur in excess. Although the jury is still out on this, it is wise to keep triglycerides at what is considered normal levels. A diet low in fat (in particular the saturated kind) and simple sugars and high in complex carbohydrates is recommended to achieve this. High alcohol consumption and excess body weight seem to increase tryglyceride levels in people prone to this condition—yet another reason to follow the healthy principles of eating that are outlined in this book!

Fats and Fatsimiles

Fat makes up about 40 percent of the North American diet. This is in contrast to the 30 percent recommended by the Canadian Cancer Society and the American Heart Association. It is recommended that this 30 percent be made up of no more than one-third from saturated fats along with a maximum of one-third polyunsaturated fats. The remainder should be from monounsaturated fats.

How does this affect our food intake and its calories? If a person consumes 2,000 calories a day, 40 per-

cent of which is fat, he or she is eating 89 grams of fat
(fat supplies nine calories per gram). To reduce fat intake
to the desirable 30 percent, a person should consume
only 67 grams of fat a day, reducing consumption by 22
grams. This can be achieved by cutting out six teaspoons
of fat.

Here are some examples of how this can be done.
Switching from whole to skim milk reduces fat by eight
grams a glass. Measuring out salad dressing instead of
pouring it on with gay abandon can save four to eight
grams. And slicing one or two ounces from a helping of
meat can slice off a generous three to eight grams.

Rating the Fats

There are three basic kinds of fats—saturated, polyunsaturated, and monounsaturated. All the fats we eat are
made up of a combination of all three and are classified
according to which one predominates. One tablespoon of
sunflower oil, for example, which contains 8.9 grams of
polyunsaturated fat, 1.5 grams of saturated fat, and 2.9
grams of monounsaturated fat, falls into the polyunsaturated group. Here is how these three fat types differ.

Saturated Fats

These are the fats that raise cholesterol in the body, and
it is these fats that most of us eat in excess. Usually solid
when at room temperature, saturated fats are mainly
found in foods of animal origin such as whole-milk dairy
products, cream, butter, and the fat on meat and poultry.
Two vegetable fats, palm oil and coconut oil, used widely
in commercial baking, in cereals, and in non-dairy whiteners, also fall into this group of fats.

In the United States, there is a trend away from these
tropical oils. Food companies are bowing to consumer
demand and, as a result, are switching to more healthful
oils. In Canada, though, the use of saturated fats and oils
in processed foods is still widespread.

Polyunsaturated
Fats

These fats, which are found mainly in vegetable oils that
do not harden at room or refrigerator temperature, have
the favourable effect of lowering blood cholesterol. But
because both LDL and HDL levels have been shown to be
lowered by polyunsaturated fats, it would be a good idea
to include a variety of oils in the diet. As well, because
the long-term effects of eating too many polyunsaturated
fats are not known, we should not consume more than
10 percent of our calories as polyunsaturated fats.

Another benefit of polyunsaturated fats is that they contain linoleic acid, an essential fatty acid that, unlike other fatty acids, cannot be produced by the body from fat, protein, or carbohydrate. Safflower, sunflower, soybean, and corn oils all contain polyunsaturated fats; so do margarines made from these oils. These fats can also be found in some nuts and seeds such as walnuts and sunflower seeds.

Monounsaturated Fats

Found in oils such as olive, peanut, and canola oils as well as in certain nuts, these are usually liquid at room temperature but turn solid when refrigerated. Because of the low level of heart disease is Mediterranean countries, where olive oil is a diet staple, it is thought that monounsaturated fats may be a contributing factors. Recent investigations have shown that these fats have no impact on blood cholesterol levels on their own, but when substituted for the saturated type may result in lowered cholesterol levels. Canola oil contains an appreciable amount of the heart-healthy omega-3 fatty acids (see page 41), so it may be a wise choice for a cooking oil.

Fats and Fiction

A little knowledge and a good dose of discrimination when choosing what you eat can go a long way toward cutting down on unwanted fats. Understanding labels on foods can also help demystify some fat facts and fallacies. For example, if the label on a package of cheese states that there are 93 calories and seven grams of fat per slice, we can deduce that, because fat contains nine calories per gram, this cheese has a total of 63 fat calories. This leaves a measly 30 calories for its good nutrients!

There has been considerable controversy over the fatty virtues and vices of butter versus margarine.

Because butter is considered a saturated fat, it contains all the nutritional hazards of other saturated fats and, therefore, we should cut down on the amount we eat.

As for margarines, they are not all they seem. When an unsaturated fat is hardened, it becomes saturated. This means that most of the fat in hard margarine winds up being saturated even though it did not start that way. Soft margarines are a better choice. Best bets are the ones with the highest level of unsaturated fat. Just add up the monounsaturated and polyunsaturated fats to get the total.

The process of hydrogenation changes liquid fats into solids. These fats then behave like saturated fats and may raise cholesterol accordingly. Reading labels on such foods as oils, margarine, shortening, and peanut butter is the best way to determine if hydrogenation has occurred. Hydrogenation also results in the formation of compounds called trans fatty acids. A recent study in the Netherlands found that these fatty acids, which are unsaturated, act in a similar way to saturated fat, in that they raise the levels of the harmful LDL cholesterol. But here's where they're worse than saturated fat—they have also been found to lower the levels of beneficial HDL cholesterol. Choose a non-hydrogenated product over one that is. But don't forget to consider the quantity. Less fat is always better, no matter what kind it is. The less hydrogenated the better, as in the case of soft margarines.

The following chart shows how to reduce your fat intake.

WAYS TO TRIM THE FAT

High-Fat Choices	Lower-Fat Alternatives	Fat Savings (tsp.)
Granola, 1 oz./30 g	100% Bran, $\frac{1}{3}$ cup/75 mL	1
Croissant	Whole-grain roll	2
Processed meat, 2 oz./60 g	Sliced chicken, 2 oz./60 g	2
Salad dressing, liberally poured	Salad dressing, measured	2–3
French fries, 10 pieces	Baked potato, 1 large	1
Beef, 6-oz./175-g serving, untrimmed	Beef, 3-oz./85-g serving, lean only	3
Milk, whole, 8 oz./250 mL	Milk, skim, 8 oz./250 g	2
Potato chips, 10 pieces	Popcorn, air-popped, 1 cup/250 mL	2
	Total	15–16

Trimming the Fat

Here are some nifty ways to reduce the amount of fat you use in cooking. You'll be surprised at how little fat you actually need for taste results that are still tops.

- Use lean meat. Trim off any excess fat before cooking.

- When buying meat, look for lean cuts. The fat content of meat is low only if meat is lean (well trimmed). Examples of lean cuts are beef—flank, round, chuck, sirloin, T-bone, and rib-eye; lamb—loin, roast, and chops; pork—leg, tenderloin, ham, and Canadian (back) bacon; and all cuts of veal.

- Remove the skin from poultry before cooking, but be careful not to overcook it, or it will become dry.

- Bake, roast, steam, or broil instead of frying to reduce the fat content.

- When roasting or baking meat, place it on a wire rack in a baking pan to let the fat drain off. Use wine or stock for basting.

- When making stews or casseroles, refrigerate them after cooking to let the fat harden on top. It is then much easier to remove than when the food is hot and the fat is floating on the liquid.

- When making stock, sauce, or gravy, follow the preceding method to remove fat from the surface.

- Use non-stick pans to sauté foods. Use a thin coating of oil by applying it with a brush or piece of waxed paper. Add stocks when sautéeing or stir-frying to stop foods from sticking to the pan.

- If the flavour of the oil is important in a particular recipe, use a good-quality oil such as virgin olive or nut oil and augment it with a flavourless vegetable oil.

- The oil called for in a recipe (except in baking) can usually be substantially reduced without negative results. Experiment with using less.

- When baking, look for recipes that are low in fat.

- If you are deep-frying foods, make sure the oil is as hot as possible without burning before adding the food. Food absorbs less oil this way.

Fibre Fanfare

The fibre furor dates back to the 1970s, when British physician Dr. Denis Burkitt discovered that people in countries where the diet was high in fibre had less intestinal cancer, diverticular disease of the bowel, hiatus hernia, appendicitis, varicose veins, and heart disease than we who exist to a great extent on refined foods.

And recent reports from bodies such as the Canadian Cancer Society and the National Cancer Institute in the United States have taken up the call, urging North Americans to increase their fibre intake. In fact, a survey on dietary fibre by the Expert Advisory Committee on Dietary Fibre (Health and Welfare Canada), published in 1985, suggested that we double the amount of fibre we consume to 20 or 30 grams a day.

What is fibre, and why is it so good for us? Fibre is the material in plant foods that is resistant to digestion by humans. Here are the ways it can contribute to the prevention of certain diseases.

Heart Disease
: Fibre can combine with bile salts, which are made partially from cholesterol, and prevent them from being absorbed. When this happens, the body takes cholesterol from the blood to manufacture more bile salts. The result is lower blood cholesterol, which helps prevent heart disease.

Diverticular Disease
: Diverticula are small bulges on the wall of the bowel caused by increased pressure and weakness of the bowel muscle. Fibre increases the bulk of bowel material while softening its texture, thereby reducing pressure on the bowel walls. Increased fibre in the diet therefore reduces stress on the bowel walls and prevents outpockets from appearing there.

Large-Bowel Cancer
: Fibre helps speed the path of waste materials through the gut. This means that waste products come into contact with the gut wall for a shorter time, thereby reducing the risk of irritation, infection, and the growth of potential cancer-causing substances.

Breast and Prostate Cancer
: Fibre has been shown to bind to the hormones estrogen and androgen, increasing their elimination through the gut. Studies have shown that this may have a protective effect against breast and prostate cancer. Fibre from linseed, oats, barley, soybean, and wheat bran seem to excel in this role.

Obesity
: Foods that are high in fibre take longer to chew and are bulkier once they are ingested. They therefore cause a

The Enlightened Eater

greater feeling of fullness than their refined counterparts and give us a feeling of satisfaction without a huge quantity of calories.

The Two Faces of Fibre

There are two kinds of fibre—soluble and insoluble. There are foods that contain one or the other and a third group that contains both.

Soluble Fibres

Soluble in water, these are gummy fibres found in pectins, gums, and mucilages—that is, in foods such as legumes (dried beans like kidney beans and lentils), apples, and grains such as oats (specifically in oat bran), bran, rye and barley.

When these foods are eaten, the soluble fibres swell and form a gel-like structure that traps nutrients like sugars and starch, which then take longer to be absorbed into the blood. This effect is beneficial for everyone, because blood sugar and thereby energy levels are stabilized, but it is particularly beneficial for diabetics.

Another benefit of soluble fibres is that they bind with bile salts. Bile salts come from cholesterol, so the higher the soluble fibre in the diet (especially from oat bran), the lower the cholesterol.

Insoluble Fibres

These consist mainly of a substance called *cellulose* and are insoluble in water. They include fibres such as wheat bran and other cereal fibres, which help promote regularity of the bowels by holding water in the stool. This makes the stool bulkier, enabling it to pass out of the body more easily. Because these fibres work in conjunction with water, a person who increases the amount of these fibres in his or her diet must also drink more water, or constipation will be the unpleasant result.

The Soluble-Insoluble Combination

Some foods contain a mixture of both types of fibre. Most notable of these are fruits and vegetables.

Fibre Tips

- Increase your fibre intake gradually, or you will have abdominal discomfort. In other words, if you eat eight bran muffins in one day, your bloated stomach is going to be a real pain!

- As with all changes in eating habits, begin gradually and adapt the changes to your tastes in foods. Eating a whole slew of unfamiliar foods at once may result in a temporary change, but chances are you'll be back eating the same old foods in no time. So if you hate hot cereal but love the flavour of rye bread, you're well advised to get soluble fibre in your favourite sandwich instead of trying to force down some rib-hugging gruel at breakfast time!

- Eat fresh fruits and vegetables rather than their juices to enjoy all their fibre potential.

- Eat whole-grain breads such as rye, whole wheat, bran, and oatmeal rather than white.

- Add nuts and seeds (in small amounts because of their high fat content) to salads and keep them handy along with dried fruit as healthful snacks.

- Use bran (either the oat or wheat variety) as a filler for hamburgers and meat loaf, a topping in casseroles, and a substitute for breadcrumbs when cooking.

- Try to eat fibres from both the soluble and insoluble groups throughout the day. For example, have oatmeal at breakfast, fruit as a morning snack, and a bran muffin in the afternoon.

Fibre: A Note of Caution

Eating too much fibre in too short a time, introducing fibre too suddenly into one's diet, and not drinking enough water (about eight glasses a day is a good idea) can result in gas and therefore bad stomach pains.

People on low-calorie diets should beware of fibre supplements designed to decrease a dieter's appetite. Someone who is dieting might already be lacking important minerals such as calcium and iron, and a fibre supplement might further decrease the absorption of the few minerals that the dieter is consuming. In keeping with the general rule, it is best to get fibre from food rather than from supplements—we don't know the dangers of consuming too much fibre.

There has also been some concern among health professionals about "non-native" fibres—fibres not inherent in one food but added to it from another. They worry that these fibres might act differently when consumed in a foreign food. For example, does the pea fibre act the same way when it is added to a "high fibre" bread as it does when it is eaten in a pea?

"Novel" fibres such as the wood fibre found in some breads are also unknown quantities. More research and detailed labelling are needed in these areas.

By making small changes in your diet, you can increase your fibre intake. Review these sources of dietary fibre and check out the sample menus that follow.

SOURCES OF DIETARY FIBRE

	Food	Amount	Calories per Serving
A Very High Source of Dietary Fibre: Greater than 7 Grams per Serving	All-Bran	$\frac{1}{3}$ cup/75 mL	90
	Bran Buds	$\frac{1}{3}$ cup/75 mL	98
	100% Bran	$\frac{1}{2}$ cup/125 mL	76
	Baked beans in tomato sauce	$\frac{1}{2}$ cup/125 mL	155
	Kidney beans	$\frac{1}{2}$ cup/125 mL	138
High Source of Dietary Fibre: 4.5–6.9 Grams per Serving	Bran Chex	$\frac{2}{3}$ cup/150 mL	91
	Corn Bran	$\frac{2}{3}$ cup/150 mL	89
	Dried peas	$\frac{1}{2}$ cup/125 mL	115
	Lima beans	$\frac{1}{2}$ cup/125 mL	138
	Navy beans	$\frac{1}{2}$ cup/125 mL	112
Moderate Source of Dietary Fibre: 2.0–4.4 Grams per Serving	40% bran cereal	$\frac{3}{4}$ cup/175 mL	93
	Cracklin' Bran	$\frac{1}{3}$ cup/75 mL	108
	Raisin Bran	$\frac{3}{4}$ cup/175 mL	115
	Shredded Wheat	$\frac{2}{3}$ cup/150 mL	102
	Total	1 cup/250 mL	100
	Wheat Chex	$\frac{2}{3}$ cup/150 mL	104
	Wheaties	1 cup/250 mL	107
	Wheat germ	$\frac{1}{4}$ cup/50 mL	100
	Bran muffin	1	120

Food	Amount	Calories per Serving
Crisp crackers, rye	2 crackers	50
Whole-wheat bread	2 slices	120
Lentils	$\frac{1}{2}$ cup/125 mL	95
Broccoli	$\frac{1}{2}$ cup/125 mL	27
Brussels sprouts	$\frac{1}{2}$ cup/125 mL	32
Carrots	$\frac{1}{2}$ cup/125 mL	24
Corn	$\frac{1}{2}$ cup/125 mL	70
Peas	$\frac{1}{2}$ cup/125 mL	62
Potato with skin	1 medium	90
Spinach	$\frac{1}{2}$ cup/125 mL	20
Apple	1 medium	80
Banana	1 medium	105
Blueberries	$\frac{1}{2}$ cup/125 mL	43
Cantaloupe	$\frac{1}{2}$ small	80
Orange	1	62
Pear	$\frac{1}{2}$	50
Prunes	2	40
Raisins	3 tbsp./45 mL	94
Raspberries	$\frac{1}{2}$ cup/125 mL	32
Strawberries	1 cup/250 mL	55

SAMPLE MENUS

	Normal	High Fibre
Breakfast	Orange juice	Fresh orange
	Refined cereal	Oat Bran
	Milk	Milk
	Egg	Egg
	White toast	Whole-wheat toast
	Beverage	Beverage
Lunch	Cream soup	Pea soup
	Sandwich on white	Sandwich on whole-grain
	Fruit-flavoured yogurt	Fresh fruit and plain yogurt
	Water	Water
Snack	Doughnut	Bran muffin
	Milk	Milk
Dinner	Baked chicken with pre-mixed crumb coating	Baked chicken with wheat germ and almond coating
	French fries	Baked potato with skin
	Iceberg lettuce salad	Spinach salad
	Broccoli, stems peeled	Broccoli, unpeeled
	Apple pie	Apple crisp with bran topping

3   The Protein Preference

Protein is the main nutrient from which our bodies grow and regenerate. Amino acids, which make up proteins, are to proteins what bricks are to a wall. Although more than 20 amino acids are known to exist in the human body, only eight are considered essential, that is, required for growth, repair, and maintenance of tissues. These essential amino acids cannot be synthesized by the body; they must come from what we eat.

Proteins that contain all these essential amino acids in proportions and amounts most useful to the body have *high biological value*. In general, animal proteins such as meat, poultry, eggs, milk, and cheese supply plentiful amounts of essential amino acids and are therefore considered excellent dietary sources of protein.

Proteins of plant origin lack or are low in one or more essential amino acids. However, nuts, seeds, dried peas and beans, lentils, and grains yield high-quality, complete protein in combination with each other and some other foods.

Comparing Proteins

Foods that contain protein do not always contain complete protein: some contain varying amounts of incomplete protein. Complete, high-quality proteins are found in meat, fish, poultry, eggs, milk in all its forms, and cheese—cottage, hard, and processed. Nuts and legumes (dried peas and beans, chick peas or garbanzo beans, lentils, and so on) yield partially incomplete proteins. And grains (wheat, oats, rye, rice, barley, quinoa, amaranth, etc.), and breads and cereals made from them, supply incomplete proteins.

Protein—Playing with a Full Deck

Vegetarians   These days a growing sector of the population is deciding to become vegetarian. However, many people are blissfully unaware of the adjustments they should be making to their new-found eating style, especially in the protein department. Telling meat to move over to make way for vegetables simply isn't good enough. A teenage convert to vegetarianism, for example, who eats the same meals as the rest of the family without the meat—namely, the protein food—is heading for trouble in the shape of an unbalanced diet.

There are, however, solutions to the problem of how to satisy the needs of carnivores and vegetarians who eat at the same table. The following protein information is also useful for anyone contemplating a meatless diet. The secret lies in complementary proteins.

Complementary
Proteins

When proteins are called *complementary*, it means that a combination of two or more of them supply all the amino acids our bodies need. Complementary proteins can be formed in two ways: by combining plant and animal protein—for example, by eating pasta with cheese—and by eating, at the same meal, two or more plant proteins that together provide the necessary amino acids. It was previously thought that these foods must be eaten together to obtain this effect. But eating a variety of foods throughout the day may be satisfactory. But for those whose diets may not be balanced, paying heed to the concept of complementary proteins may still be a good idea. A teenage girl who grabs a muffin for breakfast and a green salad for lunch would do well to dine on pasta and beans.

Eggs, milk, yogurt, and low-fat cheese are all handy foods that can be included in a meal of incomplete proteins as complements to increase protein value. Grating some cheddar or Monterey Jack on a bowl of chili or enjoying some crusty bread alongside are examples of maximizing the protein value.

Protein's Good Company
High-protein foods are a good source of several important vitamins and minerals.

COMPLEMENTARY PROTEINS

Milk products	+	Grains	=	Complete protein
Legumes	+	Grains	=	Complete protein
Milk products	+	Legumes	=	Complete protein
Nuts or seeds	+	Legumes	=	Complete protein
Nuts or seeds	+	Milk products	=	Complete protein

Iron	Many high-protein foods are high in iron. Iron comes in good amounts from meats (especially organ meats), egg yolk, dried peas and beans, lentils, nuts, and seeds. The heme iron that comes from meat is absorbed more easily by our bodies than non-heme iron, which comes from foods like egg yolk, cereals, and beans. Vitamin C helps the body absorb non-heme iron, so a fresh orange eaten along with a boiled egg is a terrific way to get the most out of that egg.
Other Minerals	High-protein foods also supply zinc, copper, phosphorus, calcium, and magnesium.
Vitamins	Significant amounts of thiamin, riboflavin, and niacin come from high-protein foods. Dried peas, beans, and lentils are important sources of folacin. Organ meats are good ways to ingest vitamin A. Vitamin B12 is found only in foods of animal origin and may be lacking in the diet of strict vegetarians (vegans) if they do not take a B12 supplement of some kind. This is discussed at greater length in Chapter 10.

Protein—Time It Right

When eating protein, the crucial factor—and where most people go wrong—is timing.

Protein is thought to be crucial for keeping us mentally alert, and trying to function without eating any protein is like attempting to drive a car without gas. The best time to fuel our bodies with protein is when we're most in need of it—at the beginning of the day. We should then restock with smaller amounts of protein at intervals throughout the day. Eating a large meal after a hard day's work, as many people do, is not the best way to treat our minds or our bodies.

Why is timing so important when eating protein? Protein foods take longer to digest than other foods, such as carbohydrates, so they help keep our blood sugar levels and, consequently, our energy levels, stable. Fewer dips in blood sugar cause fewer dips in energy levels, all of which produces sounder bodies and minds. The protein-mind connection has been attracting some attention lately. The theory is that protein increases the alertness level of the mind by its action on the brain's chemical production. Carbohydrates, eaten alone, may have a calming effect and therefore slow you down.

Traditional eating habits have not been helpful in all this. A large evening meal based on protein—a sizable main meat course—counteracts the ideal protein-eating pattern. The best way to pace your protein is to eat most of it at breakfast and lunch, tapering off your intake toward the end of the day. For example, the person who eats a green salad, slice of bread, and an apple for lunch will crave a snack a couple of hours later. However, adding a few ounces of tuna or chicken to the same lunch prevents that person's blood sugar from dropping rapidly and eliminates that craving.

As with all things, however, too much of a good thing can also be a problem. Excess protein is broken down by the body and is stored as fat. Also, a person who eats too much protein (as some high-protein weight-loss diets recommend) could upset his or her calcium balance.

Red Meat—Good Things Come in Small Packages

Nobody with a knowledge of nutrition is going to shed a tear over the demise of the ten-ounce steak that many North Americans used to consider their rightful meat portion. More and more people are realizing that a chicken breast marinated in herbs and lemon juice, then grilled and topped with a mustard sauce, can be just as satisfying as a huge slab of sirloin done on the barbecue.

There are, however, some dangers in the growing trend toward eating less red meat—a trend based mainly on a sound fear of consuming too many saturated fats. Many people who give up red meat because of its high fat content unwittingly replace it with equally fat-laden foods. Opting for the fried fish fillet instead of a burger at a fast-food chain or choosing fish in puff pastry instead of the filet mignon in a restaurant are cases in point.

What is more, giving up red meat means giving up important nutrients like iron, and they must be replaced in the rest of the diet—a fact that many who renounce red meat are not aware of. Our mothers were right when they told us to eat our liver. Liver is high in iron, but also in cholesterol, so it should be eaten in moderation. A person who gives up red meat should eat foods high in iron, such as legumes and enriched cereals, to fill that gap.

The best way to solve the legitimate concern of consuming the excess of saturated fats contained in red meat without losing out on its benefits is to eat lean meat in smaller portions. A little red meat goes a long way, and a four-ounce steak eaten with plenty of vegetables and some carbohydrate is a good source of protein and makes a satisfying meal.

Red meat takes longer to digest than white meat or fish because of its higher fat content, so it takes longer to satisfy the eater. It is therefore difficult to know when you've eaten the right amount, and if you keep eating until you're full, you will probably have eaten too much. So make a conscious effort to reduce your portions of red meat. It will help if you supplement red meat with plenty of other foods to make up a healthy, square meal.

Cooking smaller portions of red meat into stir-fries along with a bevy of tender-crisp vegetables, and serving a small amount of meat sauce with a generous helping of pasta, are a couple of painless, healthy ways to cut down on red meat.

Taste in food is a powerful factor in deciding what we eat. North Americans have been conditioned to think that a prime roast of beef, the perfect juicy burger that bulges out of its bun, and a succulent T-bone steak are the epitome of culinary delight. A change of eating habits doesn't come overnight. To make matters more difficult, fat—the culprit in all this—*does* add flavour. So if we want to eliminate or at least reduce fat and still have good taste, we must find new ways to season and enhance our food.

Fowl Fare

Poultry is an extremely healthy protein alternative to red meat. Chicken, for example, is wonderfully versatile. Not only is it superb roasted with a few herbs and perhaps a little soy sauce, but it can also be cooked cacciatore one night, done Szechuan the next, or poached in a little white wine and lemon juice with artichokes the following dinnertime.

Turkey is another good choice of poultry, but avoid fatty birds such as duck, goose, and stewing hens. To lower your fat even further, have white meat instead of dark. It is also best to remove the skin from poultry before cooking, because it is high in fat and cholesterol.

Feast on Fish

Fish is an excellent, low-fat, nutritious alternative to red meat as a source of protein. And these days fish is just beginning to overcome the bad reputation it has long had. One reason for this is our bad memories of how fish used to taste once it arrived at inland destinations without today's advanced methods of shipping and preserving freshness. Another reason is a fear of coming across bones. Still others are that most people overcook fish and have a fear of cooking it at all.

Finding a reputable fishmonger who sells fresh fish is the first step toward enjoying eating fish at home. Choosing a fresh fish yourself means finding one that does not have a strong smell, has bright eyes if the head is still attached, and has a firm texture—enough that you feel resistance when you press the flesh with a finger. And fish fillets are a simple solution to a fear of bones. You can buy packaged fillets fresh or frozen or ask your fishmonger to fillet fresh fish for you.

The next step is finding good ways to cook fish. This part is much easier than you might think. Fish is wonderfully versatile and takes only minutes to cook—perfect for today's fast-paced lifestyle.

If you don't have the time or inclination to cook fish, canned salmon and tuna are tasty alternatives. When buying these, choose the water-packed versions rather than those packed in oil. They save a lot of calories and fat. There are now also several brands of fish canned without salt—another wise choice.

Recent studies point to a particularly important benefit of eating fish. One such study conducted in Holland showed that the respondents who included a lot of fish in their diets suffered much less from heart disease than those who did not eat much fish. The particular substance in fish thought to stave off heart disease is polyunsaturated fatty acid, called *omega-3 fatty acid*.

Recent research has linked omega-3 fatty acid with improved joint pain in patients suffering from rheumatoid arthritis. It also seems to have a beneficial effect on those with ulcerative colitis. More work still needs to be done in these areas.

A good guide for judging the omega-3 fatty-acid levels in fish is its total fat content. Good sources of omega-3 are fish with more than 5 percent fat. Some saltwater examples are mackerel, salmon, sea herring, sablefish, anchovies, mullet, canned sardines, and smelts. Freshwater fish high in fat are lake trout, rainbow trout, and catfish. Fish with medium oil content are halibut, sea trout, rockfish, ocean perch, red snapper, and swordfish. Canned white albacore—the Rolls Royce of tuna fish—has a medium fat content. Other kinds of tuna have the fatty acids removed in processing. Shellfish is low in fat but higher in omega-3 fatty acid than other low-fat fish.

Fish oil supplements have been advocated by some as an alternative to eating fish itself. Banishing fish from the diet in favour of supplements may result in consuming less of other nutrients. For example, fish is rich in the mineral selenium, which may play a role in lowering the risk of certain cancers. Cod liver oil doesn't contain large amounts of these omega-3 fatty acids, so that to obtain their benefit from this source, a person would simultaneously take in toxic amounts of vitamins A and D.

Some people are rightly concerned about the effects of polluted waters where fish have been caught. Avoid fish that originate in extremely polluted bodies of water. Freshwater fish with a high fat content tend to contain the highest level of contaminants. One way to avert the problem of the contaminants in fish and still get the health benefits is to eat fish from a variety of places. If you are concerned about a specific fish, check with local government authorities. Refraining from eating raw fish and shellfish may be prudent because of the possibility of food poisoning. Reports of viral infections such as hepatitis have been linked to eating raw fish.

Meat for Lunch?

As if we needed yet another thing to worry about when it comes to eating meat! But there is good cause for concern about luncheon meats—meats that have been highly salted, smoked, and/or nitrite-cured. The worry surrounds *nitrates* and *nitrites*—compounds that are found naturally in some foods but are added to others such as bacon and many cold cuts. Nitrate is changed to nitrite in the body and can act with other substances called amines or amides to produce nitroso compounds called nitrosamines or nitrosamides. Many nitroso compounds are carcinogenic and are believed to increase the risk of stomach and other cancers.

Foods that naturally contain nitrates and nitrites also contain vitamin C, which, it is thought, blocks the conversion of nitrites to nitroso compounds. The concern is mainly over those foods to which nitrates and nitrites have been added. This leads to another controversy.

Sodium nitrate and sodium nitrite are added to cured meats for the wholesome purpose of preventing botulism poisoning. If they were not used, there might be an increase in botulism, which is fatal. Here is another case of the devil and the deep blue sea. For this reason, nitrates and nitrites are still added to meat, but in the smallest amounts possible to still be effective.

Another reason to go easy on luncheon meats is their high salt content. Stomach irritation can result from a long-term overindulgence of salt and may ultimately cause stomach cancer.

Luncheon meats are quick and easy, but they do have hazards, as we have discussed. To avoid relying on them, try the following. When cooking chicken or other lean meat, cook extra and wrap small portions of the leftovers in plastic, label with their name and date, and freeze. This gives you handy packages of unsalted, uncured, lean meat for making sandwiches. If you're too busy to do this, buy a rotisserie chicken or plain cooked turkey breast at the local deli rather than relying on salami and luncheon meats.

Love those Legumes

If there is one food group that is underrated in North America, it is legumes. Legumes are the seeds that grow inside the pods of leguminous plants. Most legumes fall into the categories of dried peas, beans, and lentils. Legumes have fabulous properties. They are a superb, inexpensive source of protein. They are packed with soluble fibres. They are loaded with B vitamins. As well, they are a source of calcium, iron, and potassium. Raw, they keep indefinitely without preservatives. Once cooked, they can easily be frozen.

It is therefore hard to understand why legumes have such a bad image on this continent and why the average person eats them so rarely. Perhaps it's because they are considered a staple in other, poorer parts of the world. Perhaps it's because they produce gas after they have been eaten!

It's important to know the protein value of legumes in order to maximize their nutritional benefits. Legumes contain complementary proteins, so they must be eaten with nuts and seeds, or grains, to bring out their full nutritional potential.

Legumes are the only protein foods that contain a substantial amount of fibre—another reason to include them in your diet. They contain soluble fibres, which slow down the rate of absorption of carbohydrate. This in turn keeps you feeling satisfied longer and prevents you from overeating. Because of their fibre content, legumes also help lower cholesterol. Dr. James Anderson, of the University of Kentucky, found that when participants consumed 17 grams of soluble fibre from either oat bran or pinto and navy beans each day, their cholesterol levels fell by a whopping 19 percent.

Legumes are a good source of B vitamins, but only when they are cooked properly. B vitamins are light-sensitive, so to avoid vitamin loss, store legumes in a dark place or in the fridge in airtight jars. They keep indefinitely this way too.

Although B vitamins are also water-soluble, it's important to soak legumes and rinse well before cooking. This method will get rid of some of the indigestible sugars that cause gas. Legumes must also be boiled to eliminate lectins, which are toxins that can cause stomachaches. When cooking beans, bring them to a brief boil, then simmer them slowly for as long as required.

If this sounds like a lot of effort, you might want to run out and buy a can of beans, but in addition to paying a higher price, you get more salt this way—something you can do without. Cooking up a batch of beans for salads, soups, or chili is worth it if you freeze it to have on hand and reheat quickly. Still, when time is of the essence, canned beans are a good second choice. Rinse them well to decrease their sodium content as well as lower the amount of the indigestible sugars.

Legumes have one last virtue—they're amazingly versatile. They absorb the flavour of the liquid they're cooked in and are thus terrific in spice-laden chili, thick soups loaded with herbs, or main-dish salads tossed with well-seasoned dressings.

Here are the most common and versatile legumes that you can include in your cooking repertoire.

Black Beans Also known as turtle beans, these are small, black-skinned, and oval in shape. They are a staple of South American cuisine and are excellent in soup or cooked with rice.

Black-Eyed Peas A tradition in the southern United States, these are a Cajun specialty when cooked with rice or just served alone with spicy seasoning.

Chick Peas Also called garbanzo beans, these are round, beige beans commonly used in Spanish, Italian, and Middle Eastern cooking. They are terrific tossed in a vinaigrette with some chopped red onion or sweet red pepper, a tasty, protein-filled addition to any salad, and superb blended with lemon juice and herbs in hummus (see page 81). They take two to three hours to cook, so it is a good idea to make a large batch at a time and freeze some.

Flageolets These are the authentic French beans to use in cassoulet.

They are pricey, small, white, kidney-shaped beans that are tasty cooked in a herb-flavoured stock or served with roast poultry or lamb.

Kidney Beans   Large and kidney-shaped, these come in both red and white. The red variety is more common and is best known as the crucial ingredient in chili con carne.

Lentils   Small and flat, these are either brown or red. The red ones turn soft and mushy when cooked, so they are best used in purées and soups. Brown lentils, which hold their shape, are ideal as a cold salad mixed with vinaigrette and some chopped onion.

Mung Beans   The green ones are the most common of these small, round beans. They can be eaten raw as sprouts and often wind up in Oriental noodles, sometimes called cellophane or glass noodles, or pasta made from mung-bean flour.

Pinto Beans   These are pink with black dots and smaller than kidney beans, with which they are more or less interchangeable.

Soybeans   These are small, oval, beige-coloured beans that are extremely nutritious and versatile. They are easiest to use in cooking once they have been processed into tofu, or bean curd.

Try them in a fabulous dip (see pages 149, 240), delicious mayonnaise (page 239), and a divine cheesecake (page 242).

Split Peas   Small and flattened on one side, these take less time to cook than most legumes. The green version is the basis for pea soup when simmered together with a ham bone and seasoning. The yellow ones can only be made into soup or curried, as in Indian dahl.

White Beans   These come in several types, most common of which are the pea and navy beans used to make baked beans. Either of these types can also be used in cassoulet, purées, and many Italian dishes using beans.

The Many Tastes of Tofu

Tofu, often known as bean curd, is made from soybeans. The beans are cooked to form a milky liquid and then processed in a manner similar to the way cottage cheese is made from cow's milk. Tofu comes in soft or firm textures and is a boon to vegetarians because of its calcium, magnesium, phosphorus, and iron content. Tofu is thought by many to be bland and tasteless, but in fact it takes on the flavours of other ingredients in the recipe.

Soft and moist in texture and lacking a definite taste of its own, tofu is amazingly versatile when it is cooked properly. Anyone who has enjoyed it in a bowl of Szechuan hot and sour soup or deep-fried in a Japanese tempura knows what I mean. And tofu cheesecake and mayonnaise are dishes that have a delicate flavour and give you superb taste and texture without the cholesterol or calories!

Tofu is available in most Chinese groceries, health food stores, and some major supermarkets. When buying tofu, look for the varieties made with calcium rather than the synthetic rennet often added for extra firmness. It comes packaged in water and should be stored in the fridge. Change this water every couple of days. Tofu will keep this way for up to two weeks, but it is best when it is fresh. It also freezes well, although its texture then becomes more crumbly.

When you cook with the soft variety of tofu, drain it well before using it in any dish. If you are adding it to a stir-fry, soup, or baked dish like lasagna, when it should be as firm as possible, press the slabs between tea towels covered with a baking sheet or cutting board topped with a two- to five-pound weight such as a couple of cans of food. Leave for 30 minutes to two hours, depending on the desired firmness.

Going Nuts for Seeds
Seeds and nuts are valuable sources of incomplete proteins. So if you use them at meals, round them out with other foods to bring out their protein potential.

One problem with nuts and seeds is that they are high in fat, and although they make a terrific protein snack when eaten between meals, it is important not to eat too many. They are often highly salted—one more reason to go easy on the quantities you eat—so buy the unsalted variety if possible. Also avoid nuts and seeds that have been roasted with oils, because the oils are likely to be the saturated type, such as coconut. A good idea is to roast your own nuts and seeds by placing them on a baking sheet with a few herbs or spices if desired (this isn't really necessary, because roasting brings out wonderful flavour) and roasting for 20 to 30 minutes at 325°F (160°C). Package them in small quantities for a fast snack and to avoid eating too many at one time.

Peanut Butter's True Nature

Peanuts are the only nut belonging to the legume group. Consumed with other proteins, peanut butter—as North American as apple pie but twice as healthful—is a terrific source of protein.

Natural peanut butter is more healthful for you than the more processed kind. Its fat is less saturated than peanut butters made from hydrogenated vegetable oils. And the natural versions do not have added sugar—another plus. All peanut butter, however, is high in fat and should not be eaten in excess.

Another hazard is the danger of consuming mouldy nuts. If you grind your own peanut butter, be careful not to include any mouldy or shrivelled nuts. Mould contains aflatoxins, which are thought to be a health risk. Therefore, peanut butter is best stored in the refrigerator. Commercial brands of peanut butter are monitored for this and should not be cause for concern.

Egg It or Leave It

There is considerable debate and confusion about the nutritional virtues and vices of eggs. Some people, worried about eggs' cholesterol content, omit them entirely from their diets; others have no concerns at all about eating them. Still others try to moderate their consumption of eggs, all the while disregarding the number they use in cooking.

Let's try to set the record straight. Although eggs are extremely high in cholesterol—215 mg per large egg—they also contain a number of valuable nutrients. Rich in protein, B vitamins, vitamin A, and iron, eggs are also too easy on the budget and versatile in cooking to be completely eliminated from our diets. Many shun eggs for breakfast to end up with high-fat cheeses, giant muffins, and the like.

Because the current recommendation from Health and Welfare Canada for cholesterol intake for the average person is about 300 mg per day, consuming one egg a day would almost eat up that ration without leaving room for other nutritious cholesterol-containing foods such as meat, fish, poultry, and dairy products. If, however, your intake of cholesterol-containing foods is extremely low, you could eat eggs more frequently. Your guide to eating eggs should be your cholesterol count, which can easily be checked by a simple blood test.

If you have not been advised to cut down on eggs,

it's prudent to moderate the number of egg yolks you eat. Egg whites, which do not contain cholesterol, need not be limited. One nifty way to stretch out your egg consumption is to add extra egg whites or milk to an omelette or other egg dish.

Calories 1
Protein *1 g
Fat *1 g
Carbohydrate *1 g

*Less than

Fish Stock

Makes about 4 cups/1 L.

Great to keep in the freezer to use in soups or fish sauces. You can get bones from the fishmonger for next to nothing. Use this recipe as a guideline for quantities, including whatever mild-flavoured veggies you have on hand.

1	tsp. vegetable oil	5 mL
1	small onion, chopped	
1	leek, chopped	
1	celery stalk, chopped	
1	carrot, chopped	
2	sprigs parsley	
1½	lb. bones of lean fish, cut into pieces	750 g
5	cups cold water	1.25 L

Heat the oil in a large, heavy saucepan and sauté the vegetables until soft. Add the parsley, fish bones, and water and bring to a boil. Reduce heat; simmer, uncovered, for 30–40 minutes, skimming off the scum at intervals. Strain and cool. Refrigerate or freeze until needed.

Calories *1
Protein *1 g
Fat *1 g
Carbohydrate *1 g

*Less than

Chicken Stock

Makes about 6 cups/1.5 L.

An absolute must to have on hand for healthy cooking. Save the bones from boned chicken to use in this, freezing them if necessary until you have a sizable batch.

4	lb. chicken bones	2 kg
2	onions, peeled and quartered	
2	carrots, scrubbed and sliced	
2	celery stalks, sliced	
1	bouquet garni (see note)	
1	clove garlic, unpeeled	

Place all the ingredients in a large stockpot with enough cold water to cover. Bring to a boil, then reduce heat. Simmer, skimming off the scum at intervals, for about 2 hours or until reduced by one-third. Strain. For stronger flavour, reduce further. Refrigerate overnight. Remove the fat from the surface.

Note: To make the bouquet garni, wrap in cheesecloth a few stalks fresh parsley, 1 bay leaf, 1 sprig fresh or 1 pinch dried thyme, and 10 whole peppercorns. Tie with string to make a small bag.

Calories	3
Protein	*1 g
Fat	*1 g
Carbohydrate	*1 g

*Less than

Beef Stock

Makes about 6 cups/1.5 L.

Browning the bones in the oven is essential for a dark, rich stock. Have your butcher chop the bones for you.

4	lb. beef bones, cut into chunks	2 kg
2	onions, peeled and quartered	
2	carrots, scrubbed and cut into chunks	
2	celery stalks, cut into chunks	
1	bouquet garni (see note under chicken stock)	
1	clove garlic, unpeeled	
1	tomato, seeded and chopped	

Roast the bones in a roasting pan at 450°F/230°C for about 30 minutes or until browned. Add the vegetables to the pan and roast until browned, about 30 minutes.

Drain the fat from the pan. Transfer the bones and vegetables to a large stockpot. Add the bouquet garni, garlic, tomato, and enough water to cover. Bring to a boil and reduce heat. Simmer, skimming the scum off the surface, for 3–4 hours or until the stock is reduced by one-third. Strain. For stronger flavour, reduce further. Refrigerate overnight. Remove the fat from the surface.

Roasted Red Pepper Sauce

Calories 16
Protein *1 g
Fat *1 g
Carbohydrate 4 g

*Less than

Makes about 1 cup/250 mL.

Once you've tried roasting peppers, you'll find yourself an addict. This sauce is enhanced by the slightly sweet, delicate flavour that results from the roasting. For a luxurious touch, add 2 tbsp./25 mL fromage blanc (see page 161), but if you are heating the sauce to serve it hot, remember not to boil it. Great with grilled, poached, or baked meat, poultry, or fish.

2	large red bell peppers	
$\frac{1}{4}$	tsp. Tabasco sauce	1 mL
$\frac{1}{2}$	tsp. white wine vinegar	2 mL
2	tbsp. dry white wine	25 mL
2	tbsp. chopped fresh basil	25 mL

Salt and freshly ground pepper to taste

To roast the peppers, place them on a barbecue grill over medium heat or under the broiler and grill, turning at intervals, until blistered and slightly charred all over—about 10 minutes. Place the peppers in a brown paper bag; seal tightly. Leave for about 10 minutes, then peel off the skin with a sharp knife. Cut in half and remove seeds, working over a bowl to catch the juice.

Process the roasted peppers, their juice, the Tabasco, vinegar, and wine in a food processor or blender until smooth. Add the basil, salt, and pepper. To serve this sauce with pasta, cook it in a saucepan until heated through. It is also excellent served cold with cold chicken or fish or hot with grilled or baked chicken or fish.

Note: This sauce makes a terrific dip for vegetables by using $\frac{1}{4}$ cup/50 mL low-fat plain yogurt instead of wine.

Calories	3
Protein	*1 g
Fat	*1 g
Carbohydrate	*1 g

*Less than

Carrot Sauce

Makes about 1 cup/250 mL or enough to serve as a sauce with chicken or fish for 4.

Great hot or cold as a sauce for grilled or poached chicken or fish. And a great way to get in some beta-carotene.

4	medium carrots, thinly sliced	
2	tsp. lemon juice	10 mL
1	tbsp. orange juice	15 mL
$\frac{1}{2}$	tsp. grated orange peel	2 mL
$\frac{1}{2}$	cup low-fat plain yogurt	125 mL
1	tbsp. finely chopped fresh coriander (also	15 mL
	called Chinese parsley or cilantro)	

Salt and freshly ground pepper to taste

Place the carrots in a saucepan with enough water to cover. Bring to a boil, then reduce heat and simmer, covered, for about 10 minutes or until tender. Drain, reserving 3 tbsp./45 mL of cooking liquid.

Process the cooked carrots, reserved cooking liquid, lemon juice, and orange juice in a food processor or blender until very smooth. Transfer to a bowl. Stir in the remaining ingredients and mix well. Cover and chill.

Calories	129
Protein	27 g
Fat	2 g
Carbohydrate	0 g

Poached Chicken Breasts

The chicken turns out juicy and tender when cooked this way. Keep some pieces individually wrapped and frozen for later use in salads and sandwiches or for when you prepare a meal for one. Great as a main dish served with the red pepper or carrot sauce (see page 50 and above). Perfect for Mexican Chicken Salad (see page 52).

3 cups chicken stock (see page 48)   750 mL
Single chicken breasts

Bring chicken stock to a boil in a saucepan. Reduce heat to low and add chicken. Steam (but do not simmer) for 7–10 minutes or until breasts are cooked through.

Calories 258
Protein 29 g
Fat 11 g
Carbohydrate 11 g

*Less than

Mexican Chicken Salad

Serves 4.

Great on a bed of shredded lettuce with a crusty roll on the side. For a meal for one, stuff some in a tortilla or whole-wheat pita pocket. Delicious the next day—if you manage to have any left over.

$1\frac{3}{4}$	cup chicken breasts, poached (see page 51), skinned, boned, and cubed	425 mL
1	cup tomatoes, coarsely chopped	250 mL
$\frac{1}{3}$	cup red onion, finely chopped	75 mL
$\frac{1}{2}$	cup avocado, chopped	125 mL
1	tbsp. jalapeno pepper, seeded and finely chopped	15 mL
2	tbsp. fresh coriander, finely chopped	25 mL
$\frac{2}{3}$	cup canned corn, drained	150 mL
$1\frac{1}{2}$	tbsp. lime juice	20 mL
1	tbsp. virgin olive oil	15 mL

Salt and freshly ground pepper to taste

Mix chicken, tomatoes, onion, avocado, pepper, coriander, and corn in a large bowl. Combine lime juice, oil, salt, and pepper in a second bowl. Pour dressing over the salad and adjust seasonings if necessary. Chill in fridge about an hour.

Calories 205
Protein 20 g
Fat 7 g
Carbohydrate 14 g

Oriental Chicken Salad

Serves 6.

Try this chicken salad for an exotic taste from the Orient. Its vibrant colours and flavours will liven up any buffet table.

1	lb. chicken breasts, skinned, boned, and cubed	500 g
8	oz. zucchini, julienned	250 g
8	oz. red pepper, julienned	250 g
8	oz. snow peas, julienned	250 g
1	cup water chestnuts, sliced	250 mL
$1\frac{1}{2}$	tbsp. vegetable oil	20 mL

Coating		
$\frac{1}{2}$	tsp. salt	2 mL
2	tsp. freshly ground pepper	10 mL
2	tsp. Chinese 5 spices (see note)	10 mL
2	tsp. ground ginger	10 mL
2	tsp. dry mustard	10 mL
1	tsp. turmeric	5 mL
1	tsp. mild curry powder	5 mL

Vinaigrette		
$\frac{1}{3}$	cup orange juice concentrate	75 mL
$\frac{1}{4}$	cup water	50 mL
4	tsp. vegetable oil	20 mL

Combine coating ingredients in a small bowl. Sprinkle mixture over chicken breasts and chill in fridge $1\frac{1}{2}$ hours. Meanwhile, prepare vinaigrette by combining orange juice concentrate, water, and oil. Set aside.

Bring salted water to boil in a saucepan. Immerse vegetables 15–20 seconds, drain, and refresh under cold water. Set vegetables aside.

Heat oil in a wok or frying pan and cook chicken about 5 minutes. To assemble salad, toss together warm chicken and vegetables, then mix in dressing. Serve at room temperature.

Note: This packaged combination is available at Oriental grocery or specialty food stores; can substitute $\frac{1}{4}$ tsp./1 mL each of ground fennel, ginger, cinnamon, and cloves.

Almond Herbed Chicken Roll-Ups

Calories 314
Protein 35 g
Fat 13 g
Carbohydrate 5 g

Serves 8.

A low-fat version of chicken Kiev, this is a big hit with children. It's crisp and juicy all at the same time.

8	single chicken breasts, skinned and boned	
$\frac{1}{2}$	tsp. dried or 1 tsp. fresh thyme	2 mL/5 mL
$\frac{1}{2}$	tsp. dried or 1 tsp. fresh oregano	2 mL/5 mL
2	tsp. dried or 1 tbsp. fresh basil	10 mL/15 mL
Salt and freshly ground pepper to taste		
2	tbsp. chopped fresh parsley	25 mL
2	tbsp. soft margarine	25 mL
1	cup whole-wheat bread crumbs	250 mL
$\frac{1}{3}$	cup wheat germ	75 mL
$\frac{3}{4}$	cup chopped almonds	175 mL
2	eggs, beaten	

Pound the chicken breasts with a mallet between two sheets of plastic wrap until they are about $\frac{1}{4}$ inch/$\frac{1}{2}$ cm thick.

Combine the seasonings in a small bowl and sprinkle them evenly over the chicken. Divide the margarine into 8 portions; place each portion near the end of each flattened chicken breast. Roll the chicken up jelly roll style, tucking in the ends to form a package.

Combine the bread crumbs, wheat germ, and almonds in a shallow dish. Place the eggs in a separate shallow dish. Dip each chicken roll in the crumb mixture, then in the egg mixture, and back in the crumb mixture, turning to coat well. Place on a lightly greased baking sheet.

Bake at 350°F/180°C for 30–40 minutes or until crisp and golden brown.

Tarragon Chicken

Serves 6.

One of the quickest and most delicious ways to cook chicken. Its incomparably rich-tasting sauce is made by reducing the vinegar and chicken stock.

4	medium onions, sliced	
$\frac{1}{4}$	cup water	50 mL
2	large tomatoes, coarsely chopped	
2	cloves garlic, minced	
1	bay leaf	
1	tsp. dried or 2 tbsp. fresh tarragon	5 mL/25 mL
1	tbsp. vegetable oil	15 mL
6	single chicken breasts, skinned and boned	
1	cup red or white wine vinegar	250 mL
1	cup homemade chicken stock (see pages 48–49)	250 mL

Salt and freshly ground pepper to taste

Place the onions and water in a large, heavy casserole. Bring to a boil, then reduce heat. Cover and simmer for 30 minutes, stirring occasionally and adding a little more water if necessary. Add the tomatoes, garlic, bay leaf, and tarragon. Cover and simmer 5 minutes longer.

Heat the oil in a large, heavy skillet. Add the chicken and brown on both sides. Transfer the chicken to the onion-tomato mixture in the casserole. Bring the mixture to a boil and reduce heat. Cover and simmer for 20 minutes or until the chicken is cooked.

Add the vinegar to the skillet in which the chicken was browned, stirring up the brown bits from the bottom of the pan with a spoon. Bring to a boil and cook over high heat until thick and syrupy—about 10 minutes. Add the stock and return to the boil. Cook over high heat until it is reduced to about $\frac{1}{4}$ cup/50 mL—about 10 minutes. Strain and add to the chicken mixture in the casserole. Remove the chicken and keep warm. Discard the bay leaf.

Purée the vegetable mixture in a food processor or blender until smooth. Return to the casserole with the chicken. Cook until heated through. Season to taste with salt and pepper. Serve with noodles, potatoes, or rice and steamed veggies.

Grilled Chicken with Caper Mayonnaise

Calories 158
Protein 27 g
Fat 4 g
Carbohydrate 2 g

Serves 4.

The mayonnaise keeps the chicken moist and juicy. A long-time favourite at my house—great barbecued for a main dish centrepiece or served up as a burger in a pita pocket.

4	single chicken breasts, skinned and boned	
3	tbsp. light mayonnaise	45 mL
1	tbsp. lemon juice	15 mL
2	tsp. Dijon mustard	10 mL
2	tsp. chopped capers	10 mL
Salt and freshly ground pepper to taste		
2	tbsp. parsley, finely chopped, for garnish	25 mL

Mix all ingredients except chicken and parsley in a bowl. Lightly coat the chicken breasts. Broil in oven for 5 minutes, turn, and broil another 5 minutes or until chicken is cooked through. Season and garnish with chopped parsley.

Lemon Artichoke Chicken

Calories 236
Protein 34 g
Fat 8 g
Carbohydrate 11 g

Serves 4.

Perfect for a quick family meal served on a bed of noodles with a green salad. Cut the chicken into chunks for a variation on this theme.

4	single chicken breasts, skinned and boned	
4	tsp. all-purpose flour	20 mL
1	tbsp. vegetable oil	15 mL
1	medium onion, finely chopped	
1	cup sliced mushrooms	250 mL
1	clove garlic, minced	
$\frac{1}{2}$	cup homemade chicken stock (see pages 48–49)	125 mL
2	tsp. lemon juice	10 mL
$\frac{1}{2}$	cup dry white wine	75 mL
1	bay leaf	
2	tbsp. finely chopped fresh parsley	25 mL
$\frac{1}{2}$	tsp. dried or 2 tbsp. chopped fresh basil	2 mL/25 mL
1	14-oz./398-mL can artichoke hearts packed in water, drained, and halved	
	Salt and freshly ground pepper to taste	
$\frac{1}{2}$	lemon, thinly sliced, for garnish	

Dredge the chicken in flour. Heat the oil in a large, heavy saucepan or skillet. Add the onion, mushrooms, and garlic; sauté until soft. Add the chicken, stock, lemon juice, wine, and bay leaf. Bring to a boil, then reduce heat and simmer, uncovered, for 10 minutes. Stir in the parsley, basil, and artichokes. Turn the chicken breasts over in the sauce. Cover and simmer 10 minutes longer or until the chicken is cooked and the sauce is slightly thickened. Season with salt and pepper and garnish with lemon.

Chicken with Lime, Ginger, and Coriander

Calories 399
Protein 32 g
Fat 10 g
Carbohydrate 44 g

Serves 4.

An elegant dish for guests, yet easy enough to prepare any time.

4	single chicken breasts, skinned, boned, and flattened	
1	cup brown rice, uncooked	250 mL
$\frac{1}{3}$	cup wild rice, uncooked	75 mL
$1\frac{1}{2}$	tbsp. vegetable oil	20 mL
Salt and freshly ground pepper to taste		

Marinade

1	tbsp. fresh ginger, peeled and finely chopped	15 mL
1	clove garlic, minced	
3	tbsp. lime juice	45 mL
2	tsp. vegetable oil	10 mL
2	red peppers, thinly sliced	
2	tbsp. coriander, finely chopped	25 mL

Combine ginger, garlic, lime juice, and oil in a large bowl. Arrange chicken breasts in marinade and chill in fridge, turning occasionally, at least 45 minutes (overnight if possible). Before cooking chicken prepare rice according to package directions.

Heat 1 tbsp./15 mL oil in a skillet and cook chicken breasts on medium-high heat for about 3 minutes per side. Season and transfer to a warm oven.

Add 1 tsp./5 mL oil to pan and cook red peppers on medium-high heat until tender but firm, about 5 minutes.

To serve, place chicken on a bed of rice and garnish with the red pepper and chopped coriander.

Calories 265
Protein 16 g
Fat 8 g
Carbohydrate 34 g

Turkish Beef Pilaf

Serves 4–6.

A flavourful example of how to reduce your portions of meat. The apricots add just a touch of sweetness to the dish. Kashi, a prepacked grain product containing seven grains and sesame seeds, provides a nice crunch plus an added bonus of fibre.

$\frac{1}{3}$	cup orange juice	75 mL
2	tsp. vegetable oil	10 mL
1	tbsp. ginger, peeled and finely chopped	15 mL
8	oz. lean steak tips, sliced into thin strips	250 g
1	6.5-oz./package Kashi (see note)	
1	cup water	250 mL
1	cup chicken stock (see pages 48–49)	250 mL
$\frac{3}{4}$	cup onions, chopped	175 mL
$\frac{1}{4}$	cup dried apricots, finely chopped	50 mL
1	tbsp. vegetable oil	15 mL
1	large carrot, diagonally sliced	
Salt and freshly ground pepper to taste		
$\frac{1}{4}$	cup green onions, finely sliced, for garnish	50 mL

Mix orange juice, 2 tsp./10 mL oil, ginger, and meat in a bowl. Marinate in fridge at least $\frac{1}{2}$ hour.

Boil the Kashi, water, and stock in a medium-sized uncovered saucepan, then reduce heat and allow Kashi to simmer, covered. Cook for 15 minutes, add onions and apricots, and continue cooking 10–15 minutes or until all moisture has evaporated.

Meanwhile, heat 2 tsp./10 mL oil in a skillet and stir-fry steak tips for about 2 minutes. Remove beef and drain. Heat 1 tsp./5 mL oil, add carrot slices, and stir-fry for about 1 minute. Return beef to skillet for 1–2 minutes, constantly stir-frying.

To serve, place meat and carrot mixture atop bed of Kashi and garnish with green onions.

Note: Kashi is available at health food stores; can substitute brown rice, bulgur, or couscous, but adjust cooking times accordingly.

Calories 259
Protein 21 g
Fat 6 g
Carbohydrate 33 g

Chili con Carne

Serves 6.

This is a fast version that can be made with canned or cooked beans. Double the quantity and freeze half for an emergency meal. My kids love to make a "chili bar" with toppings of shredded lettuce, Tomato Salsa Dip (see page 146), and different types of tortillas.

2	tsp. vegetable oil	10 mL
8	oz. lean ground beef	250 g
1	medium onion, chopped	
3	cloves garlic, minced	
1	cup carrots, sliced	250 mL
1	cup green pepper, chopped	250 mL
1	28-oz./796-mL can Italian plum tomatoes	
1	cup tomato sauce	250 mL
3	cups kidney beans, canned or cooked	750 mL
2	tsp. chili powder	10 mL
1	tsp. cumin	5 mL
1	tsp. mild curry powder	10 mL
1	bay leaf	
$\frac{1}{2}$	tsp. cayenne	2 mL

Heat oil in a large, heavy saucepan. Add the meat and cook until it is brown, stirring occasionally. Remove beef and drain fat from pan. Return beef to saucepan and add the onion, cooking until it is soft. Add garlic and cook 2 minutes. Add carrots and green peppers and cook 3 minutes more. Stir in tomatoes and tomato sauce, crushing the tomatoes with the back of a spoon. Add kidney beans and bring mixture to a boil. Add seasonings, then simmer, covered, for about 30 minutes. Discard the bay leaf before serving.

Basic Poached Fish

A simple and quick way to prepare fish. Make two meals at one time. Tonight, try it hot with Presto Tomato Sauce (see page 98) and noodles. Tomorrow, serve it cold with Cucumber Sauce (see page 63) or Watercress Sauce (see page 63).

Poaching	1	cup water	250 mL
Liquid 1	2	tbsp. lemon juice	25 mL
		Salt and freshly ground pepper to taste	

Add all ingredients to a saucepan and bring to a boil. Reduce heat to low and add fish. Steam but do not simmer. Cook approximately 10 minutes per inch/25 cm thickness of fish. Do not overcook.

Poaching	4	cups water	1 L
Liquid 2	2	tbsp. lemon juice	25 mL
	1	medium onion, cut in half	
	1	carrot	
	$\frac{3}{4}$	celery stalk	
	4	cloves	
	12	peppercorns	

Place all ingredients in a shallow pan and bring to a boil. Reduce heat and simmer for 20 minutes. Remove vegetables, add fish, and steam but do not simmer. Cook approximately 10 minutes per inch/25 cm thickness of fish. Do not overcook.

Note: Strain liquid through cheesecloth or fine strainer. Freeze fish stock for poaching fish again or for use in soups or other recipes.

Basic Grilled Fish

Do as the fisherfolk do and cook fish the simplest way—over hot coals or an open fire. You can barbecue or broil any fish with superb results if you follow this basic method, which requires only a little oil for brushing on the fish.

- If the fish has been in the fridge, bring it to room temperature before grilling.

- Clean and descale the fish with a sharp knife. Do not remove the tail or head until the fish is cooked.

- Season the fish inside and out with a little salt, plenty of freshly ground black pepper, and herbs if you wish.

- Preheat the grill of a barbecue or broiler until very hot. Grill the fish over high heat so the skin sears; this way it will not break during cooking. Reduce the heat to medium. Cook the fish until it flakes with a fork—3 or 4 minutes per side for medium-sized fish. Do not overcook, or the fish will be dry.

- While the fish is cooking, brush it lightly at intervals with a little vegetable oil that has been mixed with fresh or dried herbs.

- Serve with a sauce such as Cucumber Sauce (see page 63) or Mango Salsa (page 64) on the side.

Cucumber Sauce

Calories 162
Protein 4 g
Fat 13 g
Carbohydrate 8 g

Makes 1 cup/250 mL.

Great as an accompaniment to grilled, poached, or baked fish with or without the capers.

1	cup peeled, seeded, and shredded cucumber	250 mL
½	cup low-fat plain yogurt	125 mL
2	tbsp. light mayonnaise	25 mL
2	tbsp. chopped fresh dill	25 mL
2	tsp. chopped capers (optional)	10 mL

Salt and freshly ground pepper to taste

Wrap the cucumber in a clean tea towel and squeeze out the excess water. Combine the yogurt and mayonnaise in a bowl and mix well. Stir in the cucumber and remaining ingredients. Chill. Serve with cooked fish.

Watercress Sauce

Calories 56
Protein 1 g
Fat 4 g
Carbohydrate 4 g

Serves 6 (makes 2 cups/500 mL).

A super sauce for cold fish. For a tasty dip, substitute low-fat plain yogurt for the buttermilk.

1	cup watercress, stems removed	250 mL
½	cup light mayonnaise	125 mL
½	cup buttermilk	125 mL
1	tbsp. lemon juice	15 mL
1	tbsp. fresh parsley	15 mL
1	tbsp. fresh dill	15 mL
½	tsp. tarragon	2 mL

Process all the ingredients in a food processor or blender until smooth. Refrigerate at least 4 hours before serving.

Calories 59
Protein 5 g
Fat 2 g
Carbohydrate 10 g

Mango Salsa

Serves 6.

This exquisite accompaniment is a simple, fast, and colorful way to dress up grilled fish (especially tuna) or chicken.

2	cups mango, coarsely chopped	500 mL
2	tbsp. red pepper, finely chopped	25 mL
2	tbsp. green pepper, finely chopped	25 mL
2	tbsp. green onion, finely chopped	25 mL
$1\frac{1}{2}$	tbsp. lime juice	20 mL
1	tbsp. fresh coriander, chopped	15 mL
2	tbsp. fresh parsley, chopped	25 mL
1	tbsp. virgin olive oil	15 mL
$\frac{1}{2}$	tsp. cumin	2 mL

Salt and freshly ground pepper to taste

Combine all the ingredients in a bowl and mix well. Adjust seasonings if necessary.

Calories 236
Protein 27 g
Fat 9 g
Carbohydrate 12 g

Crisp Fish Sticks

Serves 4–6.

A nourishing, low-fat creation that will have the kids coming back for seconds. A tasty, healthful substitute for frozen fish sticks.

$\frac{1}{2}$	cup low-fat plain yogurt	125 mL
1	tbsp. chopped fresh parsley	15 mL
Salt and freshly ground pepper to taste		
$\frac{1}{2}$	cup wheat germ, toasted	125 mL
$\frac{1}{2}$	cup whole-wheat breadcrumbs	125 mL
2	cups grated low-fat cheese	500 mL
1	lb. firm-fleshed fish fillets (halibut, cod, haddock, bluefish, etc.), cut into 8 1-inch/2-cm sticks	500 g

Combine the yogurt, parsley, salt, and pepper in a shallow dish and mix well.

To toast the wheat germ, cook in a heavy skillet over low heat, for 2–3 minutes or until golden brown, shaking the skillet constantly. Combine the toasted wheat germ, bread crumbs, and cheese in a separate shallow dish.

Dip each fish stick into the yogurt, then into the wheat germ mixture, coating well. Place on a lightly greased baking sheet. Bake at 425°F/220°C for 5 minutes. Turn and bake 5 minutes longer or until the coating is crisp and the fish flakes easily.

Ginger Fish with Oriental Vegetables

Calories 374
Protein 29 g
Fat 9 g
Carbohydrate 40 g

Serves 4.

A sure-fire way to convert non-fish eaters. This fast meal is great for the family and elegant enough for entertaining. Grilled boneless chicken breasts work every bit as well as fish.

1	lb. firm-fleshed fish fillets (grouper, snapper, etc.)	500 g
6	oz. rice noodles	175 g
2	tsp. vegetable oil	10 mL
1	tsp. sesame oil	5 mL
1	clove garlic, minced	
2	tsp. fresh ginger, peeled and finely chopped	10 mL
1	large carrot, diagonally sliced	
4	oz. snow peas, topped, tailed, and julienned	125 g
4	oz. button mushrooms, sliced	125 g
4	oz. oyster mushrooms, sliced	125 g
2	tbsp. chopped coriander, for garnish	25 mL

Marinade

4	tbsp. lime juice	50 mL
2	tbsp. sodium-reduced soy sauce	25 mL
$1\frac{1}{2}$	tbsp. fresh ginger, finely chopped	20 mL
2	cloves garlic	
2	tsp. sesame oil	10 mL

Combine all ingredients for marinade but pour only $\frac{1}{4}$ cup/50 mL over the fish. Marinate fish in the refrigerator for 1 hour or overnight.

Bake fish until it is just cooked and flakes, about 10–12 minutes, at 350°F/180°C. Be sure to check fish while completing noodle and vegetable preparation.

Meanwhile, cook noodles in a medium-sized pot. Heat 1 tsp./5 mL vegetable oil and 1 tsp./5 mL sesame oil in a wok or frying pan, and cook garlic and ginger until golden. Add carrots and cook 2 minutes more; add snow peas and cook for another minute. Add 1 tsp./5 mL oil if the vegetables are dry and stick to pan. Add mushrooms and cook until half their liquid evaporates, about 4 minutes. Add remaining marinade and mix well with vegetables. Finally, add noodles to the pan and stir constantly until they are well coated with sauce.

To serve, place vegetable-noodle mixture on plates and top with fish. Pour on the pan juices and garnish with chopped coriander.

Calories 223
Protein 30 g
Fat 10 g
Carbohydrate 2 g

Zesty Halibut Steaks

Serves 4.

This recipe is one from the Fisheries Council of British Columbia. It's also super tasting with salmon.

4	halibut steaks, each about 1-inch/2 cm. thick	
	cayenne	
2	cloves garlic	
2	tbsp. olive oil	25 mL
$\frac{1}{3}$	cup fresh parsley, chopped	100 mL
1	tsp. capers	5 mL
$\frac{1}{2}$	tsp. lemon zest	2 mL
$\frac{1}{4}$	cup lemon juice	50 mL

Sprinkle each halibut steak with pinch of cayenne. Sauté 1 clove garlic in oil at medium heat until golden; remove from oil. Increase heat to medium high. Sauté halibut 4 minutes each side. Add remaining clove garlic, parsley, capers, grated lemon zest, and lemon juice. Cook 1–2 minutes longer. Drizzle with pan juices and serve.

Greek Fish with a Warm Tomato Vinaigrette

Calories 228
Protein 21 g
Fat 5 g
Carbohydrate 15 g

Serves 4.

A zesty dish with a hint of licorice. Serve with brown rice on the side.

1	lb. salmon-trout or other firm-fleshed fish	500 g
1	tsp. vegetable oil	5 mL
1	tsp. virgin olive oil	5 mL
6	oz. fennel, white part only, finely chopped (see note)	175 g
2	tsp. ouzo or anisette liqueur	10 mL

Vinaigrette

2	tbsp. virgin olive oil	25 mL
3	tbsp. red wine vinegar	40 mL
1	tsp. brown sugar	5 mL
1	medium tomato, coarsely chopped	
Salt and freshly ground pepper to taste		

2	tbsp. olives, finely chopped	25 mL
2	tbsp. fresh parsley, finely chopped	25 mL

Heat 1 tsp./5 mL vegetable oil and 1 tsp./5 mL olive oil in a Dutch oven or casserole. Add fennel and cook 5 minutes on medium heat. Add liqueur and cook another minute. Place fish on top of fennel and bake, covered, at 350°F/180°C for 10–15 minutes.

Meanwhile, make the vinaigrette by heating the oil in a small saucepan, adding the vinegar and brown sugar, and cooking for 5 minutes. Add the tomatoes and heat through. Adjust seasonings.

Serve on individual plates, drizzling $1\frac{1}{2}$ tbsp./20 mL of warm vinaigrette over each portion of the fish and fennel. Garnish with the olives and chopped parsley.

Note: If fennel is unavailable, substitute celery or spinach.

Warm Salmon Salad
with Fennel and Orange

Calories 316
Protein 28 g
Fat 12 g
Carbohydrate 23 g

Serves 4.

Another delicious way of getting in those heart-healthy omega-3 fatty acids. The sauce is also wonderful on cold fish.

1	lb. salmon fillets, skinned	500 g
4	cups poaching liquid	1 L
1	tsp. vegetable oil	5 mL
$1\frac{1}{2}$	cups fennel, white part only, diced (see note)	375 mL
2	oranges, sectioned (retain any juice)	
	lettuce leaves	

Dressing

$\frac{1}{4}$	cup light mayonnaise	50 mL
$\frac{3}{4}$	cup low-fat plain yogurt	175 mL
$\frac{1}{4}$	cup orange juice concentrate	50 mL

Poach the salmon in a deep saucepan (see page 61) and cool slightly. Meanwhile, in another saucepan, heat the oil. Add the fennel and cook until soft and transparent, about 8 minutes. Add oranges and their juice and warm through, about 1 minute. Combine dressing ingredients in a small bowl.

Serve each fillet on an individual plate on a bed of lettuce leaves. Pour 2 tbsp./25 mL dressing over each fillet, then top with $\frac{1}{4}$ cup/50 mL of the fennel mixture.

Note: If fennel is unavailable, substitute celery.

Calories 173
Protein 11 g
Fat 10 g
Carbohydrate 8 g

Salmon and Spinach Gratin

Serves 3–4.

This recipe has been adapted from the Fisheries Council of British Columbia. Including the salmon bones is an easy way to boost the calcium content of the dish. Serve with rice or noodles.

10	oz. fresh spinach	284 g
1	tsp. soft margarine	5 mL
1	cup sliced mushrooms	250 mL
2	tbsp. soft margarine	25 mL
2	tbsp. all-purpose flour	25 mL
1	cup 1% milk	250 mL
2	tbsp. chopped green onion	25 mL
	freshly grated pepper to taste	
1	$7\frac{1}{2}$-oz/213-g can salmon	

Topping	2	tbsp. fresh brown breadcrumbs	25 mL
	2	tbsp. freshly grated Parmesan cheese	25 mL
	1	tbsp. chopped fresh parsley	15 mL

Remove stems from spinach; cook spinach in boiling water 3–5 minutes or until wilted. Drain thoroughly and chop coarsely; spread over bottom of 8-inch/20-cm gratin pan or shallow baking dish.

In small skillet, melt 1 tsp./5 mL margarine; add mushrooms and cook over medium-high heat, stirring often until lightly browned; spread over spinach.

In small saucepan melt 2 tbsp./25 mL margarine; stir in flour and cook, stirring over medium-low heat, for 1 minute. Add milk and whisk until mixture simmers and is smooth and thickened. Stir in green onion and pepper to taste. Flake salmon and add with well-mashed bones and juice; mix gently, then spoon over mushrooms.

Combine breadcrumbs, cheese, and parsley; sprinkle over top. Microwave at high for 3 minutes, or bake in oven at 400°F/200°C for 15 minutes or until heated through. Brown top under broiler for 2 minutes if necessary.

Calories 108
Protein 20 g
Fat 1 g
Carbohydrate 5 g

Scallops in a Pouch

Serves 4–6.

The delicate taste of scallops is enhanced by the flavour of ginger, lemon, and garlic in this aromatic creation cooked in a foil pouch for maximum flavour and nutrients. Adapted from a recipe from B.C. Fisheries.

Aluminum foil
Vegetable oil for brushing
1   lb. scallops   500 g
1   medium carrot, peeled and cut into thin
    julienne strips
1   leek (white part only), cut into thin
    julienne strips
1   celery stalk, cut into thin julienne strips
1   clove garlic, minced
1   tsp. minced fresh ginger root   5 mL
Juice of $\frac{1}{2}$ lemon
Salt and freshly ground pepper to taste

Lightly brush 1 large or 4 smaller squares of foil with the oil and place the scallops on them. Top with the vegetables, garlic, and ginger root. Sprinkle with the lemon juice, salt, and pepper. Fold the foil over and crimp the edges to seal well and form 1 large or 4 individual pouches. Place on a baking sheet.

Bake at 400°F/200°C for about 10 minutes or until the scallops are opaque. Place pouch(es) on 1 large or 4 individual plates and open at the table to let the aroma escape.

Calories 182
Protein 18 g
Fat 11 g
Carbohydrate 3 g

Super Seafood Kebabs

Serves 4–6.

The distinct flavour of orange peel combined with fresh ginger in this recipe, also from B.C. Fisheries, makes these grilled kebabs tops for taste as well as nutrition. A great way to include those omega-3 fatty acids in your diet.

Marinade		
$\frac{1}{2}$	cup orange juice	125 mL
3	tbsp. vegetable oil	45 mL
$\frac{1}{4}$	cup low-sodium soy sauce	50 mL
$\frac{1}{4}$	cup wine vinegar	50 mL
1	clove garlic, minced	
1	tsp. minced fresh ginger root	5 mL
1	tbsp. grated orange peel	15 mL
	Freshly ground black pepper to taste	

4	oz. fresh salmon steak, cut into 1-inch/2-cm cubes	125 g
4	oz. fresh halibut steak, cut into 1-inch/2-cm cubes	125 g
4	oz. monkfish, cut into 1-inch/2-cm cubes	125 g
4	oz. large shrimp, peeled and deveined	125 g

Whisk together the first 8 ingredients in a small bowl. Place the fish and shrimp in a shallow glass dish. Pour the marinade over and let sit for 2 hours in the fridge, turning once or twice.

Drain the seafood, reserving the marinade for basting. Thread the salmon, halibut, monkfish, and shrimp alternately on bamboo skewers that have been soaked in water for 1 hour.

Barbecue the kebabs on a lightly oiled grill over medium heat for 8–10 minutes, turning once. Serve with rice and salad.

Calories 208
Protein 18 g
Fat 4 g
Carbohydrate 26 g

Speedy Fish Chowder

Serves 6.

A cross between a stew and a soup, this hearty chowder is perfect served with a salad and a crusty roll.

1 $\frac{1}{2}$	tbsp. soft margarine	22 mL
$\frac{3}{4}$	cup onions, diced	175 mL
$\frac{1}{2}$	cup celery, diced	125 mL
1	cup carrots, diced	250 mL
2 $\frac{1}{2}$	cups water	625 mL
4	medium potatoes, diced	
1	tsp. thyme	5 mL
Salt and freshly ground pepper		
2	tbsp. fresh parsley, finely chopped	25 mL
1	pound fish fillets (sole, haddock, cod or whitefish), cut into small pieces	500 g
2	cups skim milk	500 mL
2	tbsp. fresh parsley, finely chopped	25 mL

Heat margarine in a large saucepan. Sauté onion until translucent. Add celery and carrots and sauté until soft. Add water, potatoes, thyme and seasonings; cover and simmer until tender—about 20 minutes. Add fish and simmer for about 10 minutes; add milk and cook until heated through. Ladle into bowls and garnish with parsley.

Calories	194	
Protein	17 g	
Fat	6 g	
Carbohydrate	13 g	

Bouillabaisse

Serves 12 as a main course.

A fish-filled concoction from the south of France that puts the day's catch to superb use, this recipe is designed to feed a crowd and can be adapted to incorporate almost any fresh fish. Great served with crusty bread and a crisp salad. Halve the recipe if you wish.

2	tbsp. virgin olive oil	25 mL
1	cup finely chopped onion	250 mL
2	cups finely chopped leeks	500 mL
2	tbsp. minced garlic	25 mL
1	cup finely diced celery	250 mL
2	cups finely diced red pepper	500 mL
1	tsp. saffron	5 mL
$\frac{1}{2}$	tsp. crushed fennel seeds	2 mL
1	bay leaf	
$\frac{1}{2}$	tsp. dried thyme	2 mL
2	tbsp. tomato paste	25 mL
6	cups fish stock (see page 48)	1.5 L
1	cup dry white wine	250 mL
1	cup chopped tomatoes	250 mL
1	lb. monkfish fillets, cut into chunks	500 g
1	lb. halibut fillets, cut into chunks	500 g
1	lb. swordfish fillets, cut into chunks	500 g
$\frac{1}{2}$	lb. large shrimp, peeled and deveined	250 g
18	littleneck clams	
2	lb. mussels, scrubbed and with beard removed	1 kg
$\frac{1}{2}$	cup chopped fresh parsley	125 mL

Heat the oil in a large, heavy pot. Add the onion, leeks, and garlic and sauté until soft. Add the celery and red pepper. Cook for 1 minute, stirring. Add the saffron, fennel seeds, bay leaf, thyme, tomato paste, stock, and wine. Bring to a boil, reduce heat, and simmer for about 10 minutes. Add the tomatoes and fish. Simmer for 2–3 minutes. Add the shrimp, clams, and mussels. Return to the boil, then reduce heat. Cover and simmer for 3–4 minutes or until the clams and mussels open. To serve, remove and discard the bay leaf. Sprinkle with parsley.

Calories 209
Protein 13 g
Fat 8 g
Carbohydrate 22 g

Clam Chowder

Serves 4–6.

If you wish, substitute about $\frac{3}{4}$ lb./375 g fresh fish fillets cut into chunks for the canned clams.

2	tbsp. soft margarine	25 mL
1	small onion, finely chopped	
2	tbsp. finely chopped green pepper	25 mL
1	clove garlic, minced	
3	tbsp. all-purpose flour	45 mL
$3\frac{1}{2}$	cups 2% milk	875 mL
2	medium carrots, peeled and finely diced	
2	celery stalks, finely diced	
2	medium potatoes, peeled and finely diced	
2	medium tomatoes, chopped	
2	5-oz./142-g cans baby clams, undrained	
2	tsp. dried chervil	10 mL

Salt and freshly ground pepper to taste

Heat the margarine in a large, heavy saucepan. Sauté the onion, green pepper, and garlic until soft. Stir in the flour and cook, stirring, over low heat for 1 minute. Whisk in the milk and bring to a boil. Add the carrots, celery, and potatoes and simmer for 20 minutes or until the potatoes are soft. Add the tomatoes and simmer 10 minutes longer. Add the clams with their juice, chervil, salt, and pepper. Cook until they are heated through.

Calories 272
Protein 14 g
Fat   5 g
Carbohydrate 47 g

Lentil Soup

Serves 4.

Use red rather than brown lentils for this rib-hugging soup, which packs a terrific protein punch, is high in soluble fibre, and turns an attractive yellow when cooked.

1	tbsp. vegetable oil	15 mL
1	cup finely chopped onion	250 mL
1	large clove garlic, minced	
1	cup red lentils, rinsed	250 mL
4	cups homemade chicken or vegetable stock (see pages 48–49 and 139) or water	1 L
1	bay leaf	
$\frac{1}{2}$	tsp. dried thyme	2 mL
1	cup finely chopped carrots	250 mL
1	cup finely chopped celery	250 mL
1	cup chopped tomatoes	250 mL

Juice of 2 limes or lemons
2   tsp. honey   10 mL
Salt and freshly ground pepper to taste

Heat the oil in a large, heavy pot. Add the onion and garlic; sauté until soft. Add the lentils, stock, bay leaf, and thyme. Bring to a boil, reduce heat, and simmer, covered, for 1 hour or until the lentils are tender. Add the carrots and celery. Return to the boil, then reduce heat. Simmer for 30 minutes or until the vegetables are soft. Discard the bay leaf. Add the tomatoes, lime juice, honey, salt, and pepper. Cook until heated through.

Calories 357
Protein 22 g
Fat 3 g
Carbohydrate 61 g

Black Bean Soup

Serves 8–10.

Thick, rich, creamy, and loaded with soluble fibre, this soup makes a complete protein meal when eaten with whole-grain bread. Dried black beans, sometimes called turtle beans, are available in most health, Mexican, or South American food stores.

1	tbsp. vegetable oil	15 mL
1	medium onion, finely chopped	
2	leeks, finely chopped	
3	cloves garlic, minced	
2	celery stalks, finely chopped	
2	cups black beans, soaked for 2 hours in 8 cups/2 L water	500 mL
1	bay leaf	
1	tbsp. ground cumin	15 mL
2	tsp. dried oregano	10 mL
$\frac{1}{2}$	tsp. dried thyme	2 mL
Pinch cayenne pepper or to taste		
$\frac{1}{4}$	cup dry sherry	50 mL
1	tbsp. lemon juice	15 mL
Salt and pepper to taste		
$\frac{1}{2}$	cup low-fat plain yogurt	125 mL
$\frac{1}{4}$	cup finely chopped fresh parsley for garnish	50 mL

Heat the oil in a large, heavy pot. Add the onion and leeks and sauté until soft. Add the garlic and celery; sauté for 1 minute over medium heat. Add the beans with their soaking liquid, bay leaf, cumin, oregano, thyme, and cayenne. Bring to a boil, reduce heat, and simmer, partially covered, for $1\frac{1}{2}$–2 hours or until the beans are soft.

Process the mixture in a food processor or blender in batches, if necessary, until smooth. Return to the pot, then stir in the sherry, lemon juice, salt, and pepper. Return to the boil.

To serve, ladle the soup into individual bowls, place a dollop of yogurt on top, and sprinkle with parsley.

Calories 120
Protein 6 g
Fat 2 g
Carbohydrate 20 g

Bean and Pasta Soup

Serves 6–8.

Popular in the Tuscany region of Italy, this soup is a great one to keep in the fridge or freezer for a quick winter meal. Because beans and pasta complement each other, this soup makes a complete protein meal that sticks magnificently to the ribs! You can substitute black-eyed peas or pinto, white pea, or navy beans for the kidney beans if you wish.

1	tsp. vegetable oil	5 mL
1	tsp. virgin olive oil	5 mL
1	onion, finely chopped	
2	cloves garlic, minced	
1	stalk celery, finely chopped	
1	carrot, finely chopped	
1	cup puréed canned or fresh tomatoes	250 mL
3	tbsp. finely chopped parsley	45 mL
2	tsp. dried basil	10 mL
$\frac{1}{2}$	tsp. dried sage	2 mL
$\frac{1}{4}$	tsp. dried hot pepper flakes	1 mL
7	cups vegetable or chicken stock (see pages 139 and 48–49)	1.75 L
1	cup dried white or red kidney beans, soaked for at least 2 hours in 3 cups/750 mL water	250 mL
1	cup elbow macaroni or other small pasta	250 mL

Salt and freshly ground pepper to taste

Heat the oils in a large pot. Add the onion and garlic and sauté until soft. Add the celery and carrot; sauté over medium heat for 1 minute. Stir in the tomatoes, parsley, basil, sage, and pepper flakes. Add the stock and beans with their soaking liquid. Bring to a boil, then reduce heat. Simmer, partially covered, for about 2 hours or until the beans are soft. Return the soup to the boil and add the macaroni. Cook until al dente and season with salt and pepper. Serve with grated Parmesan cheese on the side and plenty of crusty bread.

Zesty Rice and Bean Combo

Serves 6–8.

This one's a family favourite. If you like, you can substitute canned kidney beans, but my kids prefer the texture of the black turtle beans. I usually cook up a double batch of the beans and freeze them for next time.

1	tbsp. vegetable oil	15 mL
3	cloves garlic, minced	
1	onion, chopped	
2	cups mushrooms, sliced	500 mL
1	green pepper, seeded and diced	
1	red pepper, seeded and diced	
1	28-oz./796-mL can Italian plum tomatoes	
$2\frac{1}{2}$	cups black turtle beans, cooked	625 mL
2	cups corn kernels, fresh or frozen	500 mL
1	cup long grain rice	250 mL
$\frac{1}{4}$	cup water	50 mL
$2\frac{1}{2}$	tsp. chili powder	12 mL
$1\frac{1}{2}$	tsp. cumin	7 mL
1	tsp. dried oregano	5 mL
dash cayenne		
$\frac{3}{4}$	cup grated part-skim mozzarella cheese	175 mL
$\frac{1}{2}$	cup grated low-fat "cheddar-type" cheese	125 mL
3	tbsp. fresh coriander (cilantro), chopped	45 mL

In a large oven-proof saucepan, heat oil over medium heat. Add garlic and onion and sauté until soft. Add mushrooms and peppers; sauté another 3–4 minutes.

Cut tomatoes into quarters and add to saucepan with black beans, corn, rice, water, chili powder, cumin, oregano, and cayenne. Reduce heat and simmer, covered, for about 20–25 minutes until rice is tender.

Sprinkle cheeses on the mixture and heat in preheated 350°F/180°C oven for 15–20 minutes or until cheese melts. Sprinkle with coriander.

Chicky Tuna and Pasta Salad

Calories 270
Protein 16 g
Fat 4 g
Carbohydrate 41 g

Serves 4–6.

This salad is a hit with both kids and adults, including confirmed legume loathers. The chick pea dressing sounds unusual but tastes great—on regular tossed salads, too. A wonderful way of getting in some soluble fibre.

4	cups shell pasta, cooked and cooled	1 L
1	medium red onion, thinly sliced into rings	
1	7-oz./198-g tin water-packed tuna, drained and flaked	
1	small jar marinated artichoke hearts, drained and quartered	
2	tomatoes, sliced	

Dressing

1½	cup cooked chick peas	375 mL
2	cloves garlic, minced	
⅓	cup light mayonnaise	75 mL
5	tbsp. lemon juice	75 mL
2	tbsp. chopped fresh parsley	25 mL

In a food processor fitted with the steel blade, purée chick peas and garlic. Add remaining dressing ingredients and blend until smooth. Combine pasta, half the onion, and tuna in a large bowl and toss with $\frac{3}{4}$ cup/175 mL dressing. Serve pasta mixture on individual salad plates. Top with a generous tablespoon of dressing and garnish with tomato slices, artichoke pieces, and remaining onion rings.

Calories 122
Protein 6 g
Fat 4 g
Carbohydrate 17 g

Hummus

Serves 4–6 (makes $1\frac{1}{2}$ cups/375 mL).

Serve this Middle Eastern favourite as a spread for pita or a dip for vegetables. A splendid example of complementary proteins: the chick peas from the legume family plus tahini, which is made from sesame seeds (and is available at health food stores).

2	cups cooked chick peas	500 mL
2	cloves garlic, minced	
3	tbsp. tahini paste	25 mL
1	tbsp. light mayonnaise	15 mL
¼	cup lemon juice	50 mL
1	tsp. ground cumin	5 mL

Salt and freshly ground pepper to taste
Paprika (optional) as a garnish

In a food processor, fitted with the steel blade, purée chick peas and garlic. To this mixture add tahini, mayonnaise, lemon juice, cumin, and salt and pepper. Blend to a smooth consistency. To garnish, sprinkle with paprika.

Calories	113
Protein	6 g
Fat	3 g
Carbohydrate	16 g

Spicy Bean Dip

Serves 8–10 (makes about 4 cups).

For a taste of Mexico, serve this dip with vegetable crudités, pita chips (see p. 261) or bagel thins (see p. 262–63).

2	garlic cloves, minced	
2	19-oz./540-mL cans canellini (white kidney beans), rinsed and drained	
3	tbsp. lemon juice	45 mL
1	tsp. ground cumin	5 mL
1	tsp. chili powder	5 mL
2	tbsp. olive oil	25 mL
2	tbsp. chopped fresh coriander (cilantro)	25 mL
	Salt and freshly ground pepper	

Process the first six ingredients in a food processor or blender until puréed. Mix in coriander. Season with salt and pepper to taste.

4   Going with the Grain

If there is one food group with an undeservedly bad reputation, it is without a doubt breads and cereals. Who hasn't been told that eating too much bread or pasta will make us as rotund as a Russian rye or as voluptuous as a freshly steamed dumpling? In a nutshell, we've been led to believe that carbohydrates are fattening and not much else.

But the hard facts expose this bad image for what it is—another food myth. Carbohydrate contains four calories per gram, the same amount as protein. This is less than half the calorie count of fat, which racks up a whopping nine calories per gram. It is, in fact, the butter you smear on your bread and the cream sauce in which you lovingly douse those fettucini, not the bread and pasta themselves, that are the *real* culprits when it comes to calories.

Sure enough, if you suddenly eliminate carbohydrates from your diet, as many fad diets recommend, you will experience a sudden drop in weight. But this is loss of water, not fat, and you will regain the weight the moment you return to eating cereal and bread, not to mention cakes and cookies!

Not only are carbohydrates *not* fattening when consumed in moderation (too many calories of any food result in fat deposition), they are just plain good for you when eaten in balance with the other food groups.

The Nutrient Complex
The main nutrient in the bread and cereal food group is carbohydrate, of which there are two main types: simple sugars and complex carbohydrates. Simple sugars are easy to spot because they usually taste sweet; they include glucose, fructose, lactose, and sucrose. Complex carbohydrates do not taste sweet and are made up of long chains of sugars. In plant foods complex carbohydrates are called *starch*. Breads and cereals are also a terrific source of nutrients—namely, thiamin, riboflavin, niacin, iron, trace minerals, and fibre.

This food group is the main source of dietary fibre— either or both of the soluble and insoluble varieties, depending on the grain from which the food is made.

Whole-wheat bread, for example, is high in insoluble fibre, while oat products contain mostly soluble fibre.

Breaking Bread

When you are choosing bread on the basis of its fibre content, it is not a simple matter of one kind being more healthful than another. In deciding among whole-wheat, oatmeal, and mixed-grain breads, you must take into consideration your own constitution as well as other sources of soluble and insoluble fibre in your diet.

For example, a person who suffers from constipation should increase his or her intake of insoluble fibre and would be wise to opt for whole-wheat bread, while someone with a high cholesterol count might opt for oat-based breads. A diabetic, however, might more often choose a bread such as rye that is high in soluble fibre, while someone with a high cholesterol count should eat oatmeal because of the cholesterol-reducing effects of oat bran. Mixed-grain bread covers most nutritional angles and makes a good all-round choice. So do breads that contain nuts and seeds, which offer added protein as well as added taste.

As usual, purchasing bread is another case of "Buyer beware," and reading the label is the best way to avoid nutritional pitfalls. A dark loaf often gets its colour from the addition of caramel colouring, cocoa, or molasses and may in fact be only 60 percent whole wheat. This kind of bread gives you more sugar and less fibre for your bread-buying buck.

Breads and cereals contain protein, but only of the incomplete type, and they must therefore be consumed with complementary foods. A healthy grating of Parmesan cheese, for example, on top of your plate of pasta primavera, or your pita filled with hummus (made from chick peas), complement the proteins. There are also pastas on the market that are fortified with protein, which comes from the addition of whey to the dough. This makes them a better source of protein than the regular types.

Whole-grain foods contain larger amounts of vitamins and minerals than refined foods do. Whole-grain products are higher in vitamin B6, pantothenic acid, and folate than refined cereals, as well as vitamin E and trace minerals such as zinc, copper, and manganese.

White flour has lost some of its nutrients through processing, but the word "Enriched" on the label means that most of these nutrients have been replaced. Canadian food regulations require that white flour be enriched with iron, thiamin, riboflavin, and niacin. The fibre, however, is the important nutrient not added back to white flour after the whole grain is processed.

Sorting the Cereals—What's in the Box?

With the fibre fad in full swing these days, the battle between big food companies for your cereal dollar is heating up. And as usual in such instances, the consumer is often caught in the middle, faced with too much choice and a deluge of confusing information.

The best policy when buying cereals is to read the labels carefully and do some quick calculations, keeping personal taste preferences in mind, to find the brands that contain the most nutrients and the least fat and sugar. One important word of warning: don't let the labels "Natural" or "No preservatives added" make your decision—they do not necessarily imply the best nutrients.

The first thing to look for is the cereal's sugar content. Ingredients are listed in descending order of quantity, so if sugar is the first ingredient listed, then the cereal contains more sugar than it does grains and is not the healthiest choice. Sometimes the added sugar listed in the ingredients section is low, but there may be other sugars listed in the nutrient information. This could be natural sugar from dried fruit, which is acceptable because it contains other nutrients.

A cereal with a high sugar content might seem acceptable because it is fortified with all kinds of vitamins and minerals. Not so. Eating such a cereal is really the same as eating a bowlful of table sugar followed by a vitamin supplement. In other words, we're not talking real food!

Then there is the whole confusing issue of granola.

Something about that bowl of wholesome-looking cereal bursting with crunchy, honey-coated grains, nuts, and seeds has given this cereal a healthy hype it usually doesn't deserve. Commercial granola is, in fact, extremely high in sugar and, worst of all, saturated fat, which comes from the coconut oil it's steeped in. Labels on packaged granola subtly disguise this fact by using a tiny serving size to list nutrients and calories.

Many people assume that because most granolas are made with honey, they must be healthy. Not true. Honey is as much a simple sugar as sucrose or table sugar. The only difference is that it sticks to your teeth! (See Chapter 13.) The bottom line is that granola can be a nutritious food, but for the most part, only when it's homemade. Try our low-fat recipe on page 193 and vary it as you wish, adding more dried fruit for a sweeter taste.

Bran is another nutritional buzzword, and for people in search of high-fibre foods, so-called bran cereals can contain vastly different amounts. Once again it's a case of reading the label. Cereals labelled "100 percent bran" are made from the indigestible outer coating of the wheat kernel and yield the most fibre. Those that contain 40 percent bran are made from the outer coating as well as other parts of the wheat kernel.

Some cereals are high in sodium. If you are on a sodium-restricted diet, be aware of the sodium content of various cereals by reading their labels. Some people—for example, pregnant women—may require extra iron, so for them iron-fortified cereals can be a good idea. To enhance the absorption of iron, accompany the cereal with a food containing vitamin C, such as an orange or its juice.

There are people who, like Daddy Bear, enjoy nothing better at breakfast time than a rib-hugging bowl of steaming hot porridge. Others abhor the taste of hot cereal but live for their daily serving of breakfast-time bran buds steeped in cold milk and topped with fresh fruit. There is no right or wrong in this whole hot-cereal-versus-cold-cereal debate; it is simply a matter of taste. Both hot and cold cereals can be packed with important nutrients. By the same token, there are many products in both groups that are loaded to bursting with sugar, fats, and not much else.

So choose your cereals and read labels carefully. If a cereal is fortified with vitamin A and you already eat plenty of dairy products as well as fruit and vegetables, all of which are rich in this vitamin, this may not be the best cereal for you. If, however, your diet is low in iron, an iron-fortified product is a wise choice.

There is so much variety on the highly competitive cereal market these days that armed with all this nutritional information, your careful scrutiny of package labels should turn up at least one brand that meets your needs.

Gratifying Grains
There is another important benefit of exploiting all the possibilities of this wondrously varied food group. By eat-

SUGAR CONTENT OF POPULAR CEREALS

Less Than $\frac{1}{4}$ Teaspoon/1 mL per Serving		
Cheerios		Puffed Wheat
Cream of Wheat		Shredded Wheat
Oatmeal		Wheat Germ
Puffed Rice		

$\frac{1}{2}$–1 Teaspoon/2–5 mL per Serving		
All-Bran		Grape-Nuts
Bran Buds		Harvest Crunch
Bran Bites and Raisins		Life
Chex, Wheat, Corn, Bran, and Rice		Pep
Corn Flakes		Product 19
Corn Bran		Raisin Bran
Fibre Up		Rice Flakes
Fruit with Fiber, Apple-Cinnamon		Shreddies
		Team

1–2 Teaspoons/5–10 mL per Serving		
Familia		Muslix Five Grain Muesli
Frosted Mini-Wheats		Raisinut Bran
Just Right		Rice Krispies
Most		Total
Muslix Bran Muesli		Wheaties

Sugar Content of Popular Cereals (continued)

2–3 Teaspoons/10–15 mL per Serving	
Cap'n Crunch	Golden Grahams
Cocoa Crunchies	Honey Nut Cheerios
Cracklin' Bran	Honey Nut Corn Flakes
Cocoa Puffs	Instant oatmeal, honey and graham
Crispy Wheats 'n Raisins	
Fibre Crunch	Instant oatmeal, raisin and bran
Frosted Rice	Instant oatmeal, sugar and spice
Fruit with Fiber, Dates, Raisins and Walnuts	Lucky Charms

3 Teaspoons/15 mL or More per Serving	
Alpha Bits	Instant oatmeal, cinnamon and spice
Apple Jacks	Pacman
Boo Berry	Strawberry Shortcake
Cocoa Pebbles	Sugar-Crisp
Count Chocula	Sugar Corn Pops
Frankenberry	Sugar Smacks
Frosted Flakes	Trix
Fruit Loops	
Honey Comb	

ing more bread, potatoes, and grains, we can cut down on protein portions at meals (especially at dinnertime), thus decreasing fat and increasing our fibre intake all in one fell swoop. Another bonus is that grains and cereals are usually easier on the budget than large meat servings.

Look at it this way. It's difficult to decrease our protein consumption and simultaneously reduce calories when we eat meat and salad. If we were to eat a smaller steak, we would finish it and the salad in no time and probably leave the table hungry. But a small quantity of thinly sliced beef stir-fried with broccoli and served on a bed of rice is a lot more filling. It also contains adequate protein, minimal fat, and a whole lot of fibre.

One problem with grains and cereals has been that most of us don't know how to prepare many of the weird and wonderful varieties now on the market. Thanks to the influence of ethnic cuisines, however, we are lately getting more familiar with such exotic but simple-to-cook foods as tabbouleh (made from bulgur), which hails from the Middle East, kasha (cooked buckwheat) from Eastern Europe, and polenta (cooked cornmeal), an Italian specialty.

The Wonders of Wheat
The following grains and cereals all come from wheat.

Bulgur   Bulgur is a term commonly used for cracked wheat. Buy the whole-grain version, which comes in several different sizes. Bulgur contains B vitamins, trace minerals, and plenty of fibre. It is excellent when it is cooked like rice and served as an accompaniment to meat or fish; it also makes a terrific cold salad when it is soaked in water or stock for a couple of hours and then mixed with vegetables and fresh herbs.

Couscous   Couscous is the name used for the smallest size of cracked wheat. In North Africa, where it is a staple, couscous is traditionally steamed and served with small amounts of meat, vegetables, or both as a protein extender.

Wheat Berries   Wheat berries are the whole wheat kernel and can be eaten as a cooked cereal or baked into bread or muffins.

Wheat Germ   This is the germ of the wheat kernel and is a good source of B vitamins, iron, manganese, zinc, magnesium, phosphorus, copper, potassium, and fibre. Using wheat germ is a great way to add nutrients to food in cooking. Substitute it for breadcrumbs in burgers and casserole toppings and as a coating for baked chicken or fish. It's also easy to mix it into the topping of a fruit crumble. Toasting it lightly in the oven or in a heavy skillet on top of the stove before using it as a topping enhances its flavour. Store wheat germ in the fridge; because of its high oil content, it goes rancid easily. Only buy unrefrigerated wheat germ in a sealed jar; if it is refrigerated, it is all right to buy it in unsealed packages. But avoid the sweetened kind that is sold in jars.

Wheat Bran   Wheat bran, the outer coating of the wheat kernel, is the most concentrated form of insoluble fibre there is. But be careful not to eat too much—this can negatively affect the absorption of calcium and iron in your body.

Through the Corn Maize
The following belong to the corn family.

Cornmeal   Cornmeal is ground corn and is a great source of complex carbohydrates, B vitamins (when enriched), and trace minerals like iron and magnesium. The vitamin A content of cornmeal depends on how yellow it is: the yellower the colour, the more vitamin A it contains. Cornmeal is also a good source of incomplete protein and is therefore extremely nutritious when it is eaten with beans or dairy products. It is terrific in muffins, cornbread, polenta, and casseroles but less healthful when it is deep-fried in nachos and other such foods because of their high fat rating.

Popcorn   Popcorn is dried corn kernels and can be one of the most nutritious of all snacks if it is made with a minimum of fat and salt. The most fat-free way to pop corn is in a hot-air popper. Avoid those ready-to-use packages that come with their own pouch of fat—it contains highly saturated coconut oil. (These include those microwave pouches where you can't see the amount of fat inside.) When you pop corn in a pan, use unsaturated oil. After it has popped, add some grated cheese, herbs, or both instead of salt (see pages 264–65), and—it goes without saying—hold the melted butter!

Roll Out the Oats
Oats, which include oatmeal, rolled oats, quick-cooking oats, and oat bran, comprise a particularly important group of grains. This is because the fibre they contain is mainly the soluble type, which is beneficial in regulating

cholesterol and blood sugars. The fibre is found in the
bran portion known as oat bran.

Oat Bran   Dr. James Anderson of the University of Kentucky Medical
College has been conducting research into the benefits of
oat bran. His studies on groups of men with high cholesterol levels show that three ounces of oat bran a day lowered their cholesterol by about 9 percent. What is more,
while the "bad" LDL cholesterol decreased by this amount,
the "good" HDL cholesterol tended to increase or stay the
same.

If you combine these results with the findings of the
Lipid Research Clinics study (discussed in Chapter 2),
which are that a 1 percent reduction in cholesterol
decreases the risk of heart disease by 2 percent, you're
looking at some pretty good reasons to eat oat bran!

Oat bran can be cooked and eaten as a hot cereal
like porridge. It can also be used to replace one-third to
one-half the flour and other starch fillers called for in recipes. It is not advisable to use more than this proportion
because, unlike flour, oat bran does not contain gluten—
the protein required for texture development. Too much
oat bran makes food gummy. Because of the fibre it
contains, however, oat bran is excellent as a thickener in
vegetable purées, soups, and stews in place of cream.

Wild about Rice
When buying rice, choose either the brown or enriched
version whenever possible. Both contain B vitamins,
incomplete protein, and trace minerals, but little fibre.
Brown rice is rightly shedding its old association with hip-
pies and bean sprouts and emerging as a flavourful, versatile food. It is not only brimming with nutrients but can
also taste wonderful if used imaginatively. Because brown
rice takes longer to cook than regular rice, you can freeze
cooked packages of it to save time later.

Avoid prepackaged, seasoned rice dishes. They are
not only expensive but also high in salt and additives.
Use your imagination along with a variety of seasonings
and vegetables, and you'll find that rice has endless taste
possibilities.

Wild rice, harvested mostly by North America's native
peoples, is not actually a rice, but a type of grass. It is,
however, cooked in a similar manner and has similar
nutrients—protein, B vitamins, iron, and manganese.

Right on Rye—and Barley—and Buckwheat

Rye contains mainly soluble fibre, along with protein, B vitamins, phosphorus, and potassium. Although breads made from 100 percent rye flour do exist, most rye breads are made with a high-gluten product like wheat and only one-third to one-half rye flour, which has a low gluten content. Gluten gives bread its light texture.

Barley contains carbohydrates and trace minerals such as zinc, manganese, magnesium, phosphorus, copper, and iron, plus some B vitamins. Barley, which appears to be pretty potent in its cholesterol-lowering ability, tastes wonderful in soups and casseroles.

Often called buckwheat groats, buckwheat is a source of incomplete protein, fibre, B vitamins, and trace minerals such as iron, potassium, and phosphorus. Roasted buckwheat is called kasha, a delicious Eastern European specialty that can be a savoury dish made with onion and served alone or with meat. It is also a yummy dessert laced with nuts, seeds, and perhaps some dried fruit.

Oodles of Noodles

Pasta seems to be *the* carbohydrate food of the decade. And for good reason. Pasta is popular with all age groups. It is amazingly versatile and can be served hot doused in a multitude of sauces or cold as a summer picnic or barbecue accompaniment. Pasta comes in all kinds of shapes, sizes, and flavours. And last but not least, if it is coated in the right sauce, it is low in fat and calories.

The secret to the nutritional content of pasta is in the sauce. For years most North Americans considered pasta to be a plate of spaghetti slathered in a thick crown of often oily meat and tomato sauce that had been simmered for several hours. Not only was this sauce time-consuming to prepare, it also had an unsubtle flavour and had lost some of its nutrients but none of its fat during its lengthy simmering.

Today's trends in preparing pasta sauces are toward lighter versions that are cooked for a short time and rely on good, fresh ingredients enhanced by delicate seasoning. A tomato sauce, for example, laced with fresh basil and some freshly ground pepper tastes wonderful cooked for a few minutes, whether you're using fresh or even canned tomatoes. A fresh tomato sauce that isn't cooked at all (Italians call it *salsa cruda*) is even better, especially at peak tomato season (see page 96).

Pasta is so versatile that you could serve a different version every night of the week with all kinds of sauces—from artichoke and lemon to sliced ham with tomatoes—and never get bored. Such dishes are also a good way to encourage children to eat unpopular vegetables. After all, what eight-year-old is going to refuse broccoli or green beans when they're tossed with his or her favourite noodle and sprinkled with grated cheese?

Pasta has become the order of the day at many restaurants. But avoid menu items loaded with whipping cream. Even if your server assures you that a certain sauce contains only "a little cream," keep in mind that a couple of tablespoons of 35 percent cream likely started out as twice that amount before being reduced during cooking. Order a dish without cream—a generous grating of fresh Parmesan or Romano easily takes its place for taste. Also avoid pasta salads; they are often coated in rich, oily dressings and can be high in fats.

The discussion about fresh versus dried pasta is really a moot point because it is based on personal taste preference. The dried varieties are enriched with B vitamins and iron. Avoid prepackaged pasta meals, which tend to be high in salt and overpriced. You can also make your own pasta; if you do it right, you can produce an excellent, delicate noodle that tastes terrific. The exercise is also a good one in which to include children, who can always benefit from an enjoyable lesson in cooking.

Cooking times for pasta depend on whether it is dried, fresh, or homemade and on what shape it is. The thicker versions, such as large penne, shells, and lasagna noodles, obviously take slightly longer than spaghettini or small fusilli. The traditional way to cook pasta in Italy is until *al dente*, or "firm to the bite." The best way to test for this is to bite into a piece. And for those concerned about blood sugar regulation, there may be more than just a palate perk here—pasta cooked *al dente* seems to raise blood sugar levels more slowly than pasta that's overcooked.

Cook pasta by adding it to a large pot of boiling water. The pot cannot be too large, and you cannot use too much water. Lots of water prevents pasta from sticking; so does stirring at intervals during cooking. When the pasta has cooked, drain it in a colander or sieve. Do not rinse.

Muffin Madness

The old-fashioned, unglamorous bran muffin of yester-year was full of fibre and other nutrients. It also weighed in at a mere 120 calories or so. Not so today's upscale, trendy muffin—it has fallen prey to the crazed dreams of the marketing moguls. Spiked with chocolate chips, loaded with sugar or honey (for some reason, many consumers continue to believe the myth that honey is more healthful than sugar), and, worst of all, packed with fat, it can contain as many as 450 calories.

Some of today's gussied-up muffins contain as much as 30 to 35 grams of fat. That's the equivalent of three tablespoons of butter! And then their purveyors have the gall to call them "light!" Such so-called muffins are actually glorified cupcakes, and the only light thing about them is their texture.

The bottom line is that all muffins are not created equal. If you are trying to cut down on sugar, calories, and fat, beware of muffins that aren't basic, low-fat bran. Again, the best policy is to bake your own (see recipes on pages 194 to 199) or find a baker who makes the old-fashioned kind!

Pie in the Sky

Because pastry dough doesn't usually taste sweet and has a light texture, many people think it is lower in calories than cake. Again, this is not necessarily true. Most pastry, especially the flaky kind made with layers of dough that sandwich layers of shortening or butter, is extremely high in fat. It's commonly known that a slice of cherry pie is a pretty high-calorie food. But how many of us realize that a lot of these calories come from the pastry as well as the filling?

As for quiche, you can forget this trendy item as a "light meal." Quiche gives you the double whammy of a fat-laden cream filling as well as pastry that's a hiding place for yet more fat.

Another food that masks its calorie count under a "light" image is the increasingly popular croissant. Croissants are made by layering pastry dough with tiny pieces of butter. The result is a light-as-air delicacy that can conceal as much as three tablespoons of fat.

The Way the Cookie Crumbles

A love of cookies seems to be universal. It bridges the gaps of age, sex, race, and eating habits. To lump all cookies together in an effort to banish them from our diets would be as impossible as it is unnecessary.

Cookies are here to stay, so choose those that are low in fat and sugar but still tops for taste. But because finding commercially made cookies that fill this bill is a difficult, almost impossible, task, making your own is the best way to obtain nutritious results. An oatmeal cookie made with wheat germ, dried fruit or nuts, and whole-wheat flour, for example, can add valuable fibre, vitamins, and minerals to your diet and that of your children.

Fresh Tomato Basil Sauce

Calories 96
Protein 2 g
Fat 6 g
Carbohydrate 12 g

Serves 4–6.

Called *salsa cruda* in Italy, meaning "raw sauce," this unequalled concoction is a must when tomato season is in full swing. It can be used on pasta or with poultry or fish.

8–10	medium-ripe fresh tomatoes	
$\frac{1}{3}$	cup coarsely chopped fresh basil	75 mL
2	cloves garlic, minced	
2	tbsp. virgin olive oil	25 mL
Salt to taste		
Plenty of freshly ground black pepper		
Freshly grated Parmesan cheese		

Chop the tomatoes coarsely and combine with the remaining ingredients, except the Parmesan, in a bowl. Marinate at room temperature for 3–4 hours. Heat slightly if desired, but do not cook. Serve tossed with or on top of your favourite cooked pasta. Serve the Parmesan on the side.

Pasta with Tuna Tomato Sauce

Calories 365
Protein 19 g
Fat 4 g
Carbohydrate 64 g

Serves 6.

My daughter Farrah's dinner of choice when she's cooking, a meal-in-a-hurry that's sure to be a hit all round, especially with children.

1	recipe Presto Tomato Sauce (see page 98)	
1	7-oz./198-g can water-packed tuna, drained	
1	lb. pasta	500 g

Heat the tomato sauce in a saucepan. Add the tuna, flaked or left in chunks, according to taste. Heat through.

Cook the pasta in plenty of boiling salted water. Drain and top with the sauce. Serve with freshly grated Parmesan and a tossed salad.

Calories	51
Protein	2 g
Fat	3 g
Carbohydrate	8 g

Presto Tomato Sauce

Serves 6.

This sauce is a must to have on hand in the freezer. Freeze it in small and larger containers so you can make quick meals for one or a group. You can substitute fresh tomatoes when they're at their peak, but use canned when the quality is questionable. Zipping up the sauce with more herbs and garlic is an especially good idea when freezing.

1	tsp. vegetable oil	5 mL
2	tsp. virgin olive oil	10 mL
1	medium onion, chopped	
2	cloves garlic, minced	
$\frac{1}{2}$	red pepper, chopped	
1	28-oz./796-mL can Italian plum tomatoes	
$\frac{1}{4}$	cup fresh basil or 2 tsp. dried	50 mL/10 mL

Salt and freshly ground pepper to taste

Heat oils in a medium-sized saucepan. Sauté onion until translucent. Add the garlic and sauté until slightly golden. Sauté pepper for 2 minutes. Drain the plum tomatoes, reserving liquid, and cut them into quarters. Add tomatoes to pan along with half the reserved liquid and the basil. Bring to a boil, then reduce heat to simmer, stirring occasionally. Cook sauce until it is reduced by about one-third.

Note: This sauce can be puréed in the food processor. Can also be used as a topping for pizza.

Calories 423
Protein 18 g
Fat 5 g
Carbohydrate 77 g

Pasta with Beans

Serves 4–6.

This hearty pasta dish is an easy way to sneak some legumes into the diet. Canned kidney beans are fast, but if you prefer, cook up a batch of beans from scratch and substitute 2 cups/500 mL.

1	tbsp. olive oil	15 mL
1	medium onion, chopped	
2	cloves garlic, minced	
1	28-oz./796-mL can Italian plum tomatoes	
1	tbsp. chopped fresh basil or 2 tsp. dried	15 mL/10 mL
3	tbsp. chopped fresh parsley	45 mL
1	19-oz./540-mL can white kidney beans, rinsed and drained	
Salt and freshly ground pepper		
1	pound stout pasta (penne, shells, or rigatoni)	500 g
2	tbsp. chopped fresh parsley	25 mL
$\frac{1}{3}$	cup freshly grated Parmesan cheese	75 mL

Heat oil in a medium-sized saucepan. Sauté onion and garlic until soft. Add tomatoes (including liquid), basil and 3 tbsp. parsley. Bring to boil, reduce heat and simmer about 10 minutes, stirring occasionally. Add beans and simmer another 20 minutes. Add salt and pepper to taste.

Meanwhile, cook pasta in plenty of boiling salted water until al dente. Drain. Transfer to a warm serving platter or bowl and top with sauce. Garnish with parsley. Serve with Parmesan.

Pasta Primavera

Serves 6.

Any veggies taste magnificent cooked this way. A combination of green beans, asparagus, and red peppers is especially pleasing, but feel free to experiment.

1	recipe Presto Tomato Sauce (see page 98)	
1	lb. pasta	500 g
2	carrots, sliced diagonally $\frac{1}{4}$ inch/$\frac{1}{2}$ cm thick	
2	small zucchini, sliced diagonally $\frac{1}{4}$ inch/ $\frac{1}{2}$ cm thick	
1	cup snow peas, topped, tailed, and sliced diagonally	250 mL
1	small bunch broccoli, cut into small flowerets	
$\frac{1}{4}$	cup toasted pine nuts (see note)	50 mL
2	tbsp. chopped fresh parsley	25 mL
$\frac{1}{2}$	cup freshly grated Parmesan cheese	125 mL

Heat the sauce in a saucepan. Cook the pasta in plenty of boiling salted water. Meanwhile, steam the vegetables until they are only tender-crisp.

Drain the pasta and transfer to a warm serving platter or bowl. Pour the hot sauce over and toss lightly. Top with steamed vegetables and sprinkle with pine nuts and parsley. Serve the Parmesan on the side.

Note: To toast pine nuts, cook them in a small, heavy skillet over low heat, shaking constantly, for 3–4 minutes or until golden brown. Be careful not to burn them.

Calories 369
Protein 14 g
Fat 6 g
Carbohydrate 63 g

Pasta with Red Peppers

Serves 4.

Sweet bell peppers in all their gorgeous hues, from palest gold to ruby red, look as good as they taste in this simple recipe that's perfect for autumn when peppers peak. For a more time-consuming but quite elegant version, roast and peel the peppers before making the sauce (see page 50).

2	tsp. virgin olive oil	10 mL
2	cloves garlic, minced	
1	small onion, finely chopped	
2	large sweet peppers, red and/or golden, seeded and sliced	
2	large fresh tomatoes	
$\frac{1}{4}$	cup chopped fresh basil	50 mL
Salt and freshly ground pepper to taste		
$\frac{3}{4}$	lb. pasta	375 g
$\frac{1}{3}$	cup freshly grated Parmesan cheese	75 mL

Heat the oil in a heavy saucepan. Sauté the garlic and onion until soft. Reduce heat slightly and add the peppers; cook 1 minute longer. Add the tomatoes and cook for about 10 minutes, stirring at intervals. Add the basil just before serving. Season with salt and pepper.

Cook the pasta in plenty of boiling salted water until al dente. Drain. Transfer to a warm serving platter or bowl and top with the pepper sauce. Serve the Parmesan on the side.

Calories	117
Protein	2 g
Fat	13 g
Carbohydrate	1 g

Pesto

Makes about $1\frac{1}{4}$ cups/300 mL, or enough sauce for 1 lb./500 g pasta to serve 6.

This lower-fat version of a magnificently aromatic Italian tradition is thick and flavourful. Use as is or thin it out slightly if you wish with a little chicken stock or water. A natural for freezing, pesto is a must to have on hand to add to soups, as a sauce for pasta, or to layer on pizza. If you freeze pesto, omit the cheese and add it when you are ready to use the sauce.

3	cups loosely packed fresh basil, washed and dried	750 mL
3	cloves garlic, minced	
4	tbsp. virgin olive oil	50 mL
3	tbsp. pine nuts	45 mL
$\frac{3}{4}$	cup freshly grated Parmesan cheese	175 mL

Freshly ground black pepper to taste

Process all the ingredients in a food processor or blender until blended.

Note: To store pesto, place in a dish and cover the surface directly with plastic wrap to prevent discoloration. Keeps for 1 week in the fridge.

Calories	429
Protein	23 g
Fat	17 g
Carbohydrate	47 g

Pesto Noodle Roll-Ups

Serves 6.

A nifty rolled-up variation on a theme that's old but good.

1	10-oz./284-g package or 6 cups/1.5 L loosely packed fresh spinach, with coarse stems removed	
$\frac{1}{2}$	lb. low-fat ricotta cheese	250 g
1	cup freshly grated Parmesan cheese	250 mL
$\frac{1}{2}$	cup grated part-skim mozzarella cheese	125 mL
$\frac{1}{2}$	tsp. dried or 1 tsp. chopped fresh thyme	2 mL/5 mL
$\frac{1}{2}$	tsp. dried or 1 tsp. chopped fresh basil	2 mL/5 mL
$\frac{1}{3}$	cup chopped fresh parsley	75 mL
$\frac{1}{2}$	cup chopped green onion	125 mL
1	egg yolk	
	Salt and freshly ground pepper to taste	
12	lasagna noodles, cooked al dente	
$\frac{1}{2}$	cup pesto (see page 102)	125 mL
2	cups Presto Tomato Sauce (see page 98)	500 mL

Wash the spinach. Place in a large, heavy pot and steam in water that clings to the leaves until spinach is limp, about 30 seconds. Squeeze with your hands, reserving the liquid for use in vegetable stock. Chop the spinach.

Combine the spinach, cheeses, thyme, basil, parsley, green onion, egg yolk, salt, and pepper in a bowl. Stir to blend.

Divide the cheese mixture into 12 portions and spread evenly on each lasagna noodle. Roll up jelly roll style. Cut each roll in half with a serrated knife and place in a lightly oiled 12-cup/3-L ovenproof dish. Spoon the pesto onto each roll. Cover the dish and bake at 350°F/180°C for 20–30 minutes or until bubbly and heated through.

Cook the tomato sauce in a saucepan until heated through. Place 4 lasagna rolls on each plate on a pool of sauce or serve the sauce on the side.

Tuna Broccoli Pasta Salad

Calories 255
Protein 14 g
Fat 9 g
Carbohydrate 32 g

Serves 6 as a main course.

There's nothing like a pasta salad for summer barbecues or as a complete make-ahead lunch, as this one can be. If you are making this dish beforehand, add the tuna just before serving.

1	small bunch broccoli	
$\frac{1}{2}$	lb. stout pasta (fusilli, shells, penne, or macaroni), cooked al dente and drained	250 g
$\frac{1}{4}$	cup chopped green onion	50 mL
1	7-oz./198-g can water-packed tuna, drained and coarsely flaked	
$\frac{1}{4}$	cup chopped fresh basil	50 mL
2	cloves garlic, minced	
$\frac{1}{4}$	cup lemon juice	50 mL
3	tbsp. vegetable oil	45 mL
2	tbsp. virgin olive oil	25 mL
	Salt and freshly ground pepper to taste	
3	tomatoes, cut into wedges	

Cut small flowerets from the broccoli and cut smaller stems into thin julienne strips about 1 inch/2 cm long. Blanch the flowerets and stems by plunging them into boiling water for a few seconds or until tender-crisp. Drain and refresh under cold water. Drain again.

Toss the pasta with the broccoli, green onion, tuna, and basil in a large bowl. Whisk together the garlic, lemon juice, and oils in a small bowl. Season with salt and pepper. Pour over the salad, toss well, and garnish with the tomatoes. Serve at room temperature.

Calories 255
Protein 7 g
Fat 8 g
Carbohydrate 39 g

Garden Pasta Salad

Serves 6.

A pasta salad for all seasons. Substitute vegetables according to availability and freshness. Blanching vegetables is a personal preference, so skip this step if you wish.

10	oz. tri-coloured fusilli noodles	300 g
1	tsp. vegetable oil	5 mL
6	oz. zucchini, julienned	175 g
2	oz. radicchio, shredded (see note)	50 g
6	oz. yellow string beans	175 g

Dressing

$\frac{1}{3}$	cup wine vinegar	75 mL
3	tbsp. vegetable oil	40 mL
1	clove garlic, minced	
$\frac{1}{2}$	tsp. dried oregano	2 mL

Salt and freshly ground pepper to taste.

Cook pasta according to package directions. Drain, rinse with cold water, and add 1 tsp. oil to prevent sticking.

Bring salted water to a boil in a saucepan. Immerse zucchini and yellow beans in water for 15–20 seconds. Drain, rinse under cold water, and add shredded radicchio. Set aside.

Meanwhile, whisk together vinegar, oil, and seasonings. Mix pasta with vegetables in a large salad bowl. Pour dressing over the salad and serve.

Note: If radicchio is unavailable, add the touch of red by garnishing the salad with shredded red cabbage.

Stuffed Red Peppers with Mushroom Risotto

Calories 256
Protein 6 g
Fat 7 g
Carbohydrate 42 g

Serves 4–6 as an appetizer, 2–3 as a main dish.

The results are well worth the extra time. Serve half a stuffed pepper as an appetizer or, for a sumptuous main course, offer both halves with a green vegetable.

$1\frac{1}{2}$ tbsp. vegetable oil		20 mL
1 medium onion, finely chopped		
10 oz. button mushrooms, sliced		300 g
$1\frac{1}{2}$ cup arborio or other Italian short grain rice		375 mL
$\frac{1}{4}$ cup dry white wine		50 mL
$3\frac{1}{2}$ cups chicken or vegetable stock		875 mL
1 tsp. olive oil		5 mL
$\frac{1}{4}$ cup freshly grated Parmesan cheese		50 mL
2–3 red peppers, halved and seeded		
1 tbsp. virgin olive oil		15 mL
Salt and freshly ground pepper to taste		
2 tbsp. fresh chopped parsley, for garnish		25 mL

Heat the vegetable oil in a Dutch oven over medium-low heat. Add onion and cook until soft. Stirring constantly, add mushrooms and cook, allowing liquid to evaporate, about 12–15 minutes. Add rice, stirring until it is well coated with mushrooms; cook 5 minutes. Add wine and continue cooking, stirring until it has evaporated. Pour stock over the mixture and bake, covered, in 350°F/ 180°C oven for 15–20 minutes or until all the liquids are absorbed and the rice is creamy and firm. Stir in 1 tsp./ 5 mL olive oil and the grated Parmesan, and season to taste. Cool risotto slightly.

While risotto is still warm, stuff it into the pepper halves. Arrange peppers snugly in a casserole dish greased with 1 tbsp./15 mL olive oil. Cover. Bake in a 350°F/180°C oven for 45 minutes or until peppers are soft. Garnish with freshly chopped parsley.

Risotto with Fish

Serves 6–8.

A novel version of an Italian rice stand-by, this can also
be made with shrimp, mussels, or other seafood.

$2\frac{1}{2}$–3 cups fish or chicken stock		625–750 mL
1	tbsp. vegetable oil	15 mL
1	medium onion, finely chopped	
2	cups arborio or other Italian short-grain rice	500 mL
1	cup dry white wine	250 mL
1	lb. firm-fleshed fish (cod, halibut, monkfish, etc.)	500 g
3	tbsp. finely chopped fresh basil	45 mL
1	cup freshly grated Parmesan cheese	250 mL
Salt and freshly ground pepper to taste		
3	tbsp. finely chopped fresh parsley for garnish	45 mL

Bring the stock to a boil in a medium-sized saucepan.
Reduce heat and simmer.

Heat the oil in a large, heavy saucepan. Add the
onion and sauté until soft. Add the rice and cook, stirring,
until transparent. Add the wine and bring to a boil. Reduce heat and simmer, stirring, until the liquid is almost
absorbed, about 4 minutes. Add 1 cup/250 mL of the hot
stock. Simmer, stirring, until almost absorbed, about 10
minutes. Add 1 cup/250 mL more of the stock. Simmer,
stirring, until almost absorbed, about 10 minutes. Add the
fish and cook for about 10 minutes, gradually adding as
much of the remaining stock as is required to cook the
rice and still be absorbed. Stir in the basil, Parmesan, salt,
and pepper. Sprinkle with parsley.

Calories	443
Protein	29 g
Fat	15 g
Carbohydrate	50 g

Oriental Noodle Salad

Serves 4 as a main course.

The crunch of bean sprouts and cucumber combined with tender yet firm Chinese egg noodles, all laced with a flavorsome soy sauce dressing, make this dish nothing short of superb. Chili oil, available at most Chinese groceries along with the noodles, gives an extra hit of mouth-tingling heat.

$\frac{1}{2}$	lb. dried Chinese egg noodles	250 g
2	tbsp. sesame oil	25 mL
$\frac{1}{4}$	tsp. chili oil or to taste (optional)	1 mL
2	tbsp. low-sodium soy or tamari sauce	25 mL
2	tbsp. red or white wine vinegar	25 mL
$\frac{1}{2}$	tsp. dry mustard	2 mL
2	single chicken breasts, boned, skinned, and poached (see page 51)	
$\frac{1}{2}$	English cucumber, coarsely shredded or cut into small chunks	
$1\frac{1}{2}$	cups coarsely shredded iceberg or romaine lettuce	375 mL
$1\frac{1}{2}$	cups bean sprouts	375 mL
2	tbsp. chopped fresh coriander (also called Chinese parsley or cilantro)	25 mL

Cook the noodles in plenty of boiling salted water until al dente. Chinese noodles take much less time to cook than regular pasta—about 1 minute. Drain and place in a large bowl.

Whisk together the oils, soy sauce, vinegar, and mustard in a small bowl until well blended. Pour onto the noodles and toss well to coat. Chill.

Cut the chicken into small cubes or shred coarsely. Add to the noodles along with the cucumber, lettuce, and bean sprouts. Toss and sprinkle with coriander.

Polenta Pizza with Mushrooms

Calories 396
Protein 16 g
Fat 11 g
Carbohydrate 58 g

Serves 4.

This savoury polenta dish combines two long-time Italian favourites. For variety, substitute a thin layer of pesto sauce (see page 94) for the tomato sauce. Either way, it's a wonderful recipe for introducing polenta to the uninitiated.

$5\frac{1}{2}$	cups cold water	1.4 L
$1\frac{1}{2}$	cups yellow cornmeal	325 mL
$\frac{1}{2}$	cup freshly grated Parmesan cheese	125 mL
1	tbsp. virgin olive oil	15 mL
1	medium onion, finely chopped	
8	oz. button mushrooms, sliced	250 g
8	oz. oyster mushrooms, sliced	250 g
1	cup Pizza Tomato Sauce (see page 111; see note)	250 mL
1	cup part-skim mozzarella cheese, grated	250 mL

To prepare polenta base: Bring $3\frac{1}{2}$ cups/875 mL water to a boil in a deep saucepan. Combine remaining cold water and cornmeal in a bowl, stirring with a wooden spoon until the cornmeal becomes pastelike. Add this mixture to the boiling water, stirring constantly and scraping the paste down the sides of the saucepan. Cook 15–20 minutes, stirring constantly and vigorously, until polenta comes away from the sides of the pan. Remove from heat and add $\frac{1}{4}$ cup/50 mL grated Parmesan cheese and 1 tsp./5 mL olive oil.

Place polenta on a greased baking sheet and flatten to form a round pizza shape, about 1 inch/2 cm thick. Cool at room temperature.

Meanwhile, heat 2 tsp./10 mL olive oil in a frying pan and sauté onions until translucent. Add mushrooms and cook until all moisture has evaporated. Remove mushrooms from frying pan and cool them in a bowl.

To assemble, spread tomato sauce over polenta base and top with the cooked mushroom mixture. Sprinkle grated mozzarella on top along with remaining grated Parmesan. Bake at 350°F/180°C for 15–20 minutes or until cheese melts. Slice and serve.

Note: If you wish, prepare extra tomato sauce to serve on the side.

Whole-Wheat Pizza Dough

Calories 701
Protein 20 g
Fat 17 g
Carbohydrate 120 g
(per pizza)

Makes enough dough for two 9-inch/23-cm pizzas.

Pizza is one of the most nutritious, versatile, and popular foods in existence. Fancy it up with artichokes and roasted peppers or go the traditional route with green peppers and mushrooms. This crust is simple to make and freezes well.

$\frac{3}{4}$	cup lukewarm water	175 mL
1	tsp. granulated sugar	5 mL
1	envelope (1 tbsp./15 mL) dry yeast	
2	tbsp. vegetable oil	25 mL
$\frac{1}{2}$	tsp. salt	2 mL
$1\frac{1}{2}$	cups whole-wheat flour	375 mL
1	cup all-purpose flour	250 mL

Combine the water, sugar, and yeast in a small bowl. Set aside for 5–15 minutes or until foamy. Stir in the oil and blend well.

Combine the salt and flours in a large bowl. Stir in the yeast mixture to form a soft dough that pulls away from the sides of the bowl. Turn the dough onto a floured surface and sprinkle with a little flour. Knead for about 5 minutes or until the dough is smooth and elastic, adding a little more all-purpose flour if required. Place the dough in a large, lightly oiled bowl. Cover with a clean tea towel and let rise in a warm place for 40 minutes to 1 hour or until the dough has doubled in bulk.

Punch the dough down. Knead for about 1 minute, adding a little flour if it is sticky. Cut the dough in half. Roll each piece of dough on a lightly floured surface using a rolling pin or stretching with your hands to form a 9-inch/23-cm round of dough.

Place the dough on lighly oiled baking sheets or pizza pans. Top with Pizza Tomato Sauce (see page 111), grated part-skim mozzarella, and your favourite toppings.

Bake at 450°F/230°C for about 15 minutes or until the crust is brown on the bottom.

Note: For a thicker, softer crust, cover the rolled dough rounds with a clean towel and let them rest on a baking sheet in a warm place for about 30 minutes before adding the toppings.

Pizza Tomato Sauce

Calories 100
Protein 4 g
Fat 2 g
Carbohydrate 18 g
(per $\frac{1}{2}$ cup/125 mL)

Makes about $2\frac{1}{4}$ cups/550 mL, or enough for four 9-inch/23-cm pizzas.

The secret to this rich and smooth sauce is long, slow simmering and sieving out the seeds. Well worth the time and effort, this sauce freezes well.

1	28-oz./796-mL can Italian plum tomatoes	
$1\frac{1}{2}$	tsp. virgin olive oil	7 mL
1	small onion, finely chopped	
2	cloves garlic, finely chopped	
1	$5\frac{1}{2}$-oz./156-mL can tomato paste	
1	tsp. brown or white sugar	5 mL
1	tsp. dried oregano	5 mL

Good pinch each dried basil and thyme
Salt and freshly ground pepper to taste

Process the tomatoes in a food processor or blender until puréed. Strain through a sieve to remove the seeds.

Heat the oil in a heavy saucepan. Add the onion and garlic; sauté until soft. Add the puréed tomatoes, tomato paste, sugar, oregano, basil, and thyme. Bring to a boil, reduce heat, and simmer, uncovered, for about 1 hour or until thick. Season with salt and pepper. Cool before spreading on pizza dough.

Calories 160
Protein 4 g
Fat 4 g
Carbohydrate 27 g

Tabbouleh

Serves 6–8 as a side dish.

A delicious and refreshing variation of the popular Middle Eastern dish. Kashi is a prepacked grain product that contains seven grains plus sesame seeds. This version is loaded with fibre.

$2\frac{1}{2}$	cups (1 package) cooked Kashi	625 mL
$\frac{1}{2}$	cup dates, finely chopped	125 mL
$\frac{1}{2}$	cup onion, finely chopped	125 mL
2	tbsp. sesame seeds, toasted	25 mL
$\frac{1}{3}$	cup fresh parsley, finely chopped	75 mL
$1\frac{1}{2}$	tbsp. virgin olive oil	20 mL
3	tbsp. lemon juice	40 mL

Salt and freshly ground pepper to taste

Combine Kashi, dates, onion, sesame seeds, and parsley in one bowl. Mix well. Whisk together oil, lemon juice, salt, and pepper in a second bowl. Pour dressing over salad, mix well, and chill before serving.

Note: Kashi is available in health food stores. If you can't find it, substitute the traditional bulgur (medium).

Calories 119
Protein 4 g
Fat 6 g
Carbohydrate 14 g

Kasha Pilaf

Serves 6 as a side dish.

A specialty of Eastern Europe. This tasty version combines the nutty flavour of buckwheat with the crunch of almonds. Serve as a side dish with meat, chicken, or fish.

2	tsp. vegetable oil	10 mL
1	medium onion, finely chopped	
1	cup toasted buckwheat (kasha)	250 mL
1	egg, lightly beaten	
$1\frac{3}{4}$	cups water or stock	425 mL

Salt and freshly ground pepper to taste

$\frac{1}{2}$	cup slivered almonds, toasted	125 mL

Heat the oil in a Dutch oven and sauté the onion until soft. Add the kasha and egg. Cook, stirring, over medium heat until the egg sets, about 2 minutes. Add the water and bring to a boil. Cover and place in the oven at 350°F/180°C. Bake for about 20 minutes or until the liquid is absorbed. Season with salt and pepper. Sprinkle with the almonds.

Note: Toasted buckwheat, or kasha, is available in health food stores and specialty sections of supermarkets.

Eggplant Bulgur Casserole

Calories 103
Protein 4 g
Fat 3 g
Carbohydrate 18 g

Serves 4–6 as a main course.

A yummy, high-fibre, meatless meal. Perfect protein when served with yogurt.

2	medium eggplants (about $1\frac{1}{2}$ lb./750 g), cut into small cubes	
2	tsp. vegetable oil	10 mL
1	medium onion, chopped	
2	cloves garlic, minced	
1	green pepper, cut into small cubes	
1	cup medium bulgur	250 mL
2	cups tomato juice	500 mL
$\frac{1}{2}$	tsp. dried oregano	2 mL
$\frac{1}{2}$	tsp. dried basil	2 mL
	Salt and freshly ground pepper to taste	
$\frac{1}{4}$	cup chopped green onion	50 mL
$\frac{1}{2}$	cup low-fat plain yogurt	125 mL

Add the eggplant to a saucepan of boiling water and cook for about 2 minutes. Drain well.

Heat the oil in a large Dutch oven. Add the onion, garlic, and green pepper; sauté until soft. Stir in the bulgur, eggplant, tomato juice, oregano, and basil and bring to a boil. Cover and bake at 350°F/180°C for about 30 minutes, stirring once halfway through cooking. Season with salt and pepper and sprinkle with the green onion. Serve with the yogurt.

Couscous with Chicken and Vegetables

Calories 333
Protein 36 g
Fat 8 g
Carbohydrate 27 g

Serves 6.

A Middle Eastern whole-grain creation laced with the delicate aromas of cumin and coriander. This recipe has three parts—stewed vegetables, steamed couscous, and grilled or barbecued chicken. But don't be deterred: it's worth the effort.

1	tbsp. vegetable oil	15 mL
1	medium onion, chopped	
1	leek, chopped	
1	celery stalk, diced	
1	green pepper, diced	
2	medium carrots, sliced	
2	small white turnips, diced	
2	cups chicken stock	500 mL
1	cup chopped fresh tomatoes	250 mL
1	cup cooked chick peas (use canned if you wish)	250 mL
1	tsp. ground coriander	5 mL
1	tsp. ground cumin	5 mL
$\frac{1}{2}$	tsp. paprika	2 mL
$\frac{1}{4}$	tsp. cayenne pepper or to taste	1 mL
1	small zucchini, sliced	
	Salt and freshly ground pepper to taste	
1	cup couscous (not quick-cooking)	250 mL
$\frac{1}{4}$	cup water or skim milk	50 mL
6	single, boneless chicken breasts, skinned	
	Fresh parsley sprigs for garnish	

Heat the oil in a large, heavy saucepan and sauté the onion and leek until soft. Add the remaining vegetables (except zucchini), stock, tomatoes, and chick peas. Then add the coriander, cumin, paprika, and cayenne. Bring to a boil, then reduce heat; simmer for 30 minutes. Add the zucchini and cook 15 minutes longer or until the vegetables are tender. Season with salt and pepper.

Soak the couscous for 10 minutes in a bowl in water to cover. Place in a steamer lined with a tea towel and steam for 30 minutes. Spread on a baking sheet, separating the grains with a fork. Pour the water or milk over, stirring to coat the grains. Bake at 350°F/180°C for 15 minutes.

Grill the chicken for 3–4 minutes per side or until just cooked. Serve the chicken, vegetables, and couscous on separate warm platters garnished with parsley.

Zucchini Cornmeal Bran Squares

Calories 45
Protein 1 g
Fat 2 g
Carbohydrate 5 g

Makes about 48 appetizer squares.

A cocktail nibble without the usual calories. Or, in larger servings, a lovely savoury bread.

1	cup all-purpose flour	250 mL
1	cup oat bran	250 mL
$\frac{1}{2}$	cup cornmeal	125 mL
2	tbsp. freshly grated Parmesan cheese	25 mL
2	tbsp. granulated sugar	25 mL
2	tsp. baking powder	10 mL
$\frac{1}{2}$	tsp. salt	2 mL
1	cup grated zucchini	250 mL
$\frac{1}{4}$	cup chopped green onion	50 mL
2	tsp. dried basil	10 mL
1	cup low-fat plain yogurt	250 mL
2	eggs	
$\frac{1}{2}$	cup soft margarine, melted	125 mL

Combine flour, oat bran, cornmeal, cheese, sugar, baking powder, and salt in a large bowl. Mix together in a second bowl the zucchini, green onion, basil, yogurt, eggs, and margarine. Stir zucchini mixture into the dry ingredients. Combine quickly until dry ingredients are just moistened. Pour into a lightly greased 13 × 9 inch/3 L baking pan.

Bake at 350°F/180°C for 20–35 minutes or until a toothpick inserted into centre comes out clean. Cut into small squares.

Calories 146
Protein 5 g
Fat 6 g
Carbohydrate 21 g

Health Bread

Makes about 12 slices.

A savoury multi-grain fibre bread that's simple and quick because it requires no yeast. It freezes very well and is delicious toasted.

$\frac{1}{2}$	cup oat bran	125 mL
$\frac{1}{2}$	cup rolled oats	125 mL
$\frac{1}{2}$	cup rye flour	125 mL
$\frac{3}{4}$	cup all-purpose flour	175 mL
$\frac{1}{2}$	cup whole-wheat flour	125 mL
$\frac{1}{4}$	cup sesame seeds (see note)	50 mL
1	tbsp. granulated sugar	15 mL
2	tsp. baking powder	10 mL
1	tsp. baking soda	5 mL
$\frac{1}{4}$	tsp. salt	1 mL
3	tbsp. soft margarine	45 mL
$1\frac{1}{2}$	cups buttermilk	375 mL
1	slightly beaten egg white	
1	tsp. dill weed (see note)	5 mL

Combine oat bran, rolled oats, flours, sesame seeds, sugar, baking powder, baking soda, and salt. Cut in margarine with a pastry blender or two knives until mixture resembles coarse meal. Stir in buttermilk to make a soft dough. (It should separate from the sides of the bowl.)

Turn dough onto a lightly floured surface. Knead until smooth, about twelve strokes. Place dough a on lightly greased baking sheet. Flatten to a large circle about 3 inches/7 cm thick. Brush top with egg white. Sprinkle with dill weed.

Bake at 350°F/180°C for 40–45 minutes or until a toothpick inserted into centre comes out clean.

Note: Vary recipe by replacing sesame seeds with poppy or caraway seeds and dill weed with other herbs (oregano, basil, tarragon, rosemary, etc.).

Savoury Oat Bran Coating Mix

Calories 309
Protein 17 g
Fat 16 g
Carbohydrate 37 g
(entire recipe)

Makes about $\frac{3}{4}$ cup/175 mL.

This coating is suitable for chicken pieces, fish fillets, and vegetable slices such as zucchini or eggplant. Works well too as a casserole topping.

$\frac{1}{4}$	cup fine dry bread crumbs	50 mL
$\frac{1}{4}$	cup oat bran	50 mL
2	tbsp. freshly grated Parmesan cheese	25 mL
2	tbsp. sesame seeds	25 mL
$\frac{1}{8}$	tsp. salt	.5 mL
$\frac{1}{8}$	tsp. freshly ground black pepper	.5 mL
$\frac{1}{4}$	tsp. garlic powder	1 mL
$\frac{1}{4}$	tsp. paprika	1 mL
1	tbsp. chopped fresh parsley (1 tsp./5 mL dried)	15 mL

Combine all ingredients in a small bowl. If not using right away, transfer to a tightly covered container and store in the refrigerator.

To coat meat, fish, or vegetables, dip pieces into low-fat plain yogurt, then into coating mix. Bake on lightly greased baking sheet until done. (Refer to standard cookbook for individual baking times.)

Oat Bran Dessert Topping

Calories 539
Protein 8 g
Fat 25 g
Carbohydrate 83 g
(entire recipe)

A variation on the Savoury Oat Bran Coating. Use this crumb topping for fresh fruit crisp (apple or peach slices, raspberries, blueberries, rhubarb, etc.).

$\frac{1}{4}$	cup rolled oats	50 mL
$\frac{1}{4}$	cup oat bran	50 mL
2	tbsp. sesame seeds	25 mL
$\frac{1}{2}$	tsp. ground nutmeg	2 mL
2	tsp. ground cinnamon	10 mL
2	tbsp. brown sugar	25 mL
2	tbsp. soft margarine, chilled	25 mL

Combine first six ingredients in a small bowl. Cut in the margarine with a pastry blender or two knives until coarse crumbs form.

Arrange fruit in a lightly greased baking pan, sprinkle on the topping, and bake at 350°F/180°C for 35–40 minutes.

Note: If using rhubarb, add $\frac{1}{4}$ cup/50 mL granulated sugar to 2 cups of cut-up rhubarb.

Pear and Raisin Oat Bread

Calories 155
Protein 3 g
Fat 6 g
Carbohydrate 25 g

Makes about 20 slices.

Another great way to boost your fibre and iron intake. The pear gives a distinctive flavour, but other fruits are also superb.

$1\frac{1}{4}$	cups whole-wheat flour	300 mL
$\frac{3}{4}$	cup oat bran	175 mL
$\frac{1}{2}$	cup wheat germ	125 mL
1	tsp. baking soda	5 mL
1	tsp. baking powder	5 mL
1	tsp. ground cinnamon	5 mL
$\frac{1}{2}$	tsp. ground nutmeg	2 mL
$\frac{1}{4}$	tsp. salt	1 mL
$\frac{2}{3}$	cup honey	150 mL
1	egg, lightly beaten	
$\frac{1}{3}$	cup vegetable oil	75 mL
$\frac{1}{2}$	cup low-fat plain yogurt	125 mL
2	medium pears, peeled and finely chopped (about $1\frac{1}{2}$ cups/375 mL)	
$\frac{1}{2}$	cup golden raisins	125 mL
Topping		
2	tbsp. oat bran	25 mL
2	tbsp. sesame seeds	25 mL
1	tbsp. brown sugar	15 mL
2	tbsp. soft margarine	25 mL

Combine flour, oat bran, wheat germ, baking soda, baking powder, spices, and salt in a large bowl. Combine honey, egg, oil, and yogurt in a small bowl. Stir honey mixture into flour mixture until combined. Stir in chopped pears and raisins. Pour into a greased 9 × 5 × 3 inch/ 2 L loaf pan. Combine oat bran, sesame seeds, and brown sugar; cut in margarine. Sprinkle topping evenly over batter.

Bake at 375°F/190°C for 35–40 minutes or until a toothpick inserted into centre comes out clean. Cool for 10 minutes, then remove from the pan. Cool on a wire rack.

Calories 172
Protein 3 g
Fat 7 g
Carbohydrate 25 g

Lemon Loaf

Makes about 18 slices.

Perfect tea-time or snacking fare with lots of fibre and plenty of taste and texture.

$\frac{3}{4}$	cup all-purpose flour	175 mL
$\frac{3}{4}$	cup whole-wheat flour	175 mL
$\frac{3}{4}$	cup granulated sugar	175 mL
1	tbsp. baking powder	15 mL
$\frac{1}{2}$	tsp. salt	2 mL
2	eggs, lightly beaten	
$\frac{1}{2}$	cup soft margarine, melted	125 mL
$\frac{1}{2}$	cup water	125 mL
3	tbsp. lemon juice	45 mL
	Grated peel of 1 lemon	
1	cup homemade granola (see page 183)	250 mL

Topping

1	tbsp. all-purpose flour	15 mL
1	tbsp. brown sugar	15 mL
$1\frac{1}{2}$	tsp. soft margarine	7 mL
	Grated peel of $\frac{1}{2}$ lemon	
2	tbsp. homemade granola (see page 183)	25 mL

Sift together the flours, sugar, baking powder, and salt in a large bowl.

Combine the eggs, margarine, water, lemon juice, and lemon peel in a medium-sized bowl. Add this mixture to the dry ingredients, stirring just until moistened. Stir in the granola. Pour into a lightly greased and floured 9 × 5 × 3 inch/2 L loaf pan.

To make the topping, use a fork to blend together the flour, sugar, and margarine in a small bowl. Stir in the lemon peel and granola. Sprinkle this mixture on top of the cake batter.

Bake at 350°F/180°C for 45 minutes or until a toothpick comes out clean. Cool for 10 minutes, then remove from the pan. Cool on a wire rack.

Citrus Carrot Bread

Makes about 18 slices.

What a great way to eat those veggies!

$1\frac{1}{4}$	cups whole-wheat flour	300 mL
1	tsp. cinnamon	5 mL
$\frac{1}{2}$	tsp. baking powder	2 mL
$\frac{1}{2}$	tsp. baking soda	2 mL
$\frac{1}{4}$	tsp. salt	1 mL
2	eggs, lightly beaten	
Grated peel of 1 orange and 1 lemon		
$\frac{1}{4}$	cup unsweetened orange juice	50 mL
1	tbsp. lemon juice	15 mL
$\frac{1}{4}$	cup liquid honey	50 mL
$\frac{1}{4}$	cup vegetable oil	50 mL
1	cup shredded carrots	250 mL
$\frac{1}{2}$	cup chopped walnuts	125 mL
$\frac{1}{2}$	cup raisins	125 mL

Sift together the first five ingredients in a large bowl.

Beat the eggs, orange and lemon peel, orange juice, lemon juice, honey, and oil in a medium-sized bowl. Stir this mixture into the dry ingredients just until the mixture is moistened. Stir in the carrots, walnuts, and raisins. Pour the batter into a lightly greased and floured 9 × 5 × 3 inch/2 L loaf pan.

Bake at 350°F/180°C for about 1 hour or until a toothpick comes out clean. Cool for 10 minutes, then remove from the pan. Cool on a wire rack.

Calories 131
Protein 3 g
Fat 4 g
Carbohydrate 21 g

Nutty Apricot Bread

Makes about 18 slices.

You'd be nuts not to like this super-healthy snacking cake filled with dried fruit and nuts.

1	cup whole-wheat flour	250 mL
1	cup all-purpose flour	250 mL
1	tbsp. baking powder	15 mL
1	tsp. baking soda	5 mL
$\frac{1}{2}$	tsp. salt	2 mL
$\frac{1}{2}$	tsp. cinnamon	2 mL
$\frac{1}{2}$	tsp. ground ginger	2 mL
$\frac{1}{2}$	cup granulated sugar	125 mL
1	cup chopped dried apricots	250 mL
$\frac{1}{2}$	cup chopped walnuts	125 mL
1	egg	
$\frac{1}{4}$	cup vegetable oil	50 mL
$\frac{3}{4}$	cup unsweetened orange juice	175 mL
$\frac{1}{2}$	cup skim milk	125 mL
	Grated rind of 1 orange	

Sift together the first seven ingredients in a large bowl. Stir in the sugar, apricots, and walnuts.

Beat the egg in a medium-sized bowl. Slowly whisk in the oil, orange juice, milk, and orange rind. Pour into the centre of the flour mixture. Stir only until the mixture is moistened. Pour the batter into a lightly greased and floured 9 × 5 × 3 inch/2 L loaf pan.

Bake at 350°F/180°C for about 1 hour or until a toothpick inserted into centre comes out clean. Cool for 10 minutes, then remove from the pan. Cool on a wire rack.

Calories 126
Protein 3 g
Fat 5 g
Carbohydrate 19 g

Bonanza Banana Bread

Makes 18 slices.

Kids will go bananas over this one. Mash those overripe bananas and store them in the freezer until you have the time to make this. It'll be gone in no time!

(Carob and chocolate chips tally in at similar fat levels. Use carob chips for caffeine- and chocolate-sensitive individuals. It's only the powders, carob and cocoa, that are low in fat.)

$1\frac{1}{2}$	cups whole-wheat flour	375 mL
2	tsp. baking powder	10 mL
$\frac{1}{4}$	tsp. baking soda	1 mL
$\frac{1}{2}$	tsp. salt	2 mL
$\frac{1}{2}$	tsp. cinnamon	2 mL
Pinch nutmeg		
$\frac{1}{2}$	cup granulated sugar	125 mL
$\frac{1}{4}$	cup wheat germ	50 mL
2	eggs	
$\frac{1}{3}$	cup vegetable oil	75 mL
1	cup ripe, mashed bananas	250 mL
$\frac{1}{2}$	cup carob or chocolate chips	125 mL

Sift together the first six ingredients in a large bowl. Stir in the sugar and wheat germ; mix well.

Beat the eggs, oil, and mashed bananas together in a medium-sized bowl. Pour into the centre of the dry ingredients and stir only until the mixture is moistened. Stir in the carob or chocolate chips. Pour the batter into a lightly greased and floured 9 × 5 × 3 inch/2 L loaf pan.

Bake at 350°F/180°C for 50–60 minutes or until a toothpick inserted into centre comes out clean. Cool for 10 minutes, then remove from the pan. Cool on a wire rack.

Tart Lemon Curd

Makes $1\frac{1}{4}$ cups/300 mL, or enough for 1 pie or 24 tarts.

A low-cholesterol version of an old favourite. Serve as a sauce over fresh fruit or as a pie or tart filling.

2	tbsp. soft margarine	25 mL
$\frac{2}{3}$	cup granulated sugar	150 mL
1	tbsp. grated lemon rind	15 mL
1	tbsp. cornstarch	15 mL
$\frac{2}{3}$	cup fresh lemon juice (about 2 large lemons)	150 mL
1	egg, beaten	

Melt margarine in a small, non-aluminum saucepan over low heat. Combine sugar, lemon rind, and cornstarch in a small bowl. Add to margarine, stirring well. Add lemon juice, bring to a boil, then cook over medium heat, stirring constantly, about 1 minute. Gradually stir one-quarter of hot mixture into beaten egg; add to remaining hot mixture. Cook, stirring constantly, 2 minutes or until mixture thickens. Cover and chill.

Double Oat Pastry

Makes enough for 1 pie or 24 tarts.

Fill this versatile pastry with the Tart Lemon Curd (see above) or top it off with fresh berries, peaches, apricots, etc., and a dollop of yogurt.

1	cup rolled oats	250 mL
$\frac{1}{2}$	cup oat bran	125 mL
$\frac{1}{4}$	tsp. baking soda	1 mL
$\frac{1}{3}$	cup packed brown sugar	75 mL
$\frac{1}{3}$	cup soft margarine	75 mL

Combine oats, oat bran, baking soda, and brown sugar in a bowl. Stir to blend. Cut in margarine with a pastry blender or two knives. Pat into a 9-inch/23-cm pie plate.

Bake at 375°F/190°C for 12–15 minutes or until golden brown.

Note: For tarts, pat pastry into 24 2-inch/5-cm tart pans.

Apple 'n' Oat Almond Bars

Makes about 35 bars.

These fruity bars have the double bonus of soluble fibre from the oat bran and the apple.

$\frac{1}{2}$	cup soft margarine	125 mL
$\frac{1}{2}$	cup granulated sugar	125 mL
3	egg whites	
$1\frac{1}{2}$	cups graham wafer crumbs	375 mL
1	cup oat bran	250 mL
2	tsp. baking powder	10 mL
$\frac{1}{2}$	tsp. ground allspice	2 mL
$\frac{1}{2}$	tsp. ground cinnamon	2 mL
$\frac{1}{2}$	tsp. salt	2 mL
1	cup skim milk	250 mL
2	cups peeled and finely chopped tart apple (2–3 medium apples)	
$\frac{1}{4}$	cup slivered almonds	50 mL
1	tsp. icing sugar	5 mL

Beat margarine and sugar in a large bowl until creamy. Add egg whites, one at a time, beating well after each addition. Stir graham crumbs, oat bran, baking powder, spices, and salt into creamed mixture along with milk until blended. Stir in apple and almonds. Spread batter in a lightly greased 13 × 9 inch/3 L baking pan.

Bake at 350°F/180°C for 35–40 minutes or until a toothpick inserted into centre comes out clean. Cool before dusting with sugar just before serving.

Calories 77
Protein 2 g
Fat 4 g
Carbohydrate 11 g

5   The Garden of Eden

Fruits and vegetables are included in the same food group because they contain similar nutrients. And a pretty impressive list they are: vitamin A, vitamin C, thiamin, folacin, iron, trace minerals (potassium, iodine, copper, and zinc), carbohydrate, and fibre.

Vitamins for Vitality

The yellowish-orange pigment in fruits and vegetables comes from carotene, also known as provitamin A. Carotene also exists in green vegetables, but its colour is masked by the green chlorophyl. Carotene is converted by the body into physiologically active vitamin A.

Fruits and vegetables are the prime sources of vitamin C—another important vitamin. (See the discussion in Chapter 1.) However, many of the foods we depend on for a natural source of vitamin C are seasonal and thus not always easily available. So many products are fortified with it—in particular, fruit and vegetable juices and drinks. But this practice also has its nutritional hazards.

Fruit drinks fortified with vitamin C may or may not be made with any real fruits or vegetables, so that the only vitamin or mineral they often contain is vitamin C. Unfortunately, such beverages often contain less wholesome ingredients—namely, sugar, colouring, and flavouring. The addition of water, common in many of these drinks, makes them a waste of your food dollar. For example, orange drink contains only vitamin C. Orange juice, on the other hand, contains vitamin C, vitamin A, B vitamins like folic acid, and minerals such as potassium, phosphorus, iron, magnesium, and zinc.

Folacin is an important B vitamin found in vegetables like asparagus, beets, broccoli, Brussels sprouts, and spinach. Fruits that contain folacin include avocados, cantaloupe, and oranges. Iron, a vital mineral, is supplied by such dried fruits as apricots, dates, prunes, and raisins. It also exists in vegetables like lima beans, beet greens, peas, and spinach.

Fibre: A Higher Frequency

The foods in the fruit and vegetable food group are extremely important because they often contain both soluble and insoluble fibres in combination. Here are a few tips on how to maximize the fibre content of these foods:

- Eat raw fruits and vegetables as often as you can.

- Whenever possible, don't peel fruits or vegetables; otherwise, you are throwing away valuable fibre along with the peel. The peel also acts as a barrier against vitamin and mineral loss from exposure to air and water.

- Given the choice between raw fruits and vegetables and their juices, opt for the whole product—it contains more fibre than juice does. Anyone who has used a juicing machine has likely noticed the fruit and vegetable fibre left behind in the machine's filter. Puréeing fruit and vegetables is fine; it does not remove fibre the way juicing does.

Fill the Gap

One reason to increase the amount of fibre in your diet is that high-fibre foods fill you up without loading on the calories. And the fruit and vegetable group is a terrific source of this benefit. Adding a large spinach salad, doused in a low-fat yogurt dressing laced with herbs, and a stalk of perfectly steamed broccoli to your evening meal is worth its weight in satisfaction at minimal caloric expense.

Fruits and vegetables are also high in another filling substance that is particularly low in calories—water. Water fills you up more quickly than whipped cream, and without the unfortunate caloric side effects. Imagine eating a large four- to six-ounce wedge cut from a heavy head of cabbage. Its volume would take up a sizable space in your stomach and fill you up more than a calorie-dense protein food such as a piece of meat.

Another reason to eat plenty of fruit and veg is that the more you eat of them, the less you'll eat of protein foods like meat that tend to be comparatively high in fat. A good time to eat a lot of foods from this food group is at your evening meal, when you need fewer calories and less fuel.

Radical Behaviour

Vitamin C, beta carotene, and vitamin E have been linked together in their role as anti-oxidants. These nutrients appear to counter the effects of substances called *free radicals*.

Free radicals result from normal wear and tear on the body's cells, as well as from environmental pollution

Avocados	Apricots
Beet greens	Cantaloupe
Broccoli	Mangoes
Carrots	Nectarines
Chard	Papayas
Escarole	Peaches
Kale	Persimmons
Mustard greens	Plantain
Pumpkin	
Spinach	
Squash, winter	
Sweet potatoes	
Watercress	

such as cigarette smoke, and appear to be a culprit in aging and many diseases.

For example, oxidation (exposure to oxygen) by free radicals can change circulating blood cholesterol into the form that clogs arteries, increasing the risk of heart attack and stroke.

The evidence is not clear-cut, so in the meantime, it's prudent to eat a diet rich in nutrients that combat these damaging substances.

An Apple a Day . . .

There is some indication that certain fruits and vegetables can help prevent certain cancers. There appear to be numerous compounds that may be responsible for this, many as yet undiscovered, so taking supplements rather than eating the foods themselves is not advisable.

Cruciferous vegetables may reduce the risk of colon cancer. They include cauliflower, cabbage, broccoli, Brussels sprouts, kohlrabi, rutabagas, turnips, and kale. Researchers at Johns Hopkins University have isolated one substance in broccoli, sulforaphane, that appears to have potent anti-cancer effects.

It is not known whether it is the vitamin A or another substance in carotene-containing foods that may help prevent cancer of the lung, mouth, larynx, bladder, and esophagus. Vitamin A tablets, therefore, are not the

Blueberries	Asparagus
Cantaloupe	Beet greens
Grapefruits	Broccoli
Guavas	Brussels sprouts
Honeydew melons	Cabbage
Kiwi fruit	Cauliflower
Lemons	Chard
Limes	Kale
Loganberries	Lima beans
Lychees	Mustard greens
Mangoes	Peppers, green and red
Oranges	Spinach
Papayas	Tomatoes
Raisins	Turnips
Red currants	Watercress
Strawberries	

Juices from the above or
enriched with vitamin C

answer. Eating foods rich in beta-carotene, however, is certainly a good idea.

It is thought that vitamin C might reduce the incidence of gastric and esophageal cancers. It may also have another benefit—inhibiting the formation in the body of nitroso compounds, which are carcinogenic.

The type of fibre that seems to provide some protection against cancer has not yet been identified. The best way to cover all the fibre angles, therefore, is to eat a good variety of fruits and vegetables.

Don't Hold the Onions

Dr. Victor Gurewich, professor of medicine at Tufts University, Boston, observed that his patients who'd had heart attacks seemed to have low levels of the beneficial HDL cholesterol.

Dr. Gurewich found that when 50 of his patients ate 100 grams of raw onion a day over a two-month period, their HDL levels rose an average of 30 percent. Unfortunately, cooking the onions seemed to lessen this effect, and not all onions are created equal. The white and yellow types appear to be more potent in this HDL-elevating effect than the red sweet ones.

Garlic appears to have the same properties. Researchers are looking at the effects of garlic and onions on lowering the risk of breast and stomach cancer. They may also be beneficial in regulating blood pressure. All of the active ingredients have not yet been determined and may not be found in the supplements. Don't hold the onions!

Saving Graces
Fruits and vegetables are the most vulnerable of all foods to nutrient loss during storage and cooking. Most often it is vitamin C and some B vitamins that are lost. Here are some tips on how to treat this food group with nutritional tender, loving care:

- Store vegetables in plastic bags or crispers in the fridge.

- Do not wash or trim produce before storing. Nutrient loss occurs because peeling, slicing, and scraping damages cells and releases enzymes that rapidly reduce vitamin content. It is therefore not a good idea to wash, peel, and slice vegetables in the morning for your evening dinner in order to speed up preparation—you will be losing valuable nutrients on a regular basis. However, doing this on the odd occasion for a dinner party is acceptable.

- Whenever possible, don't peel fruits or vegetables before cooking. Skin and peel are the barriers that prevent nutrients from leaching into the cooking water.

- It isn't advisable to add baking soda to the water when cooking vegetables to intensify their colour. This destroys some of the thiamin.

- Vitamin C and some B vitamins are most easily lost when you are cooking fruits and vegetables because they leach into the water. The best way to avoid this can be summed up in one word—*minimalism*. Use as little cooking liquid as possible, and cook foods—covered—for as short a time as possible. Steaming and microwaving are the two best methods. Using the cooking liquid from vegetables in soups and sauces saves valuable nutrients from being thrown down the sink. Covering foods exposed to air before consuming them is another good idea. Eating them raw is, of course, tops!

- When you refrigerate foods, cover them whenever possible to minimize exposure to air, which causes vitamin loss. An opened can of juice, for example, loses its vitamin C after four days, even in the fridge. If you have trouble finishing a large can of juice in this length of time, buy smaller containers of it.

- Leaving cut-up celery, carrots, and other vegetables sitting in a glass of water in the fridge for easy snacking is not the great idea it might seem. Although vegetables stay crisp this way, they also lose most of their water-soluble vitamins, along with their nutrients, to the air and water. A better way to store raw veggies for quick snacks is to cut them up, then store them in a plastic bag or plastic wrap—without water. Even this won't preserve all the nutrients, so make sure you get them from other foods in your diet.

- When you choose fresh fruits and vegetables, use this simple rule of thumb: if the item looks fresh, it has likely retained its nutrients. If it is past its prime, so is its nutritional quality. For this reason, fruits and vegetables that have been frozen at their peak of freshness are a better choice than "fresh" ones of dubious freshness.

- When freezing your own fruits and vegetables, be sure to package them in airtight plastic bags or containers, not to defrost and then refreeze them, and to keep your freezer at the optimum temperature. When buying frozen vegetables, avoid those with calorie-laden sauces. Frozen fruits that don't contain added sugar are a better idea than their sugary counterparts.

- It's a good idea to blanch fruits and vegetables by plunging them into boiling and then cold water before freezing (consult a basic cookbook for instructions); this process destroys certain enzymes that cause the quality of such products to deteriorate.

- Although frozen fruits and vegetables are often a good choice, canned foods from this group have serious drawbacks. Canned fruits and vegetables are tempting because they are so easy to use, but they usually contain a lot of salt and sometimes less fibre due to peeling and trimming. Rinsing canned vegetables can remove some salt, but it washes away flavour and nutrients too. Of course, items like canned artichokes and canned tomatoes are wonderfully handy replacements for the real, fresh thing, which in both cases is strictly seasonal. Canned tomatoes in particular are almost indispensable for much of the year for making pasta sauces and other stand-bys. Buying the new low-salt versions is a good idea. Fruits canned in water or their own juice are a better choice than those canned in syrup. The main thing to remember is that canned fruits and vegetables should not be used exclusively as sources of these foods.

High-flying Fats—Proceed with Caution

Just as they can be one of the most nutrition-packed of all foods, vegetables can also be sneaky carriers of some substances we can do without—namely, hidden fats.

This is particularly common with vegetable dishes served in restaurants. Items that appear to be a wise nutritional choice are often prepared in such a way that they come to the table laden with hidden fats. Ratatouille, for example, is often made with large amounts of oil, which is easily absorbed by the eggplant, zucchini, and mushrooms. When cooking this dish at home, however, you can grill or fry the same vegetables using only small amounts of oil with healthier as well as tastier results.

Vegetables that have been coated in batter, deepfried, or both are also the bearers of bad nutritional news. And onion rings and french fries don't even try to hide the fats!

Another instance where a potentially nutritious vegetable intake can have dubious benefit is at the salad bar, and the main culprit here is the dressings. When you add salad dressing from one of those oversized ladles, be careful not to go the whole hog. Pour on a small amount. Marinated salads are already dressed and contain a lot of fat, so avoid them or eat them in moderation. When ordering a salad from a menu, ask for the dressing to be served on the side. Not only does this usually make the salad taste better (so many restaurants drown their salads in dressing), but it is also much healthier and lower in calories. In general, it is wise to check out a salad bar first to see how fresh the salads are; if they're not, they will have lost a lot of their nutrients. Old salad dressings could also be a cause of food poisoning.

When you make a salad at home, serve the dressing separately. And when you garnish cooked vegetables, don't smear them with butter. A dollop of unflavoured yogurt topped with a spoonful of freshly snipped herbs is more healthful and tastes delicious.

Honey-Mustard Tuna Salad

Calories 277
Protein 32 g
Fat 9 g
Carbohydrate 19 g

Serves 2 as a main dish with crusty bread.

This new twist to the traditional Niçoise salad keeps the tuna, omits the olives, and adds a nifty honey-mustard dressing that can also be used on almost any salad combo.

Dressing

$\frac{1}{2}$	cup low-fat plain yogurt	125 mL
1	tbsp. light or tofu mayonnaise (see page 239)	15 mL
2	tsp. honey	10 mL
1	tsp. lemon juice	5 mL
2	tsp. prepared mustard	10 mL
1	tsp. finely chopped fresh parsley	5 mL
1	green onion, chopped	

Salt and freshly ground pepper to taste

1	7-oz./198-g can water-packed tuna, drained	
1	cup sliced mushrooms	250 mL

Leaf lettuce

1	tomato, cut into wedges	
1	hard-boiled egg, sliced	

Blend the dressing ingredients in a food processor or blender until smooth. Chill.

Combine the tuna and mushrooms in a bowl. Line each plate with lettuce. Top with the tuna mixture and garnish with the tomato and egg. Drizzle the dressing over the top.

Calories 199
Protein 12 g
Fat 15 g
Carbohydrate 6 g

Tomato Salad Caprese

Serves 4 as an appetizer.

Eaten with a loaf of crusty Italian bread, this salad makes a heaven-sent lunch or light supper that's nutritious, low in calories, and bursting with flavour—especially in late summer, when field tomatoes and fresh basil are at their peak. Bocconcini can be found at Italian cheese stores. If unavailable, use part skim-milk mozzarella.

2	large or 3 medium, ripe, fresh field tomatoes	
6	oz. (4 balls) bocconcini cheese	175 g
2	tbsp. extra-virgin olive oil	25 mL
$\frac{1}{4}$	cup snipped fresh basil	50 mL

Salt and plenty of freshly ground black pepper to taste

Slice the tomatoes and bocconcini about $\frac{1}{4}$ inch/$\frac{1}{2}$ cm thick. Arrange the tomatoes on a serving platter or plates so that they slightly overlap. Place the bocconcini slices on top of each tomato slice. Drizzle with the oil and sprinkle with the basil, salt, and pepper.

Calories 187
Protein 4 g
Fat 8 g
Carbohydrate 29 g

Spinach Orange Salad

Serves 4.

An iron-clad creation with a delicious, fruity dressing.

4	large navel oranges	
2	small red onions, sliced into rings	
1	tsp. red or white wine vinegar	5 mL
2	tbsp. vegetable oil	25 mL
1	clove garlic, minced	

Salt and freshly ground pepper to taste

4	cups loosely packed fresh spinach, washed, dried, and with coarse stems removed	1 L

Peel the oranges and slice them thinly crosswise over a shallow dish to catch their juice. Chill the orange slices for

30 minutes. Soak the onion rings in cold water to cover for 30 minutes to remove their sharp taste.

Whisk together $\frac{1}{4}$ cup/50 mL of the reserved orange juice with the vinegar, oil, and garlic. Season with salt and pepper. Drain the onions. To serve, arrange the orange and onion slices on a bed of spinach. Drizzle with dressing.

Calories	128
Protein	4 g
Fat	3 g
Carbohydrate	22 g

Fruity Carrot Salad

Serves 4 as a side salad or appetizer.

Seeing in the dark never looked this good!

$\frac{1}{4}$	cup raisins	50 mL
2	tbsp. unsweetened pineapple juice (from can of tidbits)	25 mL
1	cup drained unsweetened pineapple tidbits	250 mL
4	medium carrots (about 4 cups/1 L), peeled and shredded	
4	tsp. light or tofu mayonnaise (see page 239)	20 mL
$\frac{1}{3}$	cup low-fat plain yogurt	75 mL

Soak the raisins in the pineapple juice in a small bowl for a few minutes. Then combine the pineapple tidbits, carrots, and raisins with their soaking liquid in a salad bowl.

Whisk together the mayonnaise and yogurt in a small bowl. Add to the carrot mixture and toss well.

Hearts of Palm with a Citrus Vinaigrette

Calories 159
Protein 3 g
Fat 9 g
Carbohydrate 20 g

Serves 4–6.

This super salad for special occasions is an adaptation of a recipe from Mark's Place, a remarkable restaurant in North Miami, Florida. The chef, Mark Militello, uses fresh hearts of palm in his recipe, so use them too if you manage to hunt them down.

1   14-oz./398-g can hearts of palm, drained and sliced into $\frac{1}{2}$-inch/1-cm rounds
1   14-oz./398-g can artichoke hearts, drained and quartered
12 cherry tomatoes, halved
$\frac{1}{2}$ green pepper, chopped

Vinaigrette

$\frac{2}{3}$	cup freshly squeezed orange juice	150 mL
$\frac{1}{4}$	cup extra virgin olive oil	50 mL
3	tbsp. balsamic vinegar	40 mL
$1\frac{1}{2}$	tbsp. Dijon mustard	20 mL
1	tbsp. honey	15 mL
1	tsp. mint (optional)	5 mL

Salt and freshly ground pepper to taste

Whisk all vinaigrette ingredients in a bowl. Combine hearts of palm and artichokes in a second bowl. Pour half the vinaigrette over the hearts of palm mixture and marinate 1 hour or overnight. Add remaining ingredients and serve the salad slightly chilled.

Buttermilk Salad Dressing

Calories 208
Protein 6 g
Fat 16 g
Carbohydrate 10 g
(entire recipe)

Makes about $\frac{3}{4}$ cup/175 mL.

Get the calcium and other goodies of buttermilk and yogurt but hardly any fat in this refreshing dressing, which is perfect for coleslaw or assorted blanched vegetables.

1	clove garlic, minced	
1	tbsp. chopped green onion	15 mL
$\frac{1}{4}$	tsp. dried mustard	1 mL
$\frac{1}{4}$	tsp. paprika	1 mL
$\frac{1}{2}$	tsp. dried or 1 tsp. chopped fresh tarragon	2 mL/5 mL
1	tsp. white wine vinegar	5 mL
1	tbsp. vegetable oil	15 mL
$\frac{1}{4}$	cup buttermilk	50 mL
$\frac{1}{2}$	cup low-fat plain yogurt	125 mL

Salt and freshly ground pepper to taste

Process all the ingredients except the yogurt, salt, and pepper in a food processor or blender until smooth. Pour into a bowl, then stir in the yogurt until blended. Season with salt and pepper. Store in an airtight jar in the fridge. Dressing keeps in the fridge for about 1 week.

Cottage Blue Cheese Dressing

Calories 263
Protein 19 g
Fat 17 g
Carbohydrate 7 g
(entire recipe)

Makes about 1 cup/250 mL.

A low-fat, top-notch version of an all-time favourite, this dressing is great on a spinach salad or one made with romaine and chopped nuts. Its extra protein makes it a terrific choice for a main-dish salad. Try to use a creamy, low-fat cottage cheese, not a dry one. You don't have to skimp if you're watching your fat intake.

$\frac{1}{4}$	cup loosely packed, crumbled blue cheese	50 mL
$\frac{1}{3}$	cup 2% cottage cheese	75 mL
$\frac{1}{3}$	cup low-fat plain yogurt	75 mL
1	tsp. lemon juice	5 mL
1	clove garlic, minced	
$\frac{1}{4}$	tsp. Worcestershire sauce	1 mL

Freshly ground pepper to taste

Process the blue cheese and cottage cheese in a food processor or blender until smooth. Pour into a bowl and stir in the remaining ingredients. Mix until blended. Store in an airtight jar in the fridge.

Fabulous Feta Salad Dressing

Calories 41
Protein 1 g
Fat 4 g
Carbohydrate 1 g
(per tablespoon)

Makes about 2 cups/500 mL.

A zesty dressing with the calcium and bite of feta combined with the Mediterranean flavour of oregano. It's good on any salad but superb on one made with fresh, ripe tomatoes and cucumber slices. This recipe makes quite a bit of dressing, so halve it if you like.

$\frac{3}{4}$	cup loosely packed, crumbled feta cheese	175 mL
$\frac{3}{4}$	cup low-fat plain yogurt	175 mL
2	cloves garlic, minced	
1	tsp. dried or 2 tsp. chopped fresh oregano	5 mL/10 mL
$\frac{1}{4}$	cup freshly grated Parmesan cheese	50 mL
Dash Worcestershire sauce		
2	tbsp. virgin olive oil	25 mL
$\frac{1}{4}$	cup vegetable oil	50 mL
Freshly ground pepper to taste		

Process all the ingredients except the oils and pepper in a food processor or blender until smooth. Add the oils in a thin stream, then process again until the dressing is well blended and slightly thickened. Store in an airtight jar in the fridge.

Poppy Seed Salad Dressing

Calories 47
Protein 1 g
Fat 5 g
Carbohydrate 1 g
(per tablespoon)

Makes about 2 cups/500 mL.

A dressing that's full of flavour with just a hint of sweetness. Works equally well as a dip.

6	oz. tofu	175 g
1	small onion, finely chopped	
1 $\frac{1}{2}$	tbsp. Dijon mustard	20 mL
2	tbsp. poppy seeds	25 mL
$\frac{1}{4}$	cup frozen orange juice concentrate	50 mL
$\frac{1}{2}$	cup + 2 tbsp. vegetable oil	125 mL
3	tbsp. vinegar	45 mL
2	tbsp. cold water	25 mL

Salt and freshly ground pepper to taste

Process tofu, onion, and mustard in a food processor or blender until smooth. Add remaining ingredients and continue processing until well mixed.

Vegetable Stock

Makes about 5 cups/1.25 L.

A must for vegetarians to use in soups and sauces and a great idea for anyone who wants to maximize the nutrients of veggies. Save half-used onions and celery leaves to make this stock. Avoid strong vegetables like cabbage, turnips, and cauliflower, which will overpower the flavour.

1	tsp. vegetable oil	5 mL
1	cup chopped onion	250 mL
1	cup chopped leeks	250 mL
1	cup chopped celery	250 mL
1	cup chopped carrots	250 mL
1	cup chopped tomatoes	250 mL
1	bouquet garni (see page 49)	
8	cups cold water	2 L

Heat the oil in a large, heavy stockpot. Add the onion and leeks; sauté until soft. Add the remaining ingredients and bring to a boil. Reduce heat and simmer, uncovered, for 45 minutes or until the vegetables are tender. Strain. Store in the fridge or freeze in plastic containers.

Calories	52
Protein	3 g
Fat	1 g
Carbohydrate	9 g

Cucumber and Dill Soup

Serves 4.

This refreshing soup will keep you cool as a cucumber.

1	medium English cucumber, sliced	
2	tbsp. shallots, chopped	25 mL
2	tbsp. fresh parsley, chopped	25 mL
2	tbsp. fresh dill, chopped	25 mL
2	tbsp. lemon juice	25 mL
$\frac{3}{4}$	cup low-fat plain yogurt	175 mL

Salt and freshly ground pepper to taste
Fresh mint leaves for garnish

Sprinkle salt on cucumber slices, sit slices in colander to drain for $\frac{1}{2}$ hour, then rinse them and pat dry. Purée cucumbers, shallots, parsley, and dill in a food processor or blender. Transfer purée to a large bowl, add lemon juice and yogurt, and mix well. Season with salt and pepper. Serve well chilled, garnished with mint leaves.

The Enlightened Eater

Carrot Soup

Serves 6.

The taste combination of carrots and orange juice sets this soup apart from most others. What's more, it's loaded with beta-carotene. Substitute $\frac{1}{2}$ tsp./2 mL dried ginger for fresh ginger root if you wish.

1	tbsp. vegetable oil	15 mL
1	tsp. finely chopped fresh ginger root	5 mL
1	medium onion, chopped	
9	medium carrots, scrubbed and thinly sliced	
3	cups vegetable or chicken stock	750 mL
1	cup unsweetened orange juice	250 mL
Salt and freshly ground pepper to taste		
2	tbsp. chopped fresh parsley for garnish	25 mL

Heat the oil in a large, heavy saucepan. Add the ginger root and onion; sauté until soft. Add the carrots and stock and bring to a boil. Reduce heat and simmer, uncovered, for 25 minutes or until the carrots are tender.

Process the carrot mixture in a food processor or blender until smooth. Return to the saucepan and add the orange juice, salt, and pepper. Cook until heated through. To serve, sprinkle each bowl of soup with parsley.

Calories	87
Protein	4 g
Fat	3 g
Carbohydrate	13 g

Zucchini Soup

Serves 6–8.

This flavourful soup is just as good made with broccoli or cauliflower and is out of this world made with green beans. Keep a batch in the freezer, but don't add the milk until you heat the soup.

1	tbsp. vegetable oil	15 mL
2	medium onions, finely chopped	
1	leek, finely chopped	
7–8	unpeeled, medium zucchini (about 2 lb./ 1 kg), thinly sliced	
$3\frac{1}{2}$	cups vegetable or chicken stock	875 mL
2	bay leaves	
$\frac{1}{2}$	tsp. dried or 1 tbsp. chopped fresh thyme	2 mL/15 mL
$\frac{1}{2}$	tsp. dried or 1 tbsp. chopped fresh oregano	2 mL/15 mL
$\frac{1}{2}$	tsp. dried or 1 tbsp. chopped fresh basil	2 mL/15 mL
1	cup 2% milk	250 mL
Salt and freshly ground pepper to taste		

Heat the oil in a large, heavy saucepan. Add the onions and leek and sauté until soft. Add the zucchini, reserving about 12 slices for garnish. Add the stock, bay leaves, thyme, oregano, and basil. Bring to a boil, then reduce heat and simmer, covered, for about 30 minutes. Discard the bay leaves.

Process the zucchini mixture in a food processor or blender until smooth. Return to the saucepan. Add the milk and cook until heated through. Season with salt and pepper. To serve, garnish each bowl with zucchini slices.

Note: If using fresh herbs, add them with the milk at the end of the cooking time.

Calories	63
Protein	2 g
Fat	1 g
Carbohydrate	14 g

Tomato Orange Soup

Serves 6.

Lucy Waverman, a Toronto food writer, has used this recipe in her cooking school for many years. It's unsurpassed when made with ripe tomatoes fresh from the field at peak season. This soup tastes great hot or cold and is extremely low in calories yet high in vitamins and minerals. This recipe involves no sautéeing in fat; all the veggies are poached. The delectable results speak for themselves.

4	cups homemade chicken stock (see pages 48–49)		1 L
2	lb. fresh or 1 28-oz./796-mL canned tomatoes, peeled, seeded, and chopped (see note)		1 kg
1	tbsp. tomato paste		15 mL
1	medium onion, finely chopped		
1	carrot, finely chopped		

Juice and finely grated peel of 1 orange

1	bay leaf		
1	tsp. dried or 1 tbsp. chopped fresh basil		5 mL/15 mL
1	tbsp. frozen unsweetened orange juice concentrate (undiluted) or to taste		15 mL

Pinch sugar
Salt and freshly ground pepper to taste
Fresh basil leaves or chopped parsley for garnish

Bring the chicken stock to a boil in a large, heavy saucepan. Add the tomatoes, tomato paste, onion, carrot, orange juice, orange peel, and bay leaf. Return to the boil, then reduce heat and simmer, uncovered, for about 20 minutes or until the carrots are tender. Discard the bay leaf.

Process the tomato mixture in a food processor or blender until smooth. Return to the saucepan. Add the basil, orange juice concentrate, sugar, salt, and pepper and cook until heated through. Can be served hot or cold. Garnish with basil or parsley.

Note: The tomato peel and seeds provide extra fibre, so include them if desired.

Calories	68
Protein	3 g
Fat	1 g
Carbohydrate	15 g

Gazpacho

Serves 6.

A cold soup *par excellence* that tastes just as good without the lashings of olive oil used in the Spanish original. Avoid using a brand of thick tomato juice for this. If the soup turns out too thick, add a little water.

2	large tomatoes, finely chopped	
2	green peppers, finely chopped	
2	red peppers, finely chopped	
1	English cucumber, finely chopped	
1	medium Spanish onion, finely chopped	
1	clove garlic, minced	
1	tbsp. lemon juice	15 mL
2	tbsp. red wine vinegar	25 mL
3	cups tomato juice	750 mL

Pinch cayenne pepper
Salt and freshly ground pepper to taste
Croutons for garnish (see note)

Set aside 1 tomato, green pepper, and red pepper, half of the cucumber, and 2 tbsp. of the onion.

Process the remaining vegetables and onion with the garlic, lemon juice, vinegar, and tomato juice in a food processor or blender until fairly smooth. Transfer to a large bowl. Season with the cayenne, salt, and pepper; stir in the reserved chopped vegetables. Chill. Serve with croutons.

Note: To make croutons, rub sliced bread (preferably stale) with a cut garlic clove. Cut into small cubes. Place on a baking sheet and bake at 350°F/180°C for 10 minutes or until golden brown and crisp.

Calories	82
Protein	3 g
Fat	5 g
Carbohydrate	7 g

Artichoke Spinach Dip

Makes about 3 cups/750 mL. Serves 6–8 as an appetizer.

Canned artichoke hearts work well in this silky-smooth dip packed with vitamins and minerals.

1	14-oz./398-mL can artichoke hearts packed in water	
1	10-oz./300-g package (about 8 cups/2 L loosely packed) fresh spinach, cooked, squeezed dry, and chopped	
1	small onion, finely chopped	
2	cloves garlic, minced	
2	tsp. dried or 2 tbsp. chopped fresh dill	10 mL/25 mL
$\frac{1}{4}$	cup chopped fresh parsley	50 mL
$1\frac{1}{2}$	cups low-fat plain yogurt	375 mL
$\frac{1}{3}$	cup light mayonnaise	75 mL
1	tsp. Dijon mustard	5 mL
2	tbsp. chopped fresh chives	25 mL
2	tbsp. lemon juice	25 mL

Salt and freshly ground pepper to taste

Process the first six ingredients in a food processor or blender until puréed. Combine the remaining ingredients except the salt and pepper in a medium-sized bowl. Add the artichoke mixture and mix well. Season with salt and pepper. Chill, covered. Serve with crackers, toast, pita triangles, or raw vegetable crudités.

Tomato Salsa Dip

Calories 18
Protein 1 g
Fat *1 g
Carbohydrate 4 g

*Less than

Makes about $2\frac{1}{2}$ cups/625 mL. Serves 6 as an appetizer or sauce.

This makes a refreshing dip served with crackers or raw veggies and is great on tacos or as a sauce to go with cold meat, fish, or chicken.

2	large, ripe, fresh tomatoes, chopped	
$\frac{1}{3}$	cup finely chopped red onion	75 mL
$\frac{1}{4}$	cup finely chopped green pepper	50 mL
$\frac{1}{2}$	tsp. minced, seeded jalapeno pepper (canned or fresh)	2 mL
1	tbsp. lime juice	15 mL
	Salt and freshly ground pepper to taste	

Combine all the ingredients in a bowl and mix well. Chill.

Avocado Pâté

Calories 105
Protein 4 g
Fat 8 g
Carbohydrate 6 g

Makes about 3 cups/750 mL. Serves 6–8 as an appetizer.

Worth every calorie for its abundance of vitamins and minerals as well as the protein and calcium of the cottage cheese and yogurt.

1	small onion, finely chopped	
1	clove garlic, minced	
1	green pepper, finely chopped	
$\frac{1}{2}$	cup 2% cottage cheese	125 mL
$\frac{1}{2}$	cup low-fat plain yogurt	125 mL
2	ripe avocados, peeled and mashed	
	Juice of 1 lime	
2	drops Tabasco or hot pepper sauce	
	Pinch chili powder	
	Salt and freshly ground pepper to taste	

Combine the onion, garlic, green pepper, cottage cheese, and yogurt in a bowl. Mix well. Mash the avocados with the lime juice with a fork in a separate bowl. Add to the cheese mixture. Stir in the Tabasco and chili powder and mix well. Season with salt and pepper.

Chill. Cover the surface of the pâté directly with plastic wrap to prevent it from turning brown. Serve with crackers or raw vegetable crudités.

Calories	57
Protein	2 g
Fat	2 g
Carbohydrate	10 g

Eggplant Antipasto

Makes about 2 cups/500 mL. Serves 6 as an appetizer.

Eggplant, garlic, raisins, and pine nuts work together to give this nutritious appetizer a harmonious blend of taste and texture. Use as a spread or dip for snacking or as a prelude to a meal.

1	medium eggplant (about $\frac{3}{4}$ lb./375 g)	
2	cloves garlic, peeled and slivered	
1	tomato, chopped	
2	tbsp. raisins	25 mL
1	tsp. low-sodium soy sauce	5 mL
1	tsp. lemon juice	5 mL
1	tsp. virgin olive oil	5 mL
Freshly ground black pepper to taste		
2	tbsp. toasted pine nuts (see page 100)	25 mL
Lettuce leaves		
3	tbsp. chopped fresh parsley for garnish	45 mL
$\frac{1}{4}$	cup chopped green onion for garnish	50 mL

Halve the eggplant lengthwise. Make several slits in the flesh and insert the garlic slivers. Place on a baking sheet and bake at 350°F/180°C for 45 minutes or until tender.

Remove the eggplant from the oven and let it cool. Peel it and finely chop the flesh. Place in a bowl and add the tomatoes and raisins.

Whisk together the soy sauce, lemon juice, oil, and pepper in a small bowl. Pour this over the eggplant mixture and mix well. Cover and refrigerate overnight.

Before serving, stir in the pine nuts. Place on an attractive plate on a bed of lettuce leaves and garnish with parsley and green onion. Serve with warmed pita or toast triangles.

Calories	95
Protein	4 g
Fat	3 g
Carbohydrate	17 g

Ratatouille

Serves 6–8 as a side dish.

A wondrous, herb-laced creation from Provence that is incredibly versatile. Serve it hot with meat or fish or cold and topped with a hot poached egg as a superb summer lunch.

4	tsp. virgin olive oil	20 mL
2	medium onions, chopped	
3	cloves garlic, minced	
1	medium eggplant (about $\frac{3}{4}$ lb./375 g), cubed	
3	small zucchini (about 1 lb./500 g), cubed	
1	small green pepper, cubed	
1	small red pepper, cubed	
1	28-oz./796-mL can Italian plum tomatoes or 2 lb./1 kg fresh tomatoes, chopped	
3	tbsp. tomato paste	45 mL
3	tbsp. dry red wine (optional)	45 mL
$1\frac{1}{2}$	tsp. dried or 3 tbsp. chopped fresh basil	7 mL/45 mL
$1\frac{1}{2}$	tsp. dried or 3 tbsp. chopped fresh oregano	7 mL/45 mL
$\frac{1}{2}$	tsp. dried or 1 tbsp. chopped fresh thyme	2 mL/15 mL

Salt and freshly ground pepper to taste

Heat the oil in a large, heavy saucepan. Add the onions and garlic and sauté until soft. Add the eggplant and zucchini and cook over medium heat, stirring, for about 10 minutes. Add the green and red peppers, tomatoes, tomato paste, and wine. Bring to a boil, reduce heat, and simmer for about 10 minutes. Add the herbs and simmer 5–10 minutes longer or until the vegetables are tender but not mushy. Season with salt and pepper.

Note: For a super main course, place 1 cup/250 mL warmed ratatouille in individual ovenproof dishes. Top with a raw egg, sprinkle with 3 tbsp./45 mL grated low-fat cheese, and bake at 350°F/180°C for 10–15 minutes or until the cheese melts and the egg sets.

Calories	67
Protein	5 g
Fat	3 g
Carbohydrate	7 g

Spinach Tofu Dip

Makes about $2\frac{1}{2}$ cups/625 mL. Serves 6 as an appetizer.

My daughter Alyssa always asks me to make this dip when she's having friends over but insists I don't reveal the ingredients—she's afraid that the kids won't touch it. By the way, there's never any left. A great way to get children to eat their veggies, and sensational with the pita chips (see page 261). Be sure to use the soft tofu.

1	10-oz./300-g package frozen chopped spinach, thawed	
6	oz. tofu, pressed to remove water	175 g
2	shallots, quartered	
$1\frac{1}{2}$	tbsp. Dijon mustard	20 mL
1	tbsp. lemon juice	15 mL
2	tbsp. light mayonnaise	25 mL
$\frac{3}{4}$	cup low-fat plain yogurt	175 mL

Salt and freshly ground pepper to taste

Squeeze spinach to remove excess liquid. Process all ingredients in a food processor or blender until smooth. Adjust seasonings.

Calories	30
Protein	3 g
Fat	1 g
Carbohydrate	3 g

Broccoli Purée

Serves 4–6 as a side dish.

The colour and taste combination makes this purée a super dress-up for a chicken or fish dish.

1	head broccoli, washed and coarsely chopped	
2	tbsp. low-fat plain yogurt	25 mL
$\frac{1}{4}$	cup freshly grated Parmesan cheese	50 mL

Pinch nutmeg
Salt and freshly ground pepper to taste

Steam broccoli until firm but tender, about 10–12 minutes. Drain. Purée in a food processor or blender, then blend in yogurt, 2 tbsp./25 mL Parmesan, and seasonings. Place purée in casserole dish and keep warm. Sprinkle the remaining grated Parmesan on top and serve.

Carrot Purée

Serves 6–8 as a side dish.

You don't need whipping cream to make a silky-smooth vegetable purée that's bursting with flavour. Here's one example using our low-fat fromage blanc instead of cream.

$1\frac{1}{2}$	lb. carrots, scrubbed and sliced	750 g
3	tbsp. fromage blanc (see page 161)	45 mL
$\frac{1}{2}$	cup skim or 2% milk	125 mL

Salt and freshly ground black pepper to taste

Steam the carrots until soft. Process together with the fromage blanc and milk in a food processor or blender until smooth. Season with salt and pepper. Serve at once or chill and reheat gently over low heat when needed.

Note: Substitute almost any vegetable you like for the carrots—green beans, squash, and broccoli all work well. For a delicious change, try puréeing turnip or parsnip with cooked fruit such as apples or pears.

Red Cabbage Casserole

Serves 6 as a side dish.

The acid in the yogurt helps the red cabbage retain its gorgeous purple hue. This healthful, low-cal dish is excellent with roast meat or poultry.

1	tbsp. vegetable oil	15 mL
1	small head red cabbage (about 7 cups/ 1.75 L), coarsely shredded	
1	tsp. paprika	5 mL
$\frac{1}{2}$	cup low-fat plain yogurt	125 mL

Salt and freshly ground pepper to taste

$\frac{1}{2}$	cup slivered almonds, toasted	125 mL

Heat the oil in a heavy casserole with a lid. Add the cabbage and paprika and cook over medium heat, stirring, for about 5 minutes. Stir in the yogurt. Cover and bake at 325°F/160°C for about 30 minutes. Season with salt and pepper and sprinkle with almonds. Serve with a dollop of yogurt if you wish.

Eggplant and Goat Cheese Sandwich

Calories 195
Protein 16 g
Fat 12 g
Carbohydrate 6 g

Serves 4.

This recipe is an adaptation of the Eggplant and Goat Cheese "Oreo" created by Bob Bermann of Toronto's Avocado Club restaurant. Include a mixed salad and some crusty bread for a splendid lunch.

8	round slices eggplant, $\frac{1}{2}$ inch/1 cm thick	
8	oz. fresh goat cheese	250 g
1	tbsp. each fresh chopped parsley, chives, basil, thyme	15 mL each
	Red Pepper Sauce (see page 50)	
2	tbsp. pine nuts	25 mL

Lightly salt eggplant in colander, and allow slices to sit for $\frac{1}{2}$ hour. Rinse off the salt and pat the eggplant dry. Broil eggplant slices on a lightly greased baking sheet, 2 minutes per side. Cool.

Prepare cheese mixture by combining cheese and herbs until smooth. Spread cheese evenly on four slices of eggplant, then top each combination with another eggplant slice. Bake sandwiches at 400°F/180°C for 5–8 minutes or until cheese just begins to melt. Serve on individual plates, encircling each sandwich with 3 tbsp./40 mL red pepper sauce. Garnish with pine nuts.

Bruschetta

Makes about 50–60 bite-sized crisps. Serves 10–12 as appetizers.

Much better finger food than the usual fat-laden cocktail nibbles, and a heaven-sent appetizer in summer, when tomatoes are at their peak. Prepare the sauce in advance if you can—the flavour gets better with time.

$\frac{1}{2}$	recipe Fresh Tomato Basil Sauce (see page 96)	
1	cup part-skim mozzarella cheese, grated	250 mL
60	pita chips (see page 261)	

Prepare the Fresh Tomato Basil Sauce and allow time for the flavours to meld. Place 1 tsp./5 mL sauce on each pita chip followed by a sprinkling of 1 tsp./5 mL mozzarella. Bake at 350°F/180°C for 5 minutes.

Sautéed Cherry Tomatoes

Serves 4 as a side dish.

When you're searching for a side dish that's chock full of flavour and colour, look no further than this fast and delicious recipe.

20	cherry tomatoes	
2	tsp. virgin olive oil	10 mL
2	cloves garlic, minced	
3	tbsp. chopped fresh parsley	40 mL
Salt and freshly ground pepper to taste		

Heat the oil in a heavy skillet. Add the garlic and the cherry tomatoes and sauté over medium-high heat, stirring gently, until tomatoes are just heated through or the first one splits open. Do not overcook. Sprinkle the parsley on the tomatoes and season with salt and pepper.

Low-Fat French Fries

Calories 123
Protein 2 g
Fat 5 g
Carbohydrate 18 g

Serves 1.

Baking is the trick to these yummy fries that should satisfy anyone of any age without going overboard on the fat content. Use this recipe as a guide, doubling or tripling the amounts according to your requirements.

1   medium potato, scrubbed and cut into
    french fry pieces
1   tsp. vegetable oil   5 mL
Paprika for sprinkling

Pat the potato pieces dry with a paper towel. Toss in a bowl with the oil to coat. Place on a lightly greased baking sheet and sprinkle lightly with paprika for added browning. Bake at 450°F/230°C for 20–30 minutes or until golden brown, turning at intervals.

Sautéed Cucumber

Calories 31
Protein 1 g
Fat 3 g
Carbohydrate 2 g

Serves 4 as a side dish.

An unusual, healthful vegetable side dish that will make you wonder why you never thought of it before. Leave the peel on for extra fibre; peel it off for elegant occasions.

2   tsp. vegetable oil   10 mL
1   whole cucumber, seeded and cut into
    $\frac{1}{4}$-inch/$\frac{1}{2}$-cm slices
3   tbsp. chopped fresh dill   45 mL
Salt and freshly ground pepper to taste

Heat the oil in a heavy skillet. Add the cucumber and sauté, stirring, over medium heat until tender-crisp—3–5 minutes. Add the dill, salt, and pepper.

Calories	82
Protein	1 g
Fat	*1 g
Carbohydrate	21 g

Three-Fruit Salad

Serves 4.

*Less than

Peaches, grapes, and blueberries taste as wonderful as they look in this colourful fruit salad.

2	tbsp. unsweetened orange juice	25 mL
2	tsp. lime juice	10 mL
Pinch ground cardamom		
1	tsp. granulated sugar	5 mL
2	ripe peaches, peeled, pitted, and sliced	
1	cup halved seedless green grapes	250 mL
1	cup blueberries	250 mL
Fresh mint leaves for garnish		

Combine the orange juice, lime juice, cardamom, and sugar in a small bowl. Stir until the sugar is dissolved. Place the fruit in a medium-sized glass bowl and pour the juice mixture over. Toss gently to coat the fruit with the dressing. Chill, then garnish with mint leaves before serving.

Calories	164
Protein	2 g
Fat	3 g
Carbohydrate	35 g

Ginger Fruit Compote

Serves 4–6.

Spice up your life with this gingered fruit compote. Lovely from the fridge, but served warm it's pure heaven.

1	cup unsweetened pineapple juice	250 mL
12	dried apricots, cut into quarters	
$\frac{1}{4}$	cup muscat raisins	50 mL
$\frac{1}{4}$	cup candied ginger, finely chopped	50 mL
2	medium apples, cubed	
2	medium pears, cubed	
$\frac{1}{4}$	cup slivered almonds, toasted, for garnish	50 mL

Combine pineapple juice, apricots, raisins, and candied ginger in a heavy saucepan fitted with a lid. Bring to a

The Enlightened Eater

boil, then reduce heat and simmer, uncovered, for 5 minutes. Using a slotted spoon, transfer the apricots, raisins, and candied ginger to a serving bowl.

Add the apples and pears to the liquid in the saucepan. Bring to a boil, then cover and simmer for 5 minutes or until fruit is barely soft. Add this mixture to the cooked dried fruits. Sprinkle slivered almonds on the fruit just before serving.

Calories 114
Protein 2 g
Fat 1 g
Carbohydrate 27 g

Sunshine Fruit Salad

Serves 6.

This fruit salad is great on its own, but you can dress it up with mango sause (see page 156). Substitute whatever fruits suit your fancy.

1	nectarine, coarsely chopped	
1	pear, coarsely chopped	
2	kiwis, peeled and sliced on the diagonal	
2	oranges, peeled and sectioned	
$\frac{3}{4}$	cup cantaloupe, cubed	175 mL
$\frac{2}{3}$	cup seedless grapes, halved	150 mL
$\frac{1}{2}$	cup blueberries	125 mL
1	banana, sliced	
2	tbsp. desiccated coconut	25 mL
1	tsp. vanilla extract	5 mL

Combine all fruit in a salad bowl, mixing gently so that pieces are coated with juice of the oranges. Sprinkle coconut on the salad. Add the vanilla. Allow to stand 20 minutes.

Calories   12
Protein   *1 g
Fat   *1 g
Carbohydrate   3 g
(per tablespoon)

*Less than

Mango Sauce

Makes about 1 cup/250 mL.

This sauce, best when made from very ripe mangoes, is sublime on frozen yogurt, Cottage Cheese Pancakes (see page 175, or a fresh fruit salad.

1	cup mango, peeled and coarsely chopped	250 mL
2	tbsp. low-fat plain yogurt	25 mL
1	tbsp. kirsch or other liqueur (optional; see note)	15 mL

Purée mango in a food processor or blender. Transfer to a bowl and add yogurt and liqueur, mixing well.

Note: The liqueur should enhance the flavour of the mango, not compete with it.

Calories   142
Protein   *1 g
Fat   *1 g
Carbohydrate   35 g

Mango Sorbet

Serves 6.

Almost any soft-fleshed fruit works well in this nicest of ices, which is high in vitamins, minerals, and fibre. To purée the mangoes, peel, cut away the flesh from the stone, then process in a food processor or blender until smooth.

¾	cup granulated sugar	175 mL
¾	cup water	175 mL
1	tbsp. lemon juice	15 mL
1	tbsp. orange or peach liqueur (optional)	15 mL
3	cups mango purée (from about 3 large mangoes)	750 mL

Combine the sugar and water in a small saucepan. Bring to a boil, stirring, and boil for 2 minutes. Cool, then transfer to a medium-sized stainless steel bowl or metal pan.

Stir in the remaining ingredients and mix well. Cover with plastic wrap and freeze until firm.

Remove the sorbet from the freezer. Place in a food processor or blender and process until the mixture is slushy but firm. Return to the freezer until needed. To serve, remove from the freezer about 15 minutes before serving time.

Strawberry and Peach Sauce

Makes about $1\frac{3}{4}$ cups/425 mL.

Use fresh strawberries when they're at their peak or frozen unsweetened ones when you want a taste of early summer. The sweetness of the sauce will vary with strawberries, so try it before you sweeten it.

8	oz. strawberries	250 g
$\frac{3}{4}$	cup fresh peaches, peeled, or canned peaches packed in juice or water	175 mL
1–2 tsp. honey (see note)		5–10 mL

Purée fruit in a food processor or blender. Taste for sweetness, add honey if needed, and mix well.

Note: Those who are counting calories can substitute an equivalent amount of sweetener.

Calories   136
Protein   1 g
Fat   * 1 g
Carbohydrate 33 g

*Less than

Raspberry Sorbet

Serves 6.

A tangy variation on the sorbet theme.

¾	cup granulated sugar	175 mL
¾	cup water	175 mL
1	tbsp. orange, raspberry, or blackcurrent liqueur	15 mL
2	10-oz./300-g packages frozen unsweet-ened raspberries, thawed and puréed (see note)	

Follow the method for mango sorbet substituting raspber-ries for mangoes.

Note: To purée the raspberries, process in a food proces-sor or blender until smooth. To remove the seeds, strain the purée through a fine sieve. The seeds, which give added fibre, can be left in if you wish.

Calories   138
Protein   1 g
Fat   * 1 g
Carbohydrate 34 g

*Less than

Sorbet Bombe

Serves 12.

The perfect healthful dessert to serve to friends at a din-ner party. This beautiful bombe is bound to be a hit!

1   recipe mango sorbet (see pages 156–57)
1   recipe raspberry sorbet (see above)
Fresh raspberries and mint leaves for garnish

Remove the sorbets from the freezer. Place the mango sorbet in a food processor or blender and process until slushy but firm. Line an 8-cup/2-L mould or stainless steel bowl evenly with the sorbet and place in the freezer.

Process the raspberry sorbet in a food processor or blender until slushy but firm. Remove the mango sorbet from the freezer. Fill the hollow in the mango sorbet with the raspberry sorbet. Cover with plastic wrap and return to the freezer.

To serve, place the bottom of the mould in a larger

bowl of hot water for a few seconds or until the bombe loosens. Run a knife around the edge and invert onto a large serving plate. Leave it in the fridge for 15–20 minutes before serving. Garnish with raspberries and mint leaves.

Poached Pears with Raspberry Sauce

Calories 145
Protein *1 g
Fat *1 g
Carbohydrate 34 g

*Less than

Makes 8 small servings.

A classic recipe for good reason. Be careful to choose ripe pears for this dish.

3	cups unsweetened apple or orange juice	750 mL
3	tbsp. granulated sugar	45 mL
1	tsp. vanilla	5 mL
1	tsp. finely grated fresh ginger root	5 mL
4	ripe pears, peeled, halved, and cored	

Fresh mint leaves for garnish

Sauce

1	10-oz./300-g package frozen unsweetened raspberries, thawed	
3	tbsp. honey	45 mL
2	tbsp. orange or raspberry liqueur (optional)	25 mL

Combine the juice, sugar, vanilla, and ginger root in a large skillet. Bring to a boil and cook, stirring, until the sugar dissolves. Reduce heat. Place the pears in the skillet in a single layer and simmer over low heat until tender— 8–10 minutes. Remove the skillet from the heat and allow the pears to cool in the syrup.

Place all the ingredients for the sauce in a food processor or blender and process until smooth. Strain the mixture through a fine sieve to remove the seeds.

To serve, pour a pool of raspberry sauce onto individual plates. Top with the pear halves and garnish with mint.

Note: Those who are counting calories can substitute an equivalent amount of sweetener for the honey in the raspberry sauce.

Calories	121
Protein	3 g
Fat	1 g
Carbohydrate	26 g

Peach Crêpes

Makes 8 crêpes.

Elegant, tasty, and low in calories. Use pears, apples, or plums instead of peaches if you wish.

Crêpes	$\frac{1}{2}$	cup skim or 2% milk	125 mL
	$\frac{1}{2}$	cup all-purpose flour	125 mL
	2	egg whites	
	1	tsp. vegetable oil	5 mL
	1	tsp. baking powder	5 mL

Filling	4	ripe peaches, peeled, pitted, and chopped	
	$\frac{1}{3}$	cup raisins	75 mL
	$\frac{1}{2}$	tsp. cinnamon	2 mL
		Finely grated peel of 1 lemon or orange	
	$\frac{1}{4}$	cup unsweetened orange juice	50 mL
	1	tbsp. orange liqueur (optional)	15 mL
	1	tbsp. granulated sugar for garnish	15 mL

Whisk together the milk and flour in a medium-sized bowl. Whisk in the egg whites, oil, and baking powder until the batter is smooth.

Heat a small, lightly oiled crêpe pan or skillet over medium heat. Add 2 tbsp./25 mL of the batter. Tilt the pan to cover it evenly. Cook over medium heat until the crêpe is set, about 1 minute. Slide the crêpe out of the pan, cooked side down. Repeat with the remaining batter to make 8 crêpes, using a little more oil to coat the bottom of the pan if required.

Combine all the filling ingredients except the sugar in a small saucepan. Simmer gently until the peaches are just tender, about 5 minutes. Set aside $\frac{1}{3}$ cup/75 mL of the filling.

Place an equal amount of filling in the middle of the uncooked side of each crêpe. Roll up and arrange in a lightly greased ovenproof dish. Sprinkle with sugar. Bake at 350°F/180°C until heated through—5–8 minutes. Serve topped with a spoonful of reserved filling.

Calories 217
Protein 3 g
Fat 9 g
Carbohydrate 35 g

Fruit Crumble

Serves 6.

Not the traditional version, this low-fat crumble is high in fibre. Use apples, peaches, pears, plums, or whatever fruits are in season and combine them with berries for a tasty combination.

5	cups sliced fruit	1.25 L
2	tbsp. lemon juice	25 mL
1	tsp. cinnamon	5 mL
$\frac{1}{2}$	cup brown sugar	125 mL
1	cup rolled oats	250 mL
$\frac{1}{4}$	cup natural bran	50 mL
$\frac{1}{4}$	cup finely chopped walnuts	50 mL
1	tsp. cinnamon	5 mL
3	tbsp. soft margarine	45 mL

Combine the fruit, lemon juice, cinnamon, and $\frac{1}{4}$ cup/50 mL of the brown sugar in an 8-cup/2-L ovenproof dish. Mix well.

Combine the rolled oats, $\frac{1}{4}$ cup/50 mL of the brown sugar, bran, walnuts, and cinnamon in a bowl and mix well. Cut in the margarine with a pastry blender or fork until the mixture resembles coarse crumbs. Sprinkle it on top of the fruit mixture.

Bake at 350°F/180°C for about 45 minutes or until the fruit is soft and the topping is golden brown.

Note: Those who are counting calories can substitute an equivalent amount of sweetener for the $\frac{1}{4}$ cup/50 mL of brown sugar used in the fruit mixture.

6   Directives from the Dairy

Mom may not have understood exactly why she was urging you to "drink your milk," but her well-meaning solicitation happens to be based on good nutritional common sense. Milk is a source of many vital nutrients—protein, calcium, vitamin A, riboflavin, niacin, folacin, vitamin B12, and if the milk is fortified, vitamin D.

Milk and milk products are some of the best sources of calcium, a mineral whose vital importance is being recognized more and more. Calcium helps make muscles, nerves, blood, and cell membranes function properly. Calcium is stored in the bones. Should the body not have enough calcium for the functions we've just described, it compensates by taking it from the bones. Without enough calcium, bone mass decreases, and the bones can become porous. They are then more susceptible to fractures—a condition known as osteoporosis. Postmenopausal women are particularly susceptible to osteoporosis, and as a result women in general have become well aware of the relationship between calcium intake and well-being. But calcium consumption is equally important to men. Calcium, from dairy products, may be related to a lower incidence of a number of diseases that strike both men and women.

Cancer of the colon and its relationship to various nutrients is being looked at extensively. A number of studies have found that those with low intakes of calcium seemed to be at a higher risk for developing cancer of the colon than those who have consumed sufficient amounts of calcium. Vitamin D may play a role, but the verdict's not in yet. At any rate, cancer of the colon has also been linked to a high-fat diet, so boosting your calcium intake with high-fat dairy products may undo the benefit as far as cancer risk is concerned. Lower-fat products, though, may give you the best of both worlds. (This is described in more detail in Chapter 1.) The role of calcium in the prevention of heart disease and high blood pressure is also being studied.

Milk fits into today's fast-paced lifestyle because it is a food that takes little preparation but is loaded with nutrients. In order to get enough calcium in our diet without consuming milk or its by-products, our diet would be one long, intricate balancing act. For example, we would have to eat about two cups of broccoli to get the same amount of calcium as we do from one cup of milk. People who like fish would have an easier alternative—they could get the equivalent calcium from six sardines!

Getting this valuable nutrient from milk rather than popping calcium supplements can have a beneficial effect on other nutrients. A recent study from the University of Illinois found that when rats were fed diets with and without milk, those who consumed milk had better absorption of folic acid, a vitamin important for maintaining healthy blood. Another feather in milk's cap is that it may help repair damaged tooth enamel. Researchers found that after patients consumed soft drinks, minerals were lost from the tooth enamel. This was completely reversed by drinking a glass of milk or eating a piece of hard cheese.

Milk is also the main food source of the vitamin niacin. Unstable when exposed to light, the niacin in milk decreases during prolonged exposure to light. It is therefore best not to keep milk in glass or other clear containers. Vitamin A, another of milk's important nutrients, is found in its fat portion. It is removed along with the fat during the processing of low-fat milk but is then added back.

Vitamin D is added to milk to fortify it, making it one of the best sources of this vitamin. In addition, the vitamin D in fortified milk has the wonderful property of aiding in the absorption of calcium; this makes fortified milk unique: vitamin D is not added to any other dairy products. Check your milk container when you buy milk to make sure it is fortified. Why miss out on valuable vitamin freebies!

Why Some Are on the Wagon
In spite of all the virtues of milk, however, many of us don't consume enough. The reasons are many; some are valid, some aren't.

First, the invalid reasons. Many self-styled nutritionists, some popular reducing diets, and certain extreme forms of vegetarianism denounce milk as being "obscene," bad for you, and the source of almost every health problem known to man or woman. Unfortunately, they often manage to persuade people that these claims are true.

Other people don't drink milk because they consider

it too high in calories to be consumed on a regular basis. Whole milk does have a fairly high fat content, and so do cheeses made from it, not to mention those varieties of high-fat cheese made from cream. Skim milk, however, contains a mere 90 calories per eight-ounce glass and is now the basis for some extremely palatable low-fat cheeses that don't taste like waxy cardboard as their unpalatable predecessors did. So instead of avoiding all dairy products in the fear that they are fattening, simply avoid those that are high in fat.

To continue the whole-milk-versus-skim-milk discussion, compare the fat contained in two glasses of whole milk and the same amount of skim. The difference is the equivalent of four teaspoons of butter. Multiply that by seven days, and you have 28 teaspoons of butter hiding in your weekly milk ration. If you don't like the taste of skim milk, try 1 percent milk. If this isn't available, combine half skim milk with half 2 percent. Drinking 2 percent milk itself still saves 14 teaspoons of fat per week over whole milk.

Some people worry about the high saturated fat and cholesterol contents of milk products. Again, they should be concerned about only those foods made from whole milk. Reading the labels on these foods is an important first step in making better choices. The initials B.F. and M.F. stand for butterfat and milk fat, respectively. Check the percentage of butterfat in part skim-milk cheeses: amounts can vary widely. And don't let words such as "Natural" on a container of yogurt deceive you into thinking that it's bound to be healthful and therefore low in fat. The high fat content of many yogurts may be more harmful to your health than the preservatives in them.

Some strict vegetarians, called *vegans*, spurn milk and other dairy products as a matter of belief. This avoidance is a personal decision and must be respected. However, these people would be well advised to assess what nutrients they are losing by avoiding milk and to make sure they find them somewhere else. (See the section on vegetarianism in Chapter 10.)

Milk Intolerance and Allergy

Many people who complain of stomach problems when they drink milk simply stop drinking it without knowing what their problem is. Milk and milk products are too important a source of nutrients to be so readily renounced. These people should have their problem diagnosed by a doctor or dietitian and then try one of the treatments that will allow them to return to drinking milk.

Adverse reactions to milk can be a result of two conditions. Some people are allergic to milk's protein and thus have a milk allergy; others cannot tolerate its lactose, or milk sugar, and have a lactose intolerance.

It is now recognized that a large number of people—about 10 percent of the population, largely from ethnic groups like Jews, Asians, and blacks—are lactose intolerant. People with lactose intolerance have trouble digesting the lactose in milk and milk products. Instead of producing the right amount of *lactase*, the enzyme that breaks down lactose in the bowel into glucose and galactose, their bodies turn lactose into lactic acid and gas. This causes lactose-intolerant people to become uncomfortably bloated and even to suffer from diarrhea after ingesting milk.

Because there is a growing awareness of this problem, there are many new products available for people suffering from lactose intolerance. For example, you can buy lactose-reduced milk (and even lactose-reduced cottage cheese in some areas); this is milk that has had the lactose predigested by the addition of lactase. You can also buy the lactase enzyme in liquid form and add it to regular milk before drinking it or in tablet form and take it before consuming any dairy product. Foods that are lactose-reduced usually taste sweeter than their regular counterparts because their sugar is in the sweeter form of glucose and galactose.

If you have been diagnosed as lactose-intolerant and you have been following a lactose-reduced diet but still show symptoms, consult a registered dietitian or doctor, who will help you examine your diet to look for hidden sources of lactose. People with lactose intolerance can usually tolerate unprocessed or natural hard cheeses better than such items as processed cheese slices. Some can tolerate yogurt, others cannot.

An allergy to the protein in milk is another story. Because the proteins vary slightly from one dairy product to another, it is important to determine which foods give you problems. People with an allergy to cow's milk should avoid it entirely, but they may not be allergic to products made from goat's milk. The symptoms of a milk allergy can also vary from stomach upset and diarrhea in one individual to hives or breathing problems in another. Again, consult a dietitian or doctor to have your symptoms diagnosed.

Pasteurization: The Raw Truth

Many people fall prey to that magical word *natural* and are led to believe that "raw" milk has some valuable properties not contained in the more common pasteurized kind. In fact, raw milk can carry bacteria like salmonella and even viruses. The *Journal of the American Medical Association* has also recently reported that people have died from consuming raw milk. Since there are no nutritional benefits to raw milk, why pass up the benefits of pasteurization, which kills bacteria and other disease-bearing organisms?

Other people don't use dairy products because they are concerned about their high salt content. These same people, however, often consume plenty of salt in other foods that are not as dense in nutrients. If you are on a low-sodium diet for medical reasons or don't like the taste of salt, choose cheese labelled low in salt. But beware: unless it is marked otherwise, it may still be high in fat.

Take It to the Limit

Here are some tips for getting the greatest benefit from milk and milk products:

- Use low-fat milk as a snack when mealtimes are far off. Milk can provide the energy you need to keep you going over those few hours.

- Try making tasty drinks using milk as a base.

- Add milk to soups instead of water.

- Add a dollop of yogurt to a bowl of cold soup.

- Use yogurt as a dip for desserts of fresh fruit. For a tasty picnic dessert, mix frozen fruit such as blueberries or strawberries with some cold yogurt. The fruit will keep the yogurt cold and make a tasty combo.

- Use yogurt as a base for vegetable dips.

- Make yogurt salad dressings, which can be poured on more generously than those high-fat versions made with oil, sour cream, and so on. This is a clever way to eat more vegetables too.

- Combine cheeses when cooking to maximize taste while minimizing fat. Use a little old cheddar for strong taste along with a low-fat cheese like mozzarella on pizza and casseroles. Parmesan is also excellent in combination with low-fat cheese because of its intense flavour, especially if you keep it in one piece in the fridge and grate it each time you use it.

- Combine grated low-fat cheeses with wheat germ or whole-wheat breadcrumbs as toppings for casseroles.

- Keep low-fat cheese in the fridge at work to eat as a snack or with a salad or bun as lunchtime protein.

- Use low-fat cheese, cubed or grated, in salads.

- Add powdered milk as a filler to soups and drinks.

- Use low-fat cheese melted on tortilla chips to make nachos or on popcorn for a nutritious snack.

- Low-fat cheese—including cottage cheese—is a terrific protein food at breakfast time.

- To store cheese, wrap it in a double layer of aluminum foil. It will dry out slightly this way but won't get mouldy. Should the cheese become dry, moisten a piece of cheesecloth or J cloth, wrap it around the cheese, then wrap foil around it. Leave it in the fridge for 12 to 24 hours—no longer, or the cheese will get mouldy—remove the cloth, and behold! A fresh piece of cheese.

- Die-hard crème fraîche fans can substitute 10 percent cream instead of whipping cream (35 percent) in the recipe on page 171.

- Cream and ice cream contain nutrients from the dairy food group but are a high-fat way of ingesting them. However, cream and ice cream are more nutritious than a "non-dairy creamer" or "non-dairy" ice creams, which are made from coconut fat and contain none of the goodness of dairy products.

Yogurt: Taste and Culture
Stories from Eastern Europe that attribute the amazing longevity of certain individuals to a diet high in yogurt have contributed to its current reputation as some kind of "wonder food" that prolongs life and cures a multitude of ailments. However, yogurt is made simply by adding a live bacterial culture to milk and then leaving it to ferment. Many people who fear taking antibiotics as medication (this is unfounded as long as antibiotics are administered properly), believe that they can replace the "good" bacteria killed off by an antibiotic by eating yogurt.

Recent research is backing up some of these claims. Yogurt containing live bacterial cultures, as opposed to yogurts made with these cultures, has been shown to be useful in treating and preventing various intestinal problems such as *salmonella* infections and the diarrhea that can often accompany a course of antibiotics. In a 1992 Finnish study involving children with intestinal infections, live-culture yogurt was shown to boost the immune system's ability to fight off the infection.

Another study by the same researchers found that when participants were fed yogurt during a bout of diarrhea, the duration was shorter. A study at Long Island Jewish Medical Center showed that regularly consuming yogurt was also beneficial in preventing vaginal yeast infections. Future research in this area should give us more answers.

But the nutritional attributes of yogurt may vary greatly. All yogurt contains appreciable amounts of calcium, riboflavin, and protein. It can, however, depending on the brand, contain high amounts of fat too. Some extremely rich, creamy yogurts rack up more than 8 percent butterfat—almost as much as half-and-half cream, which contains 10 percent; both are close rivals of sour cream for fat content. Low-fat yogurts are another matter. Some brands contain a mere 1 percent butterfat and can be perfectly tasty. To be absolutely sure of the fat content and other ingredients in the yogurt you're eating, you may wish to try making your own. It's easy and delicious.

Then there's the question of how much sweetener yogurt contains. Yogurt that is laced with honey still contains simple sugar, and some of the fruit-flavoured yogurts on the market are extremely high in sugar. The best solution is to buy low-fat, unflavoured yogurt and gussy it up yourself by adding fresh fruit and berries (unsweetened frozen or canned fruit is also good), a little low-cal sweetener, some vanilla or almond extract, or a few spoonfuls of frozen, concentrated fruit juice.

NUTRITIONAL INFORMATION FOR A 100-GRAM SERVING

Product	Calories	Fat in grams
Ice Cream		
Classic Baskin Robbins	242	12.8
Baskin Robbins International Creams	252	14.4
Beatrice	214	10.0
Häagen-Dazs Chocolate	270	20.1
Häagen-Dazs Vanilla	245	16.7
Häagen-Dazs Caramel Cone Explosion	291	19.0
Häagen-Dazs Cappuccino Commotion	291	19.0
Häagen-Dazs Triple Brownie Overload	291	19.0
Sealtest Parlour Vanilla	199	10.2
Light Ice Cream		
Baskin Robbins	203	7.2
Beatrice	191	7.0
Sealtest Parlour	177	7.3
Gelato Fresca Caffe Latte	163	6.6
Frozen Yogurt		
Baskin Robbins Yo-Lite with 2% dairy fat	140	1.3
Baskin Robbins Yo-Lite with no dairy fat	139	0.4
J. Higby	160	4.9

Product	Calories	Fat in grams
Yogen Fruz	119	3.0
Yogurty's Regular	139	1.8
Yogurty's Non-fat	119	0
Yogurty's Just 16	56	0
No Sugar Added Low-Calorie Frozen Dessert	135	2.3
Sealtest Parlour 1%	124	1.0
Baskin Robbins Sherbet	142	1.8
Baskin Robbins Ices	124	0
Gelato Fresco Passion Fruit Sorbet	120	0

Frozen Dairy Delights

When it comes to frozen desserts, you may wonder whether it really matters which one you opt for. If you rarely indulge, then go for the crème de la crème. But if you're a regular at the ice-cream counter, then maybe it's time to seek out a delectable, low-fat brand. Now, that may sound like a contradiction in terms, but when it comes to frozen desserts, manufacturers are striving to capture the nutrition-conscious market.

Premium ice creams contain about 4–6 teaspoons of fat per 100-mL scoop. As a rule, supermarket house brands of ice cream have a lower fat content than premium types. Ice milk tallies in at an even lower fat level, but the sugar's often increased to keep the product creamy.

Frozen yogurt's one of the new kids on the block. With a substantially lower fat content than ice cream, it's become a popular selection. But there's a trap—sometimes you feel so virtuous for having the low-fat product that it's easy to team it up with a giant waffle cone or load it up with nuts and hot fudge sauce!

Fromage Blanc

Makes about $3\frac{1}{2}$ cups/875 mL.

A terrific, low-fat substitute for whipping cream to use in sauces, soups, or fruit and vegetable purées.

3	cups low-fat ricotta cheese	750 mL
$\frac{3}{4}$	cup low-fat plain yogurt	175 mL

Blend the ingredients in a food processor or blender until smooth. Transfer to a jar with a tight-fitting lid and let stand at room temperature for about 6 hours or until thickened. Chill for at least 10 hours before using. Will keep in the fridge for about 2 weeks.

Crème Fraîche

Makes about 1 cup/250 mL.

This version of crème fraîche uses 10 percent instead of the usual 35 percent cream, but it tastes just as good.

1	cup 10% cream	250 mL
2	tsp. buttermilk	10 mL

Combine the cream and buttermilk in a screw-top jar and shake for about 1 minute. Let the mixture stand, covered, in a warm place until it thickens—4–24 hours, depending on the temperature. Will keep in the fridge for 2–3 weeks.

Calories	69
Protein	2 g
Fat	1 g
Carbohydrate	15 g

Frozen Berry Yogurt

Serves 8.

A refreshing, low-fat, low-calorie dessert that can be made with fresh or frozen berries.

1	10-oz./300-g package frozen unsweet- ened raspberries, thawed	
1	10-oz./300-g package frozen unsweet- ened strawberries, thawed	
3	tbsp. unsweetened orange juice	45 mL
5	tbsp. honey	65 mL
$\frac{1}{4}$	tsp. finely grated orange rind	1 mL
2	cups low-fat plain yogurt	500 mL
Fresh mint sprigs or whole berries for garnish		

Purée the berries in a food processor or blender. Add the orange juice, honey, and orange rind; process until smooth. To remove the seeds (see note), strain the purée through a fine sieve. Pour it into a bowl and stir in the yogurt. Blend well.

Pour the mixture into an 8-inch/2-L pan. Freeze until firm—3–4 hours. Remove from the freezer 15 minutes before serving. Process in a food processor or beat in a bowl with an electric mixer until slushy but firm. Spoon the mixture into serving dishes or wine glasses. Let sit in the fridge until serving time, then garnish with mint leaves or berries.

Note: Some people prefer the smoother texture of this dish when the seeds are sieved out. The seeds, however, give added fibre and can be left in if you wish.

Cottage Cheese Topping

Calories 84
Protein 8 g
Fat 1 g
Carbohydrate 10 g
(per $\frac{1}{3}$ cup/75 ml)

Makes about $1\frac{1}{3}$ cups/325 mL.

Great as an accompaniment for all kinds of desserts, especially fruit, as well as pancakes and breakfast cereals. It's also wonderful on a fruit salad plate at lunch.

1	cup 2% cottage cheese	250 mL
$\frac{1}{3}$	cup skim milk	75 mL
1	tsp. vanilla	5 mL
2	tbsp. honey	25 mL

Blend all the ingredients in a food processor or blender until smooth. Cover and chill.

Note: Substitute a low-cal sweetener for the honey if you wish.

Cinnamon Yogurt Sauce

Calories 57
Protein 3 g
Fat 1 g
Carbohydrate 10 g
(entire recipe)

Makes about $\frac{1}{2}$ cup/125 mL.

The perfect topping for Cottage Cheese Pancakes (see page 175), poached or fresh fruit, or your bowl of breakfast granola.

$\frac{1}{2}$	cup low-fat plain yogurt	125 mL
$\frac{1}{2}$	tsp. cinnamon	2 mL
1	tsp. honey	5 mL
1	tsp. lemon juice	5 mL

Whisk all the ingredients together in a bowl until blended.

Note: Substitute a low-cal sweetener for the honey if you wish.

Banana Strawberry Yogurt Shake

Calories 158
Protein 6 g
Fat 2 g
Carbohydrate 33 g

Serves 2.

Boost your calcium intake with this great-tasting drink. For a thicker shake, use unsweetened frozen strawberries.

1	ripe banana, peeled and quartered	
¾	cup strawberries, halved	175 mL
¼	cup low-fat plain yogurt	50 mL
½	cup skim milk	125 mL
1	tbsp. honey	15 mL
2	tbsp. wheat germ	25 mL

Blend all the ingredients in a food processor or blender until smooth.

Note: Substitute a low-cal sweetener for the honey if you wish.

Tropical Yogurt Shake

Calories 150
Protein 6 g
Fat 1 g
Carbohydrate 31 g

Serves 2.

Without all the calories of a pina colada, here's a drink with a taste of the tropics.

½	cup canned papaya, drained (see note)	125 mL
½	cup canned pineapple, juice-packed	125 mL
3	strawberries, halved	
¼	cup low-fat plain yogurt	50 mL
½	cup skim milk	125 mL
2	tbsp. wheat germ	25 mL
1	tbsp. honey	15 mL
½	tsp. coconut extract	2 mL

Blend all the ingredients in a food processor or blender until smooth.

Note: If papaya is unavailable, substitute bananas or additional strawberries. Substitute a low-cal sweetener for the honey if you wish.

Cottage Cheese Pancakes

Calories 45
Protein 3 g
Fat 2 g
Carbohydrate 3 g

Makes 12–15 small pancakes.

The best stack of nourishing hot cakes you'll find any-where! These pancakes provide a protein-packed break-fast when they are served with a dollop of yogurt and a hefty spoonful of Strawberry and Peach Sauce (see page 157), and they score as low in fat as they do high in taste and texture. The consistency of the batter depends greatly on the moistness of the cottage cheese. Dry cottage cheese works better than creamed. If the batter is too thick, add a couple of spoonfuls of low-fat, plain yogurt; if it is too thin, add a little more flour. Drain any excess liquid from the cottage cheese before using.

1	cup 2% cottage cheese	250 mL
2	eggs	
2	tbsp. natural bran	25 mL
1	tbsp. wheat germ	15 mL
$\frac{1}{4}$	cup whole-wheat or all-purpose flour	50 mL
$\frac{1}{4}$	tsp. cinnamon	1 mL
Salt to taste		
1	tbsp. vegetable oil	15 mL

Process the cottage cheese and eggs in a food processor or blender until smooth. Combine the bran, wheat germ, flour, cinnamon, and salt in a medium-sized bowl. Mix well. Stir in the cottage cheese mixture and mix well.

Heat the oil in a large, heavy skillet over medium heat. Drop the batter into the skillet with a spoon. Cook the pancakes, one or two at a time, on both sides until golden brown.

7   Liquid Assets

Water, which makes up more than 60 percent of our body weight, is so essential that without it we would die in only a few days. Other nutrients are crucial over the long term; a lack of them takes its toll over a much longer period of time.

Many substances that are soluble in water are carried to the cells or tissues that need them by the bloodstream. Water is also the vehicle that transports nutrients through the digestive tract. At the other end of the system, this important fluid carries waste products out of the body in the urine and feces. Water also comes in handy as a lubricant that the body uses to keep the joints working smoothly and to help digest food. A lack of water in the diet is likely to cause constipation, which can be even more of a problem if a person's diet is high in fibre.

Many of the body's chemical reactions, such as breaking down carbohydrate, protein, and fat, require water. Water is also needed to keep our body temperature at the right level. If it gets too high because of heat from the environment or from a fever, perspiring is the body's way of using water to cool down and regulate its temperature. The same occurs during physical exercise.

Every day the body loses an amazing two to two and a half litres of water in urine and intestinal waste and through the lungs and skin. Thirst is the mechanism that helps the body replace this loss of important fluids. There are occasions when the thirst mechanism fails, and the result is dehydration. For example, prolonged, vigorous exercise or exercising in extreme heat can throw this mechanism off kilter, and we may not feel adequately thirsty. The dehydration that results leads in turn to a lack of fluid for producing sweat, and the body then has no way to cool itself down. In extreme cases, a further rise in body temperature causes heat prostration, which leads to a decrease in blood volume. If this is not corrected by drinking fluids, the circulatory system can collapse, possibly causing death. Exercise enthusiasts should therefore note the importance of consuming liquids as fluid replacement after a strenuous workout. (This discussion is continued in Chapter 9.)

The thirst mechanism can also be thrown off course

by the consumption of another fluid—alcohol. Alcohol causes the body to lose water simply because water is needed to get rid of it. In fact, it takes eight ounces of water to purge the body of one ounce of alcohol, so that awful "hung over" feeling is actually a serious case of dehydration. Therefore, if you do consume alcohol, it is wise to drink plenty of water at the same time.

... and Not a Drop to Drink

Fortunately for us, meeting our bodies' water requirements is not just a matter of consuming gallons of fluids. Certain foods are also terrific sources of water. Cantaloupe, for example, is 85 percent water; so are apples. Cottage cheese racks up a water count of 80 percent, while hard cheeses contain less than 37 percent. Lettuce is in the lead in the water ratings with a score of 95 percent, followed by spinach with 90 percent. Milk is also largely water—88 percent, to be exact.

Fluids such as juices, coffee, tea, soft drinks, and alcoholic beverages also contribute water to our diet. Because of some of their negative side effects, however, these drinks should be consumed only in moderation, with lots of your basic water in between.

Here are some tips for getting into the water-drinking habit:

- Order a glass of water instead of a soft drink at your next meal.

- Keep a pitcher of water flavoured with lemon slices in the fridge for a thirst-quenching cooler.

- Take a thermos of ice water to work instead of coffee, and stop by the water fountain instead of going to the cafeteria for yet another soft drink or coffee.

- When you travel by plane, load up on extra water to combat the dry environment that makes you lose fluids and become fatigued. Coffee, tea, and alcohol only add to your dehydration.

- If you're trying to lose weight, water can be a satisfying, no-calorie filler when the hungries hit.

Water—Tapping the Mineral Rites

The next question to arise is: what water should I drink—tap, filtered tap, distilled, spring, mineral, or well water?

There are many variables to consider. Underground and spring wells are both sources of mineral water.

Spring water comes from springs that are above ground. Mineral water can be naturally bubbly or artificially carbonated. Although both kinds of water contain some minerals, neither contains enough to meet a person's mineral requirements. Both mineral and spring water contain negligible amounts of fluoride, unlike tap water, to which fluoride has been added. What is more, bottled waters can be high in the mineral that most of us do *not* need more of—namely, sodium. People who are restricting their sodium intake should check the sodium content of bottled waters, which ranges from 100 to 300 mg per litre. Home water softeners can also add sodium to drinking water.

Distilled water is the condensed steam obtained from boiling water. It is free of minerals and therefore tastes rather bland. Club soda is usually tap water that has been filtered and carbonated. Different waters get their taste from their particular combination of minerals.

Tap and well water vary, depending on their environment and methods of water treatment. How well the components of these waters are monitored depends on the work of local governments and environmental groups. If you are concerned about the quality of your tap water, contact your municipal officials or local watchdog groups.

Methods of water treatment used by local authorities consist mainly of disinfection and filtration. Chlorination, a method of disinfecting water, gives rise to low levels of a group of chemicals called *trihalomethanes*, which may be carcinogenic, so further study is needed to check this possibility. Home filtration units that decrease the levels of chemicals in water can provide a solution to this, but if bacteria is allowed to grow in the filters through careless maintenance, other problems can occur.

Lead from pipes in your home can also be a concern. Lead leaches into hot water more easily than cold, so use only cold water for drinking and food preparation. Run the cold water for a few minutes first thing in the morning or if the tap hasn't been used in several hours. The lead content is highest in water that comes out when the tap is first turned on.

Be particularly careful to do this when mixing up baby formula reconstituted from powder or concentrate. A study reported in the *New England Journal of Medicine* stated that infants who drink these types of formulas get more lead per body weight than other children. And chances are that if a baby is formula fed, the first thing to be made in the day—using the more lead-concentrated water—is the baby's bottle. Taking those extra couple of minutes to flush out the pipes is well worth while.

Because bottled water harbours fewer chemicals, it is usually assumed to be the best choice of water. However, it is not regularly monitored for chemicals the way tap water is, so its quality is not guaranteed. In addition, methods of disinfecting tap water get rid of contaminants such as bacteria, which may be found in bottled water.

The bottom line is that neither tap nor bottled water is without flaws. The best route to go, therefore, is to alternate the kinds of water you drink. It is also wise to express your concern to the right authorities about the safety of tap water. The more regulations there are controlling the pollution of our waterways and the more controls there are on bottled water, the better for us all.

Caffeine Controversy

Caffeine is one of a group of compounds called *methylanxthines*. Consumed by all of us in the form of coffee, tea, and soft drinks, caffeine is, in fact, a stimulant that has become as acceptable a part of our lifestyle as the automobile and sliced bread. Because of its effect on our bodies, however, many of us are now questioning whether overindulging in caffeine could be detrimental to our health.

Caffeine is absorbed in the gastrointestinal tract. Its effects reach their peak 15 to 45 minutes after being consumed, depending on how sensitive a person is to it and on his or her size. Caffeine affects a smaller person more quickly than a larger one, a fact that explains why foods as seemingly harmless as a bar of chocolate washed down with a glass of cola can make a small child irritable and even sleepless.

How fast caffeine is eliminated from the body also varies from person to person and is especially affected by age and the presence of disease.

The stimulant effect of caffeine runs the gamut from increasing alertness in some people to anxiety, irritability, or headaches in others. It can also cause insomnia, a poor sleep pattern, or sleep that leaves a person feeling badly rested. These symptoms occur because caffeine narrows the blood vessels, thereby making the heart

CAFFEINE CONTENT OF VARIOUS FOODS AND MEDICATIONS

Item	Amount	Caffeine Content (mg)
Coffee, drip	5 oz./150 g	140
Coffee, instant	5 oz./150 g	60
Coffee, instant, decaffeinated	5 oz./150 g	3
Coffee, percolated	5 oz./150 g	110
Tea, black, brewed 1 minute	5 oz./150 g	30
Tea, black, brewed 3 minutes	5 oz./150 g	40
Tea, black, brewed 5 minutes	5 oz./150 g	45
Tea, green, brewed 5 minutes	5 oz./150 g	30
Tea, oolong, brewed 5 minutes	5 oz./150 g	40
Cocoa	5 oz./150 g	13
Cola beverages	12 oz./375 g	35–50
Baking chocolate	1 oz./30 g	35
Chocolate powder for milk	1 tbsp./15 mL	10
Anacin	1 tablet	32
Dexatrim	1 tablet	200
Dristan	1 tablet	16
Excedrin	1 tablet	65
Midol	1 tablet	32
Triaminic	1 tablet	30
Cafergot	1 capsule	100
Fiorinal	1 tablet	40

work harder to pump the blood through them. In cases of real excess or caffeine sensitivity, heart palpitations can result.

Caffeine can also cause trouble for the digestive system because it stimulates the digestive juices. This can lead to gastrointestinal irritation in predisposed individuals and can easily irritate an empty stomach.

People who are trying to watch their weight should certainly beware of caffeine because it raises blood sugar levels. This can lead to a surge of insulin and a subsequent drop in blood sugar to a level lower than before the caffeine was consumed. The result? That cup of coffee downed in order to squelch hunger pangs can lead to even greater hunger. In addition, the calories in cream and sugar slipped into cups of coffee can quickly add up by day's end. You can reduce the 40 to 50 calories in a "regular" coffee by using milk instead of cream and eliminating sugar. Avoid coffee whiteners—they are high in saturated fats and are as unhealthful as they are caloric.

Caffeine also has a diuretic effect, meaning that it causes the body to lose fluids. This can be especially harmful to people who are trying to maintain their body's fluid level because they exercise regularly or live or work in environments that are hot or dry.

And there is still more on caffeine's criminal record.

Caffeine seems to have a negative effect on other nutrients in the body, in particular calcium. High caffeine intakes have been shown to result in a negative calcium balance. Caffeine and its connection to Pre-Menstrual Syndrome is a new area of research. One study has linked high caffeine consumption with the presence and severity of PMS, which can cause irritability, anxiety, headache, fatigue, breast tenderness, and food cravings.

Last but by no means least, caffeine is addictive. If you don't believe this, just try cutting it out cold turkey and see how it feels! Symptoms of withdrawal for people who are addicted range from headaches to depression.

So how much caffeine is acceptable? Healthy adults, it seems, can safely drink 200 to 250 mg a day. That's two 5-ounce cups of perked coffee, less if you drink drip coffee. And don't forget to include soft drinks when you do your caffeine count. Pregnant and nursing women should reduce their caffeine consumption even further.

For many of us, the thought of starting the day without that ritualistic cup of coffee is hard to imagine. So if you want to cut down on your caffeine consumption, do it slowly. Try substituting decaffeinated coffee for regular, or mixing half your usual coffee with half decaffeinated. Some people worry about the chemical used to decaffeinate most coffees, methyl chloride. Studies show that it seems to be safe, but if you are still wary, try brands that are decaffeinated by the water process, which uses steam, not chemicals, to extract the caffeine. There's been some research that shows decaffeinated may raise blood cholesterol levels, but as yet this has not been proven.

Varying your beverages is also wise when trying to cut down on caffeine, and milk, water, and substituting the odd herbal tea might be to your taste. A craving for the stimulation of coffee could also be a helpful indicator of a nutritional lack. For example, skipping breakfast or lunch could be the reason for that dip in energy that makes your body cry out for a cola or coffee. Try a nutritious snack instead.

Alcohol, et al.
Drinking alcohol is such an integral part of our lifestyle, and the nutritional information on it is often so contradictory, that many people are totally confused. Should they eliminate alcohol from their diets completely or throw caution to the winds and enjoy a few beers like their friends do?

The key once again is moderation.

But it varies. One person's moderation could be another's overindulgence. Three beers a night could be moderate for one person; for another it could be two to three drinks a month. One to two drinks a day—allowing 12 ounces of beer, 5 ounces of wine, and 1.5 ounces of liquor per drink—seems to be the guide to moderate imbibing.

The liver is the place in the body where alcohol takes its sometimes deadly toll. The liver detoxifies alcohol and converts it into energy for the body to use. Excess alcohol makes the liver fatty, and continued excess causes cirrhosis. (However, a person can develop liver disease without being an alcoholic.) Although the combination of bad nutrition and excess alcohol is likely to cause changes in the liver, the liver can return to normal if the alcohol intake is lowered before permanent damage is done.

It is also thought that excess alcohol may be associated with cancer of the liver and breast. Heavy beer drinking has been associated with increased risk of rectal and colon cancer. The Canadian Cancer Society recommends that if you do drink alcohol, limit your drinking to one or two drinks a day.

For Whom the Bar Bell Tolls

Heavy drinking can have many other bad effects on our health.

Depending on the amount consumed, alcohol creates a greater need in the body for other nutrients. Although a little alcohol stimulates the appetite, too much dulls it. This explains why heavy drinkers often do not eat nutritious foods and do not eat adequate amounts. This, combined with the fact that alcohol causes some nutrients not to be used by the body, explains why many heavy drinkers suffer from malnutrition.

Although alcohol may offer the body enough calories to keep it stable, it may not meet the body's nutritional demands. In addition, the body's need for thiamin (vitamin B1) increases with the amount of alcohol that is consumed; a persistent deficiency of thiamin could result in a disease called beri beri.

Alcohol can also irritate the linings of the stomach and intestines; this can result in decreased absorption of B vitamins. Heavy drinking also seems to affect a person's selenium status. Anyone who suffers from stomach problems should monitor the effect alcohol has on them, because alcohol can be an irritant, especially on an empty stomach.

People with hypoglycemia should be aware that drinking alcohol can cause their blood sugar to fall. This can vary, depending on when the alcohol is consumed and what has been eaten, but abstinence is probably the best policy if you are not symptom-free.

There is a great deal of research going on into many aspects of alcohol consumption. Does drinking a lot of alcohol during pregnancy cause birth defects? Does excess alcohol predispose a person to bone loss, or osteoporosis? Does a lowered intake of alcohol help control high blood pressure? And on the other side of the coin, does a little wine served to the elderly in nursing homes lead to more restful sleep and a greater zest for life?

Certainly alcohol is not all bad. Its moderate use has been shown to increase HDL cholesterol levels in the blood. In predisposed people, however, even moderate consumption can raise triglyceride levels.

Then, of course, there's the matter of weight control.

ALCOHOL AND CALORIC CONTENT OF VARIOUS ALCOHOLIC BEVERAGES

Beverage	Amount	Alcohol (g)	Calories
Cider, fermented	6 oz./175 g	9.4	71
Liqueur	1 oz./30 g	7.0	64
Liquor, 80 proof (gin, rum, whiskey, vodka)	$1\frac{1}{2}$ oz./45 g	14.0	97
Liquor, 90 proof	$1\frac{1}{2}$ oz./45 g	15.9	110
Liquor, 100 proof	$1\frac{1}{2}$ oz./45 g	17.9	124
Wine, sweet dessert	$3\frac{1}{2}$ oz./100 g	15.8	153
Wine, dry table	$3\frac{1}{2}$ oz./100 g	9.9	85
Champagne, dry	4 oz./125 g	13.0	105
Beer	8 oz./250 g	8.7	99
Beer, light	8 oz./250 g	7.0–12.0	60–130
Planter's punch	4 oz./125 g	21.5	175
Martini	$3\frac{1}{2}$ oz./100 g	18.5	140
Eggnog	4 oz./125 g	15.0	335

Note: Differences in calories may be a result of carbohydrate content.

After being metabolized in the liver, alcohol yields fewer calories per gram than fat but almost twice as many as protein and carbohydrate. Within each gram of alcohol lurk seven calories, accompanied by negligible nutrients. Add the empty calories of a mixer to your drink, and you can rack up a mammoth calorie count and no appreciable nourishment before you can say "gin and tonic!"

When rating alcoholic drinks for calories, remember that light beers can contain anywhere from about 60 to 120 calories per bottle, depending on the brand. Keep in mind too that most calorie charts give the number of calories for a four- or five-ounce glass of wine, which is smaller than the amount that is often served. Note also that cooking with wine and other alcoholic beverages does not add calories to a meal because alcohol evaporates during the cooking process, leaving only its flavour. If calories are a concern, however, restrict the alcohol in your cooking to dry wine or brandy; avoid sweet liqueurs, which leave behind a lot of sugar.

Another hazard of alcohol if you are trying to lose weight is that it is more readily absorbed on an empty stomach. As your blood alcohol level rises, you likely become hungrier. This combined with your diminishing willpower, caused by the effects of the alcohol on your mind, could cause you to eat more when you're under the influence. One way you can avoid this in social situations is to alternate alcoholic drinks with non-alcoholic ones, for example, drinking a tall glass of soda with lime between beers. The extra fluid will fill you up without adding calories and reducing your mental fortitude!

Crystal Clear?
Last but not least, how you store and serve your alcoholic beverages may have an impact on your health. It is said that the fall of the Roman Empire may have been caused, in part, by lead poisoning.

Recent studies have shown that lead from a lead crystal decanter can leach into the liquid it holds, particularly if the fluid is acidic. Your port wine, brandy or other liquor can end up being laced with lead. The risk is *storing* beverages in crystal decanters, not drinking from a lead crystal goblet. Use your decanters only for serving. Pour leftover beverages back into the bottle.

8   Breakfast for Champions

You can be sure you're a convert to healthful eating when someone offers you one meal a day and you choose breakfast! If there's one thing I hope this book will teach, it's that eating a nutritious breakfast is an absolute must.

Yet in spite of the crucial role of breakfast in ensuring a balanced diet—and as a result, a healthy body and mind—many if not most people either skip this meal altogether or consider a cup of coffee and slice of toast adequate sustenance at the start of the day. Perhaps the most common reason people give for eating little or no breakfast is that they simply aren't hungry at this time of day. This is a perfect example of how "mind over matter" can become a dangerous thing.

When your mind tells you that you're tired or in a hurry to get to work, you can actually override your body's healthy craving for food until it becomes a habit. Once you learn to override your hunger, you suppress the important ability to regulate your appetite. And if you don't know when your body is hungry, then you won't know when your body is satisfied. The result is that you tend to eat foods that are convenient at times that are convenient, not when your body needs them for nourishment.

And there are more repercussions of this unhealthy syndrome. People who are not hungry at breakfast are, in contrast, usually hungry at night—the very time their bodies do not require much food. Our bodies need fuel to *start* the day, not to end it.

What can be done to save this situation? With a little effort and persistence, it is possible to get our bodies back in touch with their needs, so that they are hungry when they need the nutrients. This means listening to the requirements of our bodies instead of the power of our minds.

The simple practice of eating a substantial breakfast is the best way to change your eating pattern and teach your body how to regulate its appetite. It may be difficult at first, but after a period of sustained breakfast eating, I guarantee that you will begin to feel hungry at the start of the day.

Some people who are not used to eating breakfast will actually feel nauseated when they do. This may be because their blood sugar is low from not eating during the night. But their nausea will gradually decrease as eating breakfast becomes a habit.

Take a Minute in the Morning

There are several reasons why breakfast is the meal of prime importance.

First, there's the matter of weight control. Being the right weight is highly dependent on your ability to regulate your appetite. If you don't know when you are hungry—and most people have tricked their bodies into believing that rushing out of the house with a cup of coffee inside them is enough—then you won't know when you are full either.

In other words, downing a huge piece of chocolate cake while you're watching the late-night news may be pleasant, but it is biological nonsense when all you have ahead of you is a night's sleep. On the other hand, eating a bowl of porridge topped with nuts, fruit, and milk makes a lot of sense as a prelude to an energy-filled day.

Another reason to eat breakfast to control our weight is that our bodies run at a slower pace during sleep. This means that our metabolic rate—the rate at which our bodies burn calories—is slower after sleeping. Eating a balanced breakfast raises the metabolic rate, so our metabolism is faster after we eat a good breakfast than if we had eaten no breakfast at all. A word of warning here, however: as with everything, moderation is the key; eating too much breakfast can cause problems too.

Still on the subject of weight control, frequent, small meals are less fattening than a few big meals. In other words, the same 1,500 calories downed in one large meal may cause more fat deposition than the same number of calories consumed in six small meals. And another reason to start eating first thing in the morning—Dr. David Jenkins, of the University of Toronto, found that when participants in his study ate small meals throughout the day, they had lower blood cholesterol levels than when they ate large meals less frequently. The ideal eating pattern for losing weight and maintaining good health is to taper off meals from the beginning to the end of the day. Keep in mind the credo: Eat breakfast like a queen or king, lunch like a princess or prince, and dinner like a pauper.

Should you eat a large, late dinner one night and wake up the next morning with no appetite, stick to the preceding game plan. Eat your usual large breakfast and go easy on the rest of your meals, especially dinner. If you do miss breakfast in such an instance, it's almost guaranteed that you will want a large evening meal, and before you know it, you could be back into the breakfast-skipping syndrome!

What is more, people who eat a good breakfast have fewer cravings for empty-calorie foods later in the day— the sad fate of those unrealistically cheerful snackers on TV commercials who grab a chocolate bar as soon as the "mid-afternoon hungries" hit. Breakfast skippers are also the most likely people to long for chocolate, potato chips, and cola drinks at 4 P.M. when a nutritious snack of yogurt and fruit seems inconvenient and far less tempting.

Energize Your Day

The body's blood sugar and energy levels go hand in hand. So energy levels throughout the day can be affected by eating or not eating the right breakfast. It may be hard to believe, but a balanced intake at the beginning of the day seems to prevent drastic highs and lows in energy levels later on.

In other words, the "4 P.M. slump" can be eradicated by eating a substantial meal at 8 A.M. Also, if your energy levels are maintained throughout the day, you won't feel as exhausted at night. This is easier to understand when you picture the body functioning without breakfast as a machine running on little or no fuel. It's not surprising that it eventually cuts out. A person who goes for the first half of the day without fuel is bound to be weary by the time evening comes around.

The person who says that he or she is not a "morning person" is probably someone who doesn't make a habit of eating breakfast. But why waste those precious morning hours to sluggishness and droopy eyelids when you could be bursting with energy? Studies show that protein is a crucial breakfast ingredient—it seems to stimulate the mind and give us mental energy. This explains why children who arrive at school without eating breakfast are likely to doze off in the middle of a morning class.

Many people overcome their lack of energy in the morning, when blood sugar and energy levels are somewhat low, by means of a stimulant like caffeine. This source of energy is, however, a poor substitute for good food. Not only is it comparatively short-lived, but it is also lacking in nutrients and so addictive that the body may crave higher and higher doses. In addition, this short surge of energy is followed by a lowering of the blood sugar, which can make you feel more tired and hungry than before you had that hit of coffee, tea, or other source of caffeine.

A Family Affair

Many parents expect their children to eat a good, nutritious breakfast in the morning while they set a bad example and eat little or nothing. And some people, especially women, are so busy getting their family ready to leave home in the morning that they simply skip breakfast. This is the time when everyone most needs nourishing food in order to cope with frenzied mornings.

Instead, make breakfast a family affair. It is a good time for the family to come together, especially with everyone's busy work and school schedules during the week. Also, encourage your children to plan their own breakfasts the night before. If they are part of the decision-making process, they will be more likely to follow through by eating a more substantial morning meal.

Planning breakfast is a good idea even for adults, because it is often the most rushed meal of the day. You could prepare the makings of a tuna melt or grilled cheese sandwich the night before, then put them in the fridge ready to pop under the broiler the next morning while you're getting ready. Brown-bagging it is another nifty idea for people who are rushed in the morning. A cheese sandwich and piece of fruit eaten in the car or at your office desk is better than no breakfast at all.

Breaking with traditional breakfast foods like the fat-laden stand-by of fried eggs, bacon, and buttered toast is also a good way to get more variety into this underrated meal. Kids who eat tuna melts, pizza, or grilled cheese sandwiches in the morning are less likely to get bored with breakfast than those who are faced with the same packaged cereal every day.

Breakfast—A Choice Meal

What are the best foods to eat at breakfast?

Ideally, this meal should contain foods from all four food groups and should make up one-quarter to one-third of the day's nutrients. For many people, breakfast is the only meal eaten at home, in which case it is important to pack it with good amounts of fibre, vitamins, and minerals. The meal should also contain some of the following.

Milk and Milk Products	Choose low-fat foods from this group such as a tall glass of skim or 1% milk or a cup of low-fat yogurt. Both are also excellent whipped up into a quick blender drink with fruit. Low-fat cheese can count as a serving from this group or from the protein foods—meat, fish, poultry, and alternates.
Meat, Fish, Poultry, and Alternates	Again, go for a low amount of fat and be adventurous. The egg is not the only protein food that has a place on the breakfast table, although it is a favourite of many. Moderating your egg-yolk intake is advised because of their cholesterol content, but you can extend these with plenty of egg whites, especially in omelettes and scrambled eggs.
	Bacon and sausages should be eaten in moderation and with an eye to fat content. Side bacon is basically saturated fat, salt, nitrites, and not much more. Back, or Canadian, bacon is much leaner and is all right if it is consumed occasionally; the same is true for sausages, which are high in fat. When you cook these meats, cook them so the fat drips off.
	Why not try fish at breakfast? Along with the traditional kipper, albacore tuna, complete with its omega-3 fatty acid, is excellent on a melt (the cheese gives you the dairy component) or in a whole-wheat pita.
Breads and Cereals	Choose whole-grain breads and cereals where possible or, as second best, enriched versions of refined breads. Be careful when you select muffins, quick breads, or breakfast pastries. That good-looking Danish is probably loaded with fats as well as sugar. The same goes for most store-bought granolas (see also Chapter 4) and for the lashings of butter you might be tempted to smear on that healthy hunk of whole-wheat bread. Remember: breakfast is supposed to pep you up; lots of fat will get your day off to a sluggish start.
Fruits and Vegetables	A piece of fresh fruit is the ideal choice from this food group—a better choice than juice because of the fibre. For people who are creatures of habit and cannot start the day without a glass of juice, this is second best. Dried fruits are great additions to hot and cold cereals, especially for people who are trying to boost their iron intake.

The Chef Suggests

Eating breakfast away from home, either in a restaurant or in a hotel, presents its own set of problems. And because most dining establishments are still stuck in the bacon-and-eggs, pancakes-with-syrup, or buttered-toast-with-jam routine, it can be tricky to eat a healthful breakfast. Here are some tips:

- When ordering eggs, opt for poached or boiled rather than fried or scrambled, which are usually high in fat. If you order an omelette, see if it can be cooked with minimal butter and if it can be made with one whole egg and extra egg whites.

- Order low-fat milk.

- Order toast unbuttered, and if you want, with butter on the side. Buttering toast yourself can really reduce your fat intake. Ask for whole-wheat or other whole-grain toast or bread rather than white.

- Fresh fruit may not be listed on a restaurant menu but is often available on request.

- When you are travelling, if your hotel room has a fridge, stock it with nutritious items not offered on the breakfast menu—low-fat cheese, fresh fruit, and low-fat milk.

- For nutritional content of fast-food breakfasts, see the chart on pages 217 to 225.

What to Munch at Brunch
Brunch is becoming an increasingly popular midday meal, especially on weekends. But this pleasant custom has some unique hazards. Here is some advice on how to avoid them:

- Never go to a brunch (especially one of those lavish buffet affairs consisting of everything from lobster thermidor to Black Forest cake) starving! Don't skip breakfast in anticipation of a big brunch, especially if you have slept late, in which case your body will be even hungrier. Remember that you can always skip your evening meal.

- When you select food from a lavish brunch buffet table, remember these key words—discernment and moderation. Don't load up your plate with everything from soup to nuts. Choose small amounts of nutritious foods from all the food groups, and arrange them on your plate in an appetizing way. You can always return to the buffet for more, and you will savour your food more if you take small servings. Survey the buffet table before choosing your food, and opt where possible for dishes with the least amount of fat. A series of small, carefully chosen assortments is your best bet for brunch.

Calories 141
Protein 10 g
Fat 10 g
Carbohydrate 3 g

Scrambled Tofu

Serves 4.

A delicious way to extend eggs and minimize your cholesterol intake.

2	tsp. soft margarine	10 mL
1	clove garlic, minced (optional)	
2	cups well-drained, mashed tofu	500 mL
4	eggs, lightly beaten	

Salt and freshly ground pepper to taste
1   green onion, chopped

Heat the margarine in a heavy skillet and sauté the garlic until soft. Mix together the mashed tofu and eggs in a bowl. Add to the garlic in the skillet. Cook, stirring, over medium heat for 3–4 minutes. Season with salt and pepper and sprinkle with green onion. Serve at once.

Calories 200
Protein 6 g
Fat 9 g
Carbohydrate 27 g
(per $\frac{1}{2}$ cup/125 mL)

Great Granola

Makes 12 cups/3 L.

Lower in fat and sugar than the commercial versions, this granola is absolutely delicious and extremely high in fibre. It's also great in baking or as a topping for yogurt and fresh fruit.

5	cups rolled oats	1.25 L
1	cup chopped walnuts	250 mL
½	cup natural bran	125 mL
1	cup oat bran	250 mL
½	cup wheat germ	125 mL
¾	cup sunflower seeds	175 mL
½	cup honey	125 mL
¼	cup vegetable oil	50 mL
2	tsp. vanilla	10 mL
1	cup raisins	250 mL

Combine the first six ingredients in a large bowl. Heat the honey, oil, and vanilla in a small saucepan over low heat until blended. Pour this mixture over the dry ingredients, stirring to coat well.

Spread the mixture in a thin layer on one or two large cookie sheets. Bake at 350°F/180°C for about 20 minutes, stirring at intervals until lightly browned. Cool completely, mix in the raisins, and store in an airtight container in the fridge.

Fruity Oatmeal Muffins

Makes 1 dozen.

Use your favourite fruit, dried or otherwise, to make these delicate muffins even better.

1	cup rolled oats	250 mL
1 $\frac{1}{4}$	cups buttermilk or sour milk	300 mL
1	cup all-purpose flour	250 mL
1	tsp. baking powder	5 mL
$\frac{1}{2}$	tsp. salt	2 mL
$\frac{1}{2}$	tsp. baking soda	2 mL
1	egg	
$\frac{1}{3}$	cup brown sugar	75 mL
$\frac{1}{4}$	cup vegetable oil	50 mL
1	cup blueberries, cranberries, or raisins (see note)	250 mL

Combine the oats and buttermilk in a large bowl. Let stand. Combine the flour, baking powder, salt, and baking soda in a separate bowl. Stir well to blend.

Beat the egg, sugar, and oil together in another bowl. Stir it into the oats mixture. Add the dry ingredients and fruit, stirring just until blended. Spoon into greased muffin cups. Bake at 400°F/200°C for 18–23 minutes.

Note: If you wish, replace blueberries with $\frac{1}{2}$ cup/125 mL dried apricots or prunes soaked for 30 minutes in a little hot water, port, or fruit juice.

Orange Oat Bran Muffins

Makes 1 dozen.

Tender, light, and moist with a wonderful orange flavour plus the nutritional bonus of oat bran—the cholesterol-reducing fibre.

1	cup all-purpose flour	250 mL
1	cup oat bran	250 mL
$\frac{1}{3}$	cup granulated sugar	75 mL
1	tsp. baking powder	5 mL
1	tsp. baking soda	5 mL
$\frac{1}{4}$	tsp. salt	1 mL
$\frac{1}{2}$	tsp. cinnamon	2 mL
1	egg	
$\frac{3}{4}$	cup buttermilk or sour milk	175 mL
$\frac{1}{4}$	cup vegetable oil	50 mL
1	tbsp. grated orange rind	15 mL
2	tbsp. orange juice	25 mL
1	cup raisins or chopped dates	250 mL

Combine the first seven ingredients in a bowl and stir well to blend. Beat the egg with the buttermilk, oil, orange rind, and orange juice in a separate large bowl. Add the dry ingredients, stirring just until blended. Stir in the raisins. Spoon the mixture into greased muffin cups. Bake at 400°F/200°C for 18–23 minutes.

Banana Bran Muffins

Calories 175
Protein 3 g
Fat 6 g
Carbohydrate 31 g

Makes 12 large or 15 small muffins.

The best possible use for those overripe bananas and a favourite with kids, for whom it makes the perfect snack.

$1\frac{1}{4}$	cups all-purpose flour	300 mL
$\frac{1}{2}$	cup natural bran	125 mL
$\frac{1}{3}$	cup wheat germ	75 mL
1	tsp. baking powder	5 mL
1	tsp. baking soda	5 mL
$\frac{1}{4}$	tsp. salt	1 mL
1	egg	
$\frac{1}{3}$	cup brown sugar	75 mL
$\frac{1}{3}$	cup vegetable oil	75 mL
1	cup mashed banana (3 bananas)	250 mL
$\frac{1}{2}$	cup buttermilk or sour milk	125 mL
2	tbsp. molasses	25 mL
1	cup raisins or chopped dates	250 mL

Combine the first six ingredients in a bowl. Stir well to blend. Beat the remaining ingredients together in a separate large bowl. Add the dry ingredients, stirring just until blended. Spoon into greased muffin cups. Bake at 375°F/190°C for 20–25 minutes.

Note: Add $\frac{1}{2}$ cup/125 mL chopped nuts if you wish.

Three-Bran Refrigerator Muffins

Calories 136
Protein 3 g
Fat 3 g
Carbohydrate 25 g

Makes 5 dozen large or 6 dozen small muffins.

Have this batter on hand to bake fresh muffins that are ready when you are. This unbeatable muffin combines top-notch taste and texture with the double whammy of both insoluble and soluble fibre in the wheat and oat bran. This recipe makes *a lot*, so you might wish to halve it.

2	cups boiling water	500 mL
2	cups natural bran	500 mL
5	cups all-purpose flour (see note)	1.25 L
2	tbsp. baking soda	25 mL
1	tsp. salt	5 mL
1	cup soft margarine	250 mL
$2\frac{1}{2}$	cups granulated sugar	625 mL
$\frac{1}{2}$	cup molasses	125 mL
4	eggs	
4	cups buttermilk	1 L
2	cups All-Bran	500 mL
2	cups oat bran	500 mL
2	cups raisins	500 mL

Pour the boiling water over the natural bran in a bowl. Let stand. Meanwhile, combine the flour, baking soda, and salt in a separate bowl. Stir well to blend.

Cream the margarine, sugar, and molasses in a very large bowl until light and creamy. Add the eggs and buttermilk, beating until smooth. Stir in the natural bran. Add the flour mixture, All-Bran, and oat bran, mixing until well blended. Stir in the raisins. Spoon into greased muffin cups and bake at 400°F/200°C for 18–23 minutes.

Store unused batter in airtight containers in the fridge until you are ready to use it. This mixture keeps for up to 2 months. To use, take the batter directly from the fridge and bake the muffins at 375°F/190°C for 20–25 minutes.

Note: Substitute $2\frac{1}{2}$ cups/625 mL each of whole-wheat and all-purpose flour for 5 cups/1.25 L all-purpose if you wish.

Cheesy Cornmeal Muffins

Calories 167
Protein 9 g
Fat 6 g
Carbohydrate 18 g

Makes 1 dozen.

These mini-cornbreads make a yummy savoury snack and are great with a bowl of hot soup or chili.

1	cup all-purpose flour	250 mL
1	cup cornmeal	250 mL
3	tbsp. granulated sugar	45 mL
4 $\frac{1}{2}$	tsp. baking powder	22 mL
$\frac{3}{4}$	tsp. salt	3 mL
1 $\frac{1}{2}$	cups grated low-fat cheddar cheese	375 mL
1	egg	
1	cup milk	250 mL
$\frac{1}{4}$	cup vegetable oil	50 mL

Combine the first six ingredients in a bowl. Stir well to blend. Beat the egg, milk, and oil together in a large bowl. Add the dry ingredients, stirring just until blended. Spoon into greased muffin cups. Bake at 400°F/200°C for 18–23 minutes.

Carrot Pineapple Muffins

Calories 169
Protein 3 g
Fat 7 g
Carbohydrate 25 g

Makes 1 dozen.

Moist and tender with a hint of cinnamon.

1	cup all-purpose flour	250 mL
$\frac{3}{4}$	cup whole-wheat flour	175 mL
1	tsp. baking powder	5 mL
1	tsp. baking soda	5 mL
1	tsp. cinnamon	5 mL
$\frac{1}{2}$	tsp. salt	2 mL
1	egg	
$\frac{1}{2}$	cup liquid honey	125 mL
$\frac{1}{3}$	cup vegetable oil	75 mL
1	cup grated carrot	250 mL
1	cup crushed unsweetened pineapple with juice	250 mL

Combine the first six ingredients in a bowl. Stir well to blend. Beat the remaining ingredients together in a large bowl. Add the dry ingredients, stirring just until blended. Spoon into greased muffin cups. Bake at 400°F/200°C for 20–25 minutes.

Note: Add $\frac{1}{2}$ cup/125 mL chopped nuts or raisins if you wish.

Calories	78
Protein	3 g
Fat	3 g
Carbohydrate	11 g

Spiced Oat Pancakes

Makes 16–18 medium pancakes.

A wonderful way to spice up your mornings.

$1\frac{1}{2}$	cups skim milk	375 mL
1	cup rolled oats	250 mL
$\frac{3}{4}$	cup whole-wheat flour	175 mL
$\frac{1}{2}$	cup oat bran	125 mL
2	tbsp. brown sugar	25 mL
1	tbsp. baking powder	15 mL
1	tsp. ground cinnamon	5 mL
$\frac{1}{4}$	tsp. ground ginger	1 mL
$\frac{1}{2}$	tsp. salt	2 mL
3	egg whites	
$\frac{1}{4}$	cup soft margarine	50 mL

Combine milk and rolled oats in a large bowl; let mixture stand while you prepare the remaining ingredients. Combine flour, oat bran, brown sugar, baking powder, spices, and salt in a second bowl. Beat egg whites until soft peaks form. Add dry ingredients and margarine to oat mixture, stirring until combined. Fold in beaten egg whites.

For each pancake, pour $\frac{1}{4}$ cup/50 mL batter onto a hot, lightly greased griddle. Cook until edges dry and top is covered with bubbles. Turn and cook second side until golden brown. Serve with warm apple syrup (see page 201).

Oat Bran Breakfast Scones

Calories 116
Protein 3 g
Fat 6 g
Carbohydrate 14 g

Makes 16 scones.

A low-fat scone with some oat bran to boot.

$1\frac{1}{3}$	cups all-purpose flour	325 mL
$\frac{1}{2}$	cup oat bran	125 mL
2	tbsp. granulated sugar	25 mL
2	tsp. baking powder	10 mL
$\frac{1}{2}$	tsp. salt	2 mL
$\frac{1}{2}$	cup soft margarine, chilled	125 mL
1	egg white	
1	whole egg	
$\frac{1}{3}$	cup skim milk	75 mL
1–2	tsp. grated orange peel	5–10 mL
$\frac{1}{4}$	cup raisins or currants	50 mL
2	tbsp. milk	25 mL

Topping

1	tbsp. oat bran	15 mL
1	tbsp. granulated sugar	15 mL
$\frac{1}{2}$	tsp. cinnamon	2 mL

Combine flour, oat bran, sugar, baking powder, and salt in a large bowl. Cut in margarine with two knives or a pastry blender until coarse crumbs form. Combine egg white, egg, milk, and orange peel. Stir wet mixture plus raisins into flour mixture to form a soft dough.

Turn dough onto a lightly floured board and knead until smooth. Divide dough into 4 pieces. Pat or roll each into a circle $\frac{1}{2}$ inch/1 cm thick. Place circles on an ungreased baking sheet. Score each circle into quarters. Brush tops with milk.

Combine topping ingredients and sprinkle evenly over each scone. Bake at 400°F/200°C for about 10–12 minutes or until lightly browned.

Note: For a variation, replace orange peel and raisins with 2 tbsp./25 mL freshly grated Parmesan cheese and 1 tsp./5 mL dried oregano; omit oat bran cinnamon topping. Or, replace orange peel with lemon peel and replace raisins with chopped apricots.

Apple Syrup

Makes 2 cups/500 mL. Serves 8–10 as a topping for pancakes.

This syrup is sensational served warm on the Spiced Oat Pancakes (see page 199). Also great as a topping for cottage cheese or frozen yogurt.

2	cups unsweetened apple juice	500 mL
$\frac{1}{4}$	cup brown sugar	50 mL
2	tbsp. cornstarch	25 mL
$\frac{1}{4}$	tsp. salt	1 mL
$\frac{1}{4}$	tsp. nutmeg	1 mL

Juice of $\frac{1}{2}$ lime

Combine apple juice, brown sugar, cornstarch, salt, and nutmeg in a saucepan. Bring to a boil, reduce heat, and cook, stirring occasionally, 3–5 minutes or until thickened. Stir in lime juice.

Pita Pizza

Serves 1.

Most children never refuse pizza, so why not serve this protein-packed, simple-to-make creation at breakfast time? Have pita bread and pizza sauce on hand in the fridge or freezer, and all you have to do—or better still, your children—is grate the cheese and pop it into the oven.

3	tbsp. Pizza Tomato Sauce (see page 111)	45 mL
1	whole-wheat pita bread	
$\frac{1}{2}$	cup grated low-fat cheese	125 mL

Optional toppings (sliced mushrooms, chopped green pepper, zucchini slices, etc.)

Spread the pizza sauce over the pita. Sprinkle evenly with low-fat cheese and top with toppings if you wish. Place on a baking sheet. Bake at 450°F/230°C for about 15 minutes or until the crust is brown on the bottom and the cheese is golden brown and bubbly.

9   Fitness: Fact or Frenzy?

Eating well is the crucial first step in feeling and looking good. But this goal would be impossible without one important factor—regular physical activity.

In the days when women worked their hands to the bone cooking, cleaning, and scrubbing laundry, when men did heavy chores around the house, and when both often worked together ploughing the fields, strenuous exercise was an integral part of everyday life. Not only that, the automobile had not yet come along to relieve people of what was then a normal activity, namely, walking.

Today's lifestyle, especially for urban folk, allows little time or opportunity for good, healthy exercise. We must consciously seek it out, either by increasing our everyday activity levels or by participating in structured exercise.

Exercise Perks
The health benefits of physical exercise are many, but the most important are the prevention and, to a lesser extent, the treatment of disease.

The primary goal of exercise is to increase endurance, strength, or both. Endurance or aerobic exercise is important because it conditions the heart and lungs, thereby enhancing the capacity of the body's cardiovascular system. The use of the body's large muscles during aerobic exercise requires oxygen. This stimulates circulation, which in turn causes the heart to work harder. In order for the body to use oxygen more efficiently, aerobic activity must last for 20 to 30 minutes at a time, three to four times a week.

Activities like walking, skipping, jogging, swimming, and cycling are all considered aerobic activities, as are active sports. Sports in which there is a lot of starting and stopping, however, are not considered as effective aerobically as those in which the activity is continuous.

In order for the cardiovascular system to benefit from aerobic exercise, the heart must be working at 70 to 85 percent of its maximum rate. An easy way to determine your maximum heart rate is to subtract your age from 220. Multiplying this number by 0.7 gives you your 70 percent level. Multiplying it by 0.85 determines the *maximum* your heart rate should reach during exercise. For example, if you are 35 years old, your maximum heart rate should be 185 beats per minute (220 − 35). Your lowest heart rate during exercise should be 130 (185 × 0.7) beats per minute for aerobic benefit; your highest, 157 beats per minute (185 × 0.85). You should *never* do any exercise that increases your heart rate above 85 percent of your maximum.

There are two kinds of aerobic activity. High-intensity aerobics raise the heart rate above 70 percent of a person's maximum. Low-intensity aerobics raise a person's heart rate, but to only 60 to 70 percent of maximum. The difference lies in a person's fitness level—a high-intensity activity for a person who is not physically fit may be a low-intensity activity for someone who is.

One of the most persuasive reasons to get physically fit is that exercise, in particular the aerobic variety, has been shown to increase HDL cholesterol—the cholesterol that helps lower the risk of heart disease. Exercise is also being used in the treatment of cardiac patients to develop new circulation in areas of the body that are affected by blocked arteries, such as the heart. Exercise can help promote the development of small blood vessels, which act as alternative pathways to blocked arteries.

Exercise is beneficial for diabetics because it allows the use of blood glucose to fuel the muscles without requiring insulin. Therefore, diabetics who exercise regularly require less insulin, either from their own bodies or from injections.

It is thought that regular, weight-bearing exercise helps retain calcium in the bones. This prevents the bones from becoming thin, a process that happens in osteoporosis. Exercise is also an asset in keeping the body's joints in good shape. Good muscular control means less wear and tear on various joints. Having weak upper arm muscles, for example, could put more stress on your shoulder joints. Developing strong quadriceps in your upper leg means that you place less physical stress on your knees. But as with everything, moderation is the key. Overdoing it can make your joints tired and sore.

Regular bowel movements are another bonus of regular exercise.

Flying High
There is one benefit of exercise for which there isn't conclusive scientific proof but to which any fitness enthusiast will likely swear. This is the physical and emotional

"high," or feeling of extreme well-being, that occurs after exercising.

This does not usually occur the first time a person exercises, but rather once he or she makes it a regular activity. Some researchers believe that *endorphins*, substances produced by the body to counteract pain, could be responsible for this exercise "high." Because it is thought that the body can become addicted to a certain level of endorphins, this theory could explain the often addictive aspect of working out. It might also explain the depression that runners feel when they stop running and why a person who has stopped regular exercise for a period of time has trouble taking it up again.

If all this is true, then in order to remain motivated by the elation of exercising, and not let your body's endorphin level slide too far, it is best to exercise at least three to four times a week. Should you be forced to stop exercising for an extended period of time, return to it with more frequent workouts or swimming sessions to build up those endorphins and their accompanying good feeling.

Fight or Flight

Another major benefit of exercise is its positive effect on stress. Our bodies react in the same manner to both emotional and physical types of stress. When faced with stress, we react with a "fight or flight" readiness for action, much as animals behave when they are faced with physical danger. This situation causes our bodies to release adrenalin, which helps prepare us for action—to fight or flee. The muscles also tense up, and the blood sugar level climbs to fuel them.

Such a survival mechanism has its place in the animal kingdom, but we humans make poor use of it; we might sometimes futilely slam a door with surprising force or lift a heavy object to throw it across the room! Most often, however, we react to stress by doing little more than stewing in our own hormones; we're tense and ready for action but only able to sit and worry or pace the room. The result is often a sore neck, a headache, or both.

Enter exercise. Physical activity is a fruitful way to use our readiness for action caused by stress. And anyone who has gone to a workout class mad at the boss and come out with a much calmer perspective will testify to this! The reason is that moving our bodies with some effort gets rid of adrenalin and reduces those feelings of tension and anxiety. Naturally, this doesn't solve the core problem, but it does help us deal with the situation with a clearer head. Using long walks, jogging, or swimming as a way of combatting stress is a good habit to get into.

In the same vein, exercise can act as a physical pick-me-up. If you've had a tiring day at work and are thinking of lying down, try doing some exercises instead. A short series of stretches and some aerobics will raise your energy level and might give you the green light to go out and boogie!

Walk on the Wild Side

Walking is one of the best ways to exercise. Brisk walking and speed walking (using your arms to propel yourself) can elevate your heart rate and really benefit cardiovascular fitness training. It is also tops for burning fat. In addition, walking is not as jarring on the joints as jogging or running and does wonders for toning the muscles in the upper legs and buttocks.

As with any type of exercise, speed walking should be preceded by some stretching to help prevent muscle injury and conclude with a cooldown, which could consist of a slower pace at the end of the walk as well as a few stretches. While walking, move your arms or carry weights in your hands to help raise your heart rate.

Start your walking routine with a pace that's comfortable and slowly build up speed until you're moving at a good clip.

High Octane Fuel

When and what should you eat in relation to exercise?

Do not exercise right after eating. During a taxing degree of physical exertion, the body requires oxygen to be supplied to the muscles by the bloodstream. After eating, blood gathers in the abdominal region to aid in the digestive process. Exercising soon after eating causes excessive demand on the blood supply, which physical exertion draws to the muscles. The result can be muscle cramps, a stitch in one's side, and even digestive upset.

Avoid eating foods such as fat before exercising. They take longer to digest than other foods and cause blood to pool in the abdomen for a longer time. Avoid eating simple sugars alone as a pre-exercise snack. Unlike fats, they may digest quickly and thus not compete in the body for blood, but they can cause a surge of insulin to be re-

ESTIMATED ENERGY COST OF VARIOUS ACTIVITIES

Activity	Calories Used per Hour
Watching TV	75
Sleeping	75
Playing softball	130
Doing desk work	180
Cleaning windows	200
Gardening (raking)	200
Ironing	250
Skating	250
Playing tennis (beginner)	250
Playing table tennis	300
Playing golf (and carrying clubs)	400
Chopping wood	450
Gardening (digging)	550
Walking (4.5 mph or 7.5 km/h)	450
Jogging or walking (5 mph or 8.3 km/h)	540
Swimming (2 mph or 3.3 km/h)	550
Aerobics classes (vigorous)	550
Cycling (13 mph or 21.5 km/h)	650
Cross-country skiing	750
Rowing (vigorous)	850
Running (8 mph or 13.3 km/h)	950

Note: The above is based on the energy expended by a 150-lb/72-Kg person. People who weigh less will expend slightly less, while those who weigh more will expend more.

leased. This results in a blood sugar level that is even lower than before you ate that chocolate bar or orange, and there goes your energy! High-fibre foods are another pre-exercise no-no, because they slow down digestion, leaving less oxygen available for the muscles. They could also cause stomach upset.

Eating a snack of complex carbohydrates, however, is highly recommended. Starchy foods like whole-grain bread or pasta, eaten at least two hours before exercising, do not cause a surge of insulin. They can also be combined with a small amount of protein food for more sustained energy, as in a snack of low-fat cheese and crackers.

Thirst Quenching
Fluid replacement is important after and sometimes during athletic activity. The amount of fluid to be replaced depends on a couple of things, namely, how strenuous the activity is and the temperature of the environment. On a hot day, your body loses more fluid, and you need to drink more after or during exercise. Don't wait until you get thirsty to have some kind of drink afterward. Your body does not immediately recognize that it needs fluid, and if fluids are not replaced, dehydration can occur.

It is best not to drink just before indulging in exercise; liquid in the stomach causes blood to pool there just as food does. And sugar solutions like juice cause this to occur to a greater extent than water. However, during an extended period of activity, fluids must be replaced, but in small amounts. A maximum of eight ounces of fluid should be consumed at one time. After exercising, if you have perspired a lot, drink a couple of glasses more than your thirst demands.

Cold water is the best liquid to consume during exercise because it competes less for a share of the blood supply. Sugar solutions like juice and sports drinks should be diluted with water. Sports drinks, already somewhat diluted, are best mixed with an equal amount of water; juices should be diluted much more.

After that workout, think twice about knocking back a cool one. Alcohol is not the ideal fluid replacement because it causes fluid loss through urination. If you cannot forgo a few beers after exercising, drink a couple of glasses of water first. Beware also of drinks high in sugar; if you're trying to lose weight, a few glasses of juice could even out that "energy in–energy out" equation!

Some people worry about sodium loss during exercise. If you perspire heavily during an exercise session, some salt may need to be replaced. But moderate perspiration does not cause loss of any sodium that the body needs, because most of us already consume more salt than we need. Taking salt tablets is not a good idea for the same reason. An extra shake of the salt shaker at the next meal is adequate. People who think they need some salt replacement because they perspire excessively should consult a doctor about their salt intake.

From Famished to Fit

There are many reasons to exercise to control weight.

Studies have shown that people who diet and exercise lose more fat than those who merely diet. This is an ideal regimen—after all, the goal of dieting is to lose fat. Exercise also helps prevent loss of lean body mass during dieting. And because fat is bulkier than muscle, people who lose more fat look leaner than those who lose lean body mass as well as fat. People who exercise while dieting may even gain a little weight at first because muscle weighs more than fat. But they will likely lose inches— and who can argue with that?

Exercise also helps dieters because of its effect on their bodies' metabolic rate. The *basal metabolic rate*, or BMR, describes the energy required to sustain processes in the body and maintain body temperature. When an individual starts dieting, the body initially allows weight loss to occur. However, it soon begins to perceive this weight loss as some kind of starvation and switches on the survival mechanism by slowing down the metabolic rate. Suddenly the reducing diet becomes the maintenance intake for the body. The dieter is then faced with a choice: either reduce food consumption or increase activity in the form of exercise.

The choice seems an easy one. Who wants to keep lowering their intake of food? Not only that, people who drastically lower their caloric intake are likely to miss out on certain nutrients. In addition, lean body mass, or muscle, requires more energy than fatty tissue. This means that leaner people require more calories to maintain their weight than fatter people who weigh the same. This helps explain why men, who have more lean body mass than women, lose weight more quickly.

Studies have shown that active, slim people eat more

than sedentary, overweight people. The reason for this is partly that exercise burns calories. However, it is also thought that the metabolic rate increases for a number of hours after exercising, but only if the exercise is done on a regular basis. Research has shown that when overweight, sedentary people have their metabolic rate tested before and after an exercise session, no change in the rate occurs. But following two weeks of regular aerobic exercise, the metabolic rate will be higher after a workout for a period of 24 to 36 hours. In other words, even at rest, regular exercisers burn more calories than those who exercise sporadically.

When you first start exercising and your metabolism is slow, everything is an effort, and as a result the activity may not be very enjoyable. You end up feeling more tired when you've finished exercising than you did before you began. But when you're into a regular program and your metabolism speeds up, it's no longer a task to do the activity. It's like trying to climb a hill with a car that's stalling versus driving a car that's well-tuned. There's also quite a difference in the enjoyment level. Trying to exercise when every move is a chore is tedious. When you've finished exercising and your metabolism is higher, however, you feel energized and ready to start again the next day.

Another factor to consider in the battle of the bulge is the type of exercise. A recent study at the University of California found that swimming is not the best choice as an exercise to promote fat loss. Participants were categorized according to the type of exercise they did. Those who cycled or walked averaged a 10–12 percent weight loss while the swimmers lost no body fat. Why did the swimmers not lose any fat? The theory is that because of the cold temperature of water, the body may want to keep body fat as insulation; when exercise is done on the ground, however, the body usually wants to cool itself down and shed some of its insulation. Long-distance swimmers typically have a higher percentage of body fat than do marathon runners. This is an area that needs further research, but keep it in mind when deciding on the kind of exercise you wish to do. Swimming is an excellent exercise for cardiovascular fitness, but for those who want to lose weight, varying activities may be the best idea.

There is now a new area of research that is comparing exercise intensity and the burning of fat. It used to be thought that aerobic activities, which create a demand for oxygen by the large muscles, burned body fat. It now appears, however, that high-intensity aerobics—those that elevate the heart rate above 70 percent of a person's maximum—might not promote the burning of fat. Carbohydrate, which is stored in the liver and muscle as glycogen, is needed for fuel during high-intensity exercise. Thus a diet rich in complex carbohydrates helps fuel the body for high-intensity aerobics.

However, low-intensity aerobics—those that keep the heart rate below 70 percent of maximum—cause fat to be used as fuel. It takes about 12 minutes of low-intensity exercise before fat begins to be broken down. Therefore, in order to burn fat, a workout should be long enough to have some effect, that is, 25 to 30 minutes. Because this type of exercise does not promote cardiovascular fitness, the best idea is to combine both low- and high-intensity programs throughout the week. One goal could be to lose body fat first when you are dieting and then to concentrate on cardiovascular fitness once your body is better able to withstand the stress.

Some research shows that body weight has a *set point*. This is the weight at which the body seems to want to stay and to which some people find their body wants to return after losing weight. Exercise seems to change the set point. By exercising regularly, it appears that the body adjusts to a new, lower weight.

Another bonus of exercise is that diminished appetite usually follows. So if you are trying to reduce your food intake, go for a walk on the way home for dinner. Be warned, however, that if you are not eating properly, no amount of exercise will control your appetite. In fact, if your timing of meals is off, exercise can exaggerate the bad effects.

Where the Action Is
Here are a few tips on how to work more exercise into your life:

- Before starting on any exercise program, check whether it is the best one for you. If you have a bad back, for example, consult a doctor before joining up for aerobics classes or weight-lifting. Before joining any type of fitness club, check the instructors' qualifications, size of classes, and so on.

- Take stairs instead of an elevator whenever possible.

- If you drive to work, park your car a few blocks from where you normally park and walk the rest of the way.

- Walk small children to school instead of driving them, if the distance isn't too great. This increases activity levels for all of you.

- If your lunch hour permits, go for a 15-minute walk *before* eating lunch.

- Go on a family hike or bicycle ride on weekends instead of watching TV or going to a movie.

- If you own a bike, equip it with a carrier and use it to do shopping and other errands instead of driving.

- If you are a music lover, listen to your favourite music on your headphones while taking a brisk walk instead of lounging around.

Don't Overdo It

As with all good things, too much exercise can have negative results. For example, women who overdo it might experience a hormonal change that leads to irregular periods. This change can also affect their calcium status, as it does at menopause. Women athletes such as marathon runners should therefore be concerned about their predisposition to thinning of the bones.

Athletes should also pay attention to their consumption of iron. Iron is an essential compound of hemoglobin in the blood. Because hemoglobin is necessary for transporting oxygen, an iron deficiency can seriously impair athletic performance. Research has shown that certain types of exercise can affect an athlete's iron status. It has been found that red blood cells, which contain hemoglobin, break down when the body pounds against hard surfaces during strenuous exercise. Proper shoes, good running surfaces, and moderate distance can help protect against this breakdown. Athletes, especially those who are cutting down on their consumption of red meat, should be wary and choose a diet rich in iron.

10   Freestyle

One person's meat is indeed another's poison, and our society's eating styles reflect this timely variation on an old adage.

Today a growing number of people are choosing to live alone and must adapt their eating styles accordingly. Many others have decided to eschew meat, but finding a nourishing meatless diet, particularly one containing adequate protein, needs special care. And for the burgeoning number of elderly people, this is a time of life when eating right is a primary concern. Here are some pointers for people in these three groups.

Flying Solo

Almost one in ten people in our society lives alone. Most of these people are under 34 or over 65 years old. And the single person who stands alone by the kitchen counter eating spaghetti straight from the can at mealtime is, unfortunately, all too common.

The main nutritional concern for such people is the lack of variety in their diets. A balanced diet contains more than 50 nutrients, which have to come from a diversity of foods. The keys to achieving this balance are planning meals and carefully shopping for food. In an effort to avoid waste, many singles wind up with little or nothing in the fridge. There are, however, ways to minimize waste and still have food in the house even if you are shopping and cooking for one.

When you shop for food, it is particularly important to choose items that give good nutritional value for your dollar. One way to do this is to shop with a detailed list. Checking "best before" dates is crucial—single people have no other family members to finish the carton of yogurt that, according to the label, has only two days to go. And buying a large package of perishable food on special may not be so economical for the person who lives alone.

Storing foods carefully is another way to retain nutrients and avoid waste. A couple of good ideas are to label frozen foods and store them in see-through containers so you can tell at a glance what is in them.

Dairy products need not pose problems for singles.

Milk is cheaper bought in plastic bags and can be frozen this way. Freezing milk causes it to change in appearance because it separates somewhat, but this does not affect the taste. Skim-milk powder and small cans of low-fat evaporated milk are handy to have around. So is UHT (ultra-high temperature) milk, which can be stored at room temperature until opened, after which time it must be kept in the fridge. Cottage cheese is a versatile milk product to keep on hand for all meals and can be bought in small containers. When you buy other types of cheese, go for small packages and freeze the excess if you wish.

It's a good idea to keep canned fish, cold cooked chicken, and eggs on hand to supply the protein components of a quick meal. When you buy meat at the supermarket, ask the meat manager to sell you the portion of meat you need if no appropriate packages are available. If the item is on special in a larger amount than you need for a meal, separate it into portions at home, wrap them individually, label them with the date, and freeze them. You can also cook the whole batch and then freeze it in portions for ready-cooked, frozen meals.

Many singles, fed up with eating a couple of slices of bread and finally throwing out the rest, give up buying bread altogether. This is an instance where the freezer comes in handy. Just freeze a loaf of sliced bread and use it a slice or two at a time. Freezing muffins or buns is also a good idea. As for grains, you can cook and then freeze individual portions of slow-cooking types, such as brown rice, to warm up later.

Fruits and vegetables are often sadly lacking in a single person's household because of their short shelf life. Buying a few fresh fruits and vegetables at a time is the best solution. Frozen fruits and vegetables are convenient, especially when packaged in bags rather than boxes; they can then be taken directly from the freezer in the amounts needed. Leftover cooked vegetables can be marinated in a tasty dressing to be eaten the following day as a cold salad. It is advisable to buy juices in small containers because the vitamins in an opened container of juice last only four days.

Meatless Matters

In many countries, vegetarianism is a way of life. Sometimes the reason is religious; just as often it's simply that there is a shortage of animal meat. In North America, recent concern about eating meat, especially the red variety, along with meat's soaring prices, has led to an increased interest in vegetarianism.

There are several types of vegetarianism. Vegans are vegetarians who eat only foods of plant origin. Lacto-vegetarians eat dairy products in addition to plant foods. Lacto-ovo-vegetarians eat eggs, dairy products, and plant foods. Pesco-vegetarians exclude meat but eat fish and plants. A pollo-vegetarian is someone who does not eat red meat but eats poultry as well as plant foods.

Vegetarians, in particular those who do not eat fish or poultry, risk missing out on certain nutrients unless their diet is carefully designed. The most important of these nutrients is protein. As explained in Chapter 3, there must be a proper balance of amino acids in a meal in order for the body to use the protein those foods contain. If the protein in a particular food lacks any amino acid, then the food must be complemented with another protein that contains that amino acid. Any complete protein can accomplish this; so can an incomplete protein that contains the missing amino acid.

It is now thought that simply by eating a variety of complementary proteins throughout the entire day, a balanced diet with adequate protein can be achieved. That's assuming that the diet contains a variety of nutritious choices.

This can be a difficult task, especially for a vegetarian who eats out a lot. Vegetarian selections in many restaurants are still often limited to steamed vegetables or cheese-laden pastas and quiches.

In societies where vegetarianism is the norm, complementary proteins are built into the traditional diet. In many regions of India, legumes such as lentils cooked in yogurt are a dietary staple, and in parts of Italy so is a soup made of pasta and beans. But in North America, a vegetarian member of a family (frequently a teenager who has decided to renounce meat) often eats everything served at dinner—minus the meat. The person then faces the serious hazard of missing out on essential protein; this is a particularly bad situation for a growing teen with high nutrient requirements.

Lacto-ovo-vegetarians can balance their protein by varying the complete protein eaten at meals. They can eat an egg for breakfast, and slip yogurt into their salad dressing at dinner.

Vegans must pay more attention to their diet and their

protein intake. A simple rule to keep in mind is that similar foods lack the same amino acids. Legumes tend to lack
the amino acid methionine; grains are often low in lysine.
By combining incomplete proteins like beans and pasta,
you'll have a plateful of complete protein.

There are some other special dietary needs of which
the vegetarian should be aware.

Infants and children require increased protein in order
to grow, and this can pose problems if they are vegetarians. Soy products such as milk and tofu, as well as nut
butters, can help supply some of this extra protein. It is
also important that anyone who is still growing maintains
an adequate caloric intake; otherwise, the body begins to
break down protein for fuel, a process that could hamper
growth and the repair of tissues.

On the other hand, vegetarians, particularly teenage
vegetarians who do not eat balanced meals, are in danger of snacking on sweet, starchy foods between meals
and becoming overweight. They might then go on a diet,
which can lead to an even lower nutritional intake. The
moral for vegetarians who tend to gain weight is: be sure
to eat balanced meals that contain some complete protein and to ward off that snack attack with something
nutritious.

Vitamin B12 is another nutrient often lacking in the
vegetarian diet because it does not occur naturally in
plant foods. This vitamin is found in dairy products and
eggs, so it is the vegan who is mainly at risk here. Vegans should seek out foods fortified with vitamin B12,
such as fortified soy milk and nutritional yeasts, or take
a supplement. This is particularly important during pregnancy and breast-feeding to ensure the health of the
baby. After weaning, the vegan baby should be given a
B12 supplement. For more information on this vitamin,
see Chapter 1.

It can be tricky for vegetarians to meet their mineral
requirements, iron in particular. The iron consumed in a
vegetarian diet is non-heme iron, which the body does
not easily absorb. Iron absorption is further impeded by
high amounts of other components in the vegetarian diet,
such as phytates and oxalates. One way vegetarians can
facilitate the absorption of iron is to increase their consumption of vitamin C.

Calcium is another mineral that may be lacking in the
vegetarian diet, particularly that of vegans, who should
take special care to find good plant sources of calcium

(see Chapter 1). In addition, their absorption of calcium can be adversely affected if their diets are too high in insoluble fibre. This is of special concern to pregnant, breast-feeding, and post-menopausal women as well as adolescents, whose diets may also be low in vitamin D. They should drink fortified milk, which contains this nutrient. Although vitamin D can be manufactured if there is sufficient sunshine, it can easily be deficient in the diet of vegetarians who do not consume dairy products.

Fast Food Fixes

With the speedy pace of today's lifestyle, fast foods are becoming a bigger and bigger part of many people's diets. Often rightly frowned on as being nutritionally lacking, fast food in some shape or form is here to stay. The realistic approach, therefore, is to make some informed choices and get the most nutrition possible out of these foods. Making such choices will, one hopes, help influence the fast-food chains to improve the nutritional quality of their products.

The following tips could be helpful when deciding which fast food to feast on.

When you order a hamburger, go for the regular single patty rather than double or jumbo-sized burgers. A three-ounce beef patty is a perfectly adequate amount of protein at a meal, and this way of consuming it is high enough in fat that no one needs a double whammy! A hamburger, however, is still a better choice than a piece of fried fish or chicken. These items, because they may be fried in animal fat, are considerably higher in saturated fat.

French fries are best avoided altogether. The best choice of potato is the baked variety, with the skin intact for added fibre and without fat-laden toppings. Best toppings are steamed veggies and some grated or cottage cheese. Cheese sauce is likely to be high in fat. Avoid potato skins, which are usually deep-fried.

Don't fall for the rabbit-food-must-be-low-fat-fare myth. True, the unadorned vegetables are great, but look out for the large fat-laden dressing packets. Check out the chart for a few surprises. For example, munch on a taco salad from Taco Bell and the 61 grams of fat contained would almost devour an average woman's daily fat allowance in one fell swoop.

Watch out for regular milkshakes—they can add 300 to 400 calories to your meal. Instead drink the low-fat

NUTRIENT CONTENT OF FAST FOODS

Chain	Food	Fat (g)	Sodium (mg)	Calories
Burger King	Apple cinnamon Danish	13	305	390
	Apple pie	14	—	311
	Bacon double cheeseburger	30	932	498
	Big fish fillet sandwich	35	912	593
	Breakfast croissan'wich bagel (no meat)	15	611	305
	Broiler chicken sandwich	10	771	280
	Cheeseburger	14	679	303
	Chicken sandwich	33	1,074	596
	Chicken tenders	11	390	211
	Chunky chicken salad	4	443	142
	French fries, regular	20	238	372
	Garden salad	5	125	90
	Hamburger deluxe	19	421	335
	Onion rings	16	460	274
	Pie, apple	16	304	234
	Salad Dressing Packets			
	French	22	400	290
	1000 Island	26	403	290
	Ranch	37	316	350
	Light oil and vinegar	18	762	170
	Sausage	15	386	169
	Scrambled egg platter	26	684	429
	Shake, chocolate	10	283	376
	Shake, strawberry	10	283	373

Nutrient Content of Fast Foods (continued)

Chain	Food	Fat (g)	Sodium (mg)	Calories
	Shake, vanilla	10	263	328
	Whopper	38	799	643
Domino's	12″ Pizza, 2 slices	5	660	340
	16″ Pepperoni pizza, 2 slices	15	1,080	440
Harvey's	Apple turnover	7	150	179
	Breakfast Sausage	14	323	167
	Cheeseburger	18	950	415
	Chicken fingers (5)	12	900	240
	Chicken sandwich	16	809	419
	Double burger	26	1,036	530
	French Fries	16	9	385
	Hash browns	9	29	146
	Hamburger	19	693	379
	Hot dog	14	867	332
	Ice burger	18	74	305
	Juice, apple	2	—	80
	Juice, orange	1	—	77
	Milkshake, chocolate	11	226	321
	Milkshake, strawberry	10	197	303
	Milkshake, vanilla	10	198	305

Chain	Food	Fat (g)	Sodium (mg)	Calories
	Muffin, blueberry	6	218	254
	Muffin, bran	13	279	301
	Onion rings	14	557	288
	Pancake (1)	1	302	89
	Pancake syrup	—	1	168
	Salad	—	26	33
	Super burger	19	961	477
	Toast, plain	3	—	250
	Western sandwich	10	588	347
Kentucky Fried Chicken	Barbeque Sauce	1	450	35
	Biscuit	12	530	220
	Centre breast extra tasty crispy	19	740	330
	Centre breast hot & spicy	22	750	360
	Centre breast original recipe	14	92	260
	Chicken, fried drumstick, extra tasty crispy	14	292	205
	Chicken Little's sandwich	10	331	169
	Colonel's chicken sandwich	27	1,060	482
	Corn on the cob	3	21	176
	Crispy fries	17	761	294
	Drumstick, extra tasty crispy	12	310	190

Chain	Food	Fat (g)	Sodium (mg)	Calories
	Drumstick, hot & spicy	12	320	180
	Hot wings pieces	33	1,230	471
	Side breast, extra tasty crispy	27	710	400
	Side breast, hot & spicy	28	850	400
	Thigh, extra tasty crispy	29	520	380
	Thigh, hot & spicy	27	670	370
	Whole wing, extra tasty crispy	17	320	240
	Whole wing, hot & spicy	16	440	220
	Kentucky Nuggets (6)	18	865	284
	Coleslaw	6	177	114
	Mashed potatoes with gravy	1	370	70
McDonald's	Bacon 'n' egg McMuffin	16	879	328
	Big Mac	30	992	536
	Cheeseburger	14	595	305
	Chicken McNuggets (6)	20	487	312
	McNugget sauce			
	Barbeque	1	298	55
	Honey	Less than 1	1	74
	Hot mustard	4	254	65
	Sweet and sour	1	145	62
	Cinnamon Roll	25	350	450
	Cookies, Chocolaty Chip	15	260	289
	Cookies, McDonaldland	10	318	263
	Danish, apple	22	468	467

Chain	Food	Fat (g)	Sodium (mg)	Calories
	Danish, raspberry	22	470	475
	Egg McMuffin	14	806	306
	English muffin with butter	5	290	175
	Filet-o-fish sandwich	14	680	341
	French fries, small	12	133	247
	Hamburger	10	418	253
	Hash brown potatoes	7	146	131
	Hot cakes	8	720	359
	Low-fat apple bran muffin	2	540	255
	Low-fat milkshake, chocolate	1	263	315
	Low-fat milkshake, strawberry	1	185	309
	Low-fat milkshake, vanilla	1	172	333
	McChicken	23	836	465
	McLean deluxe	10	764	323
	McLean deluxe with cheese	15	983	380
	Pie, apple	14	228	280
	Pie, cherry	14	162	280
	Pizza, cheese personal	16	1,070	480
	Pizza, cheese 12", per slice	6	425	185
	Pizza, pepperoni personal	21	1,270	530
	Pizza, pepperoni 12", per slice	8	540	205
	Pizza, deluxe personal	22	1,340	550
	Pizza, deluxe 12", per slice	9	570	210

Chain	Food	Fat (g)	Sodium (mg)	Calories
	Quarter Pounder	22	666	421
	Quarter Pounder with cheese	31	1,179	530
	Salad, chef	2	279	55
	Salad Dressing			
	House	21	263	206
	French	14	484	152
	Vinaigrette	1	167	30
	1000 Island	18	294	187
	Salad, garden	1	39	31
	Sausage McMuffin	28	1,056	423
	Sausage McMuffin with egg	31	1,146	482
	Sausage, patty	20	488	216
	Scrambled eggs	11	181	159
	Sundae, hot caramel	2	156	262
	Sundae, hot fudge	4	203	257
	Sundae, strawberry	1	96	212
	Yogurt cone, low-fat	1	81	126
	Yogurt cone, vanilla	1	80	102
Pizza Hut (2 slices medium pizza)	Pan Pizza			
	Cheese	24	1,900	640
	Pepperoni	25	1,860	668
	Supreme	32	2,410	722
	Thin 'n' Crispy			
	Cheese	13	1,820	444
	Pepperoni	22	1,850	503
	Supreme	26	2,550	624

Chain	Food	Fat (g)	Sodium (mg)	Calories
Swiss Chalet	Baked potato	Trace	10	227
	Bar-B-Q sauce	9	106	41
	Cake, fudge nut	16	209	346
	Cake, black forest	14	218	278
	Chalet chicken soup	2	820	97
	Chalet cole slaw	1	574	56
	Chalet salad	20	760	240
	Chalet sauce	Less than 1	514	20
	Chicken Caesar	46	173	775
	Chicken salad	42	919	500
	Chicken salad amandine, warm	60	222	868
	Chicken sandwich	5	131	360
	Chicken sandwich (hot)	6	390	310
	Chicken sandwich gravy	1	202	35
	Chocolate eclair	10	113	205
	French fried potatoes	23	9	478
	Grilled chicken and rice	8	239	641
	Half back rib	72	237	200
	Half chicken	38	1,600	634
	Ice cream, vanilla	13	65	195
	Peas	Less than 1	Less than 1	44
	Pie, apple	22	292	394
	Pie, coconut	14	143	292

Chain	Food	Fat (g)	Sodium (mg)	Calories
	Quarter chicken, dark	19	800	326
	Quarter chicken, white	18	800	308
	Roll	1	n/a	116
	Syrup, butterscotch	Less than 1	81	107
	Syrup, chocolate	Less than 1	65	104
	Whip topping	3	6	40
Taco Bell	Beef Mexi-melt	15	689	306
	Burrito, bean	14	1,231	458
	Burrito, beef	21	1,394	508
	Burrito supreme	22	1,264	517
	Cheese fries	28	659	226
	Chili fries	23	556	174
	Enrichito	20	1,243	382
	Fries supreme	35	775	317
	Nachos	18	399	346
	Nachos Bell Grande	35	997	649
	Pintos 'n' cheese with red sauce	9	642	190
	Soft taco	12	554	265
	Soft Taco Supreme	16	554	312
	Steak Soft Taco	11	456	258
	Taco	11	276	183
	Taco salad	41	636	566

Nutrient Content of Fast Foods (continued)

Chain	Food	Fat (g)	Sodium (mg)	Calories
	Taco Salad, without shell	17	434	221
	Tostada with red sauce	11	596	258
Wendy's	Big Classic	33	1,085	570
	Chicken club sandwich	25	930	506
	Chili con carne	7	750	220
	Fish fillet sandwich	25	780	460
	French fries, small	12	145	240
	French toast, 2 slices	20	850	400
	Grilled chicken fillet sandwich	13	815	340
	Hamburger, single	21	890	420
	Jr. Hamburger	9	570	260
	Potato with broccoli and cheese	16	455	400
	Potato with chili and cheese	18	630	500
	Potato with sour cream and chives	23	135	500
	Potato with cheese	15	310	318
	Potato with bacon and cheese	18	1,460	520

— Values not available.

ones or low-fat milk, fruit juice, or a sugar-free drink.

Pizza can be one of the most nutritious forms of fast food. Keep the amount of fats to a minimum by avoiding meat toppings like pepperoni, sausage, and bacon. Picking them off a cooked pizza is not the answer, because the fat will have already seeped into it. Avoid high-sodium items like anchovies and olives, and load up with lots of veggies like green peppers, onions, mushrooms, and extra tomato. Some pizza places use low-fat mozzarella—an excellent idea.

Chinese fast food can be high in nutrients if you avoid fatty items like egg rolls and deep-fried, battered foods. Stir-fries are usually a better choice, especially if the chef goes easy on the oil. Steamed rice is more healthful than fried, which is usually high in sodium and fat. Ask to have the MSG omitted from your food to lower the sodium, and try seasoning food with rice vinegar instead of a salty soy sauce.

Fried chicken is a fast way to load up on unwanted fat and sodium—one piece can rack up more than 300 calories! If you do feel compelled to eat it, avoid small pieces coated in extra crispy, fat-laden batter, and choose those with a large amount of chicken compared to breading. If you have the choice, go for barbecued or rotisserie chicken and peel off the skin. But avoid the sauces that accompany all of these kinds of chicken.

Fast-food breakfasts—usually fried eggs with bacon and buttered toast—are not a good way to start the day. Instead grab a bran muffin and a piece of low-fat cheese, both of which are probably faster and more healthful to boot!

Last but not least, remember one thing. Fast-food chains are in the business of giving people what they want. If we insist on salads, baked potatoes, and meat that isn't loaded with fat but insist that they also be fast, the chains will respond by selling food that meets these requirements. It can be fast and still be good food!

Stir-Fry Heaven

The homemade stir-fry is probably the easiest, most versatile, and most healthful of fast-food meals. It is ideal for a solo lunch or dinner, takes only minutes to make, and can incorporate whatever your fridge might hold. Use our stir-fry chart along with the following pointers and recipes for sauce to come up with your favourite creation. Serve over rice or noodles.

- Cut all the ingredients into uniform sizes ahead of time and keep them close at hand. Speed is of the essence when stir-frying. Arrange them on plates in categories as shown in the chart.

- Use a wok for best results, but a large, heavy skillet will do.

- Heat the wok over medium-high heat until very hot, almost smoking. Then add 1 tsp./5 mL vegetable oil. Swirl it around the wok and heat 1 minute longer. If you wish, substitute chicken stock for oil for lower fat content.

- Add the protein ingredient from Column A. Stir-fry, tossing quickly with a slotted spoon, wok flipper, or chopsticks, for 1–5 minutes or until browned on all sides. (Shake the wok gently if you are frying tofu so it does not break.) Remove with a slotted spoon.

- Drizzle 1 tsp./5 mL oil or chicken stock into the wok and heat for 1 minute. Add the vegetables from Column B. Stir-fry for about 3 minutes or until they are tender-crisp. (It is a good idea to first blanch hard vegetables like broccoli, cauliflower, and carrots by plunging them into boiling water before adding them to the stir-fry.)

- Return the protein ingredient to the wok along with tender vegetables from Column C.

- Push the stir-fry to the sides of the wok. Add a sauce (see recipes on page 229). Cook until the sauce thickens.

- Add toppings from Column D. Toss. Serve at once.

- For a more aromatic stir-fry, add $\frac{1}{2}$ tsp./2 mL minced fresh ginger root, 1 minced garlic clove, or both to the wok before adding the protein ingredient from Column A.

A	B	C	D
Your Pick of Protein (About 3 oz./90 g)	**Veggies with Verve** (About $\frac{1}{2}$ cup/ 125 mL)	**Tender Veggies** (About $\frac{1}{4}$ cup/ 50 mL)	**Topping It Off** (About 1 tsp./ 5 mL)
Chicken, cubed or slivered	Asparagus, sliced diagonally	Bean sprouts	Toasted peanuts
Turkey, cubed or slivered	Bamboo shoots, cut into julienne strips	Bok choy leaves	Toasted sesame seeds
Lean meat, cubed or slivered	Bok choy stems, sliced diagonally	Chinese cabbage, shredded	Toasted cashews
Firm-fleshed fish, cubed	Broccoli flowerets; broccoli stems, cut diagonally	Green onion, cut into matchsticks	Toasted pine nuts
Shrimp, peeled and deveined	Carrots, cut into julienne strips	Lettuce, shredded	Toasted slivered almonds
Scallops	Celery, sliced diagonally	Spinach, shredded	Green onion, chopped
Tofu, pressed and cubed	Cauliflower flowerets		Fresh coriander (also called Chinese parsley or cilantro), chopped
	Green beans, topped and tailed		
	Green or red peppers, cubed or cut into julienne strips		
	Onion, sliced		
	Snow peas, topped and tailed		
	Turnip, cubed or cut into julienne strips		
	Water chestnuts, sliced		
	Yellow squash, cubed or cut into julienne strips		
	Zucchini, cubed or cut into julienne strips		

Note: Quantities are for one serving.

Stir-Fry Sauces

Basic Stir-Fry Sauce	¼	cup chicken or vegetable stock	50 mL
	1	tsp. low-sodium soy sauce	5 mL
	1	tsp. dry sherry	5 mL
	1	tsp. cornstarch	5 mL

Combine all the ingredients in a small bowl. Add to the stir-fry at the end of the cooking time as described in the stir-fry pointers (see page 226–27).

Szechuan Spicy Sauce Substitute chili oil for regular oil for a spicy flavour when stir-frying the ingredients. A spicy sauce can also be made by adding a pinch of minced dried chili pepper to the basic sauce.

Oyster Sauce Substitute prepared oyster sauce, available at Chinese groceries, for soy sauce in the basic sauce recipe.

Five-Spice Sauce Add a pinch of Five Spice powder, available at Chinese groceries, to the basic sauce.

Sweet and Sour Sauce Substitute pineapple juice for chicken stock in the basic sauce.

Chicken for One

Keep boneless chicken breasts, wrapped individually, in the freezer for a fast and tempting dinner. Add some rice or pasta and a salad to complete your meal.

1	tsp. vegetable oil	5 mL
1	single chicken breast, skinned and boned	

Heat oil in a small skillet on medium-high heat. Add chicken breast and cook for 2–3 minutes on each side or until golden brown. Proceed with one of the following variations.

Calories 233
Protein 28 g
Fat 11 g
Carbohydrate 5 g

Variation #1

1	tsp. vegetable oil	5 mL
$\frac{1}{4}$	green pepper, sliced	
1	small onion, sliced	

Salt and freshly ground pepper to taste

Remove chicken from skillet and keep warm. Heat 1 tsp./ 5 mL oil in skillet. Add vegetables and sauté for about 4 minutes or until soft. Season to taste, and pour vegetables and juices over the chicken.

Variation #2

Calories	228	
Protein	28 g	
Fat	11 g	
Carbohydrate	4 g	

1   tsp. vegetable oil   5 mL
2   tbsp. orange juice   25 mL
$\frac{1}{4}$ red pepper, sliced
Salt and freshly ground pepper to taste

Remove chicken from skillet and keep warm. Heat 1 tsp./ 5 mL oil in skillet. Add red pepper and orange juice. Cook for 2 minutes. Return chicken to skillet and cook, covered, for 1 minute. Turn chicken breast, cover skillet, and cook for an additional minute.

Variation #3

Calories	171	
Protein	27 g	
Fat	6 g	
Carbohydrate	*1 g	

*Less than

1   tsp. lime juice   5 mL
1   tbsp. fresh coriander, coarsely chopped   15 mL
1   tsp. lime zest, grated (optional)   5 mL
Salt and freshly ground pepper to taste

Leave chicken in skillet. Add lime juice and cook for 30 seconds. Remove from heat and add chopped coriander and lime zest.

Calories 329
Protein 23 g
Fat 12 g
Carbohydrate 20 g

Basic Meal-in-a-Pouch

Serves 1.

Baking fish, chicken, or vegetables in a pouch with your favourite seasoning and a little white wine or stock is a great way to prepare a nutritious meal that takes only minutes. It's perfect for single people who like to dine well on their own.

Foil or parchment paper
Vegetable oil for brushing

1	4-oz./125-g fish fillet or boneless, skinned chicken breast	
2	tbsp. finely chopped onion, leek, celery, fresh ginger root, or a combination of all four	25 mL
1	tsp. finely chopped fresh herbs (parsley, dill, tarragon, thyme, or basil)	5 mL
1–2	tbsp. dry white wine or fish or chicken stock	15–25 mL

Salt and freshly ground pepper to taste

Cut a square of foil or parchment paper large enough to hold the fish or meat. Brush it with oil and place the fish or meat, vegetables, and herbs on one half. Sprinkle with the wine or stock, salt, and pepper. Seal the package by crimping the edges.

Bake at 400°F/200°C for 10 minutes per 1 inch/2 cm of thickness for fish or for 20–25 minutes for chicken. To serve, place the pouch on your plate and open it at the table to release the aromas. Serve with steamed veggies, bread, rice, or potatoes.

Note: It is easy to cook your vegetables in the same pouch as the fish or chicken. Just enclose broccoli flowerets, carrot juliennes, snow peas, etc. along with a little extra wine or stock.

Low-Fat Fettuccine Alfredo

Calories 390
Protein 23 g
Fat 5 g
Carbohydrate 54 g

Serves 1.

This is as close as you can come to the silken-smooth original without using cream. A terrific way to pamper yourself when you're making dinner for one.

$\frac{1}{3}$	cup 2% cottage cheese	75 mL
2	tbsp. freshly grated Parmesan cheese	25 mL
Freshly ground pepper to taste		
3	oz. fettuccine noodles	75 mL

Blend the cottage cheese and Parmesan in a food processor or blender until smooth. Cook the mixture in a small saucepan over medium heat until heated through, stirring constantly. Do not boil, or the mixture will separate. Season with pepper.

Cook the fettuccine in plenty of boiling, salted water until al dente. Drain and toss with heated sauce.

Note: For a delicious vegetable variation on this theme, top the cooked fettuccine and Alfredo sauce with 1 cup/ 250 mL assorted veggies steamed until tender-crisp— julienned carrots, zucchini, snow peas, or broccoli flowerets.

Pronto Pasta for One

Serves 1 as a main course.

Instead of yet another frozen dinner, here's a fast and tasty dish that's perfect when you're on the run. The vegetables take almost the same time to cook as the pasta. Substitute ones that you have on hand. Broccoli, mushrooms, or snow peas work well in this recipe, but the variations are endless. If you don't have any fresh vegetables around, canned artichokes and mushrooms will do the trick.

1	tsp. virgin olive oil	5 mL
$\frac{1}{4}$	cup onions, finely chopped	50 mL
1	garlic clove, minced	
1	small carrot, diced	
$\frac{1}{4}$	cup green pepper, diced	50 mL
1	small zucchini, diced	
$\frac{1}{2}$	cup Italian plum tomatoes	125 mL
Salt and freshly ground pepper to taste		
2	oz. pasta	50 g
1	tbsp. fresh basil, finely chopped, for garnish (optional)	15 mL
2	tbsp. freshly grated Parmesan cheese	25 mL

Heat oil in a heavy saucepan. Add onions and sauté until soft. Add garlic and sauté 1 minute. Add diced vegetables and sauté for 3–5 minutes. Add plum tomatoes. Reduce heat and simmer for 8–10 minutes, uncovered. Season to taste.

Meanwhile, cook pasta in plenty of salted boiling water until al dente. Drain. Toss with vegetable mixture. Garnish with fresh basil if desired and serve with the Parmesan cheese.

Calories 446
Protein 21 g
Fat 12 g
Carbohydrate 71 g

Speedy Quesadillas

Serves 1.

Try the new dehydrated refried beans instead of the canned variety. That way you can make up just the right amount and avoid leftovers. Double, triple, or quadruple this recipe for a fast, tasty, and nutritious dinner.

$\frac{1}{2}$	cup refried beans	125 mL
3	tbsp. salsa	45 mL
2	flour tortillas	
3	tbsp. diced peppers, green or red	45 mL
2	tbsp. chopped green onion	25 mL
3	tbsp. grated low-fat cheese	45 mL
2	tbsp. chopped fresh coriander (cilantro) (optional)	25 mL

Extra salsa for serving

Preheat oven to 375°F/190°C. Mix together refried beans and salsa. Spread the mixture on one flour tortilla. Spread peppers and green onion over bean mixture. Sprinkle grated cheese over chopped vegetables and top with remaining tortilla. Spray top of tortilla with non-stick cooking spray. Transfer to a baking sheet sprayed with cooking spray and bake for 15 minutes or until golden brown. Sprinkle with coriander and serve with salsa.

Calories 208
Protein 14 g
Fat 5 g
Carbohydrate 33 g

Cheesy Baked Potato

Serves 1.

The stuffed baked potato is one of the most versatile and delicious ways to cook the noble spud. Served with a salad, this and the following two recipes are perfect for anyone needing an easy, nutritious meal. Be sure to eat the skin for extra fibre.

1	large baking potato	
1	tbsp. low-fat plain yogurt	15 mL
3	tbsp. 2% cottage cheese	45 mL
$\frac{1}{4}$	cup low-fat cheese, grated	50 mL
$\frac{1}{4}$	tsp. dried or 1 tsp. fresh basil, finely chopped	1 mL/5 mL
Salt and freshly ground pepper to taste		
1	small tomato, sliced	
1	tbsp. finely chopped green onion	15 mL

Scrub the potato and prick it with a fork. Bake at 375°F/190°C for about 1 hour or until tender. Slice in half horizontally and scoop out the pulp, leaving some attached to the skin for support.

Mash the pulp in a bowl with the yogurt, cottage cheese, and half the low-fat cheese. Mix in the basil, salt, and pepper. Divide this mixture between the potato halves. Place two slices of tomato on each half and sprinkle with the remaining low-fat cheese.

Bake on a baking sheet or in an ovenproof dish at 375°F/190°C for 20 minutes or until the cheese melts. Place under the broiler to brown if you wish. Sprinkle with green onion.

Baked Potatoes Mexicana

Calories 324
Protein 17 g
Fat 3 g
Carbohydrate 57 g

Serves 1 as main course.

South-of-the-border spuds. Add a sliced tomato salad to make a meal. Double, triple, or quadruple the recipe if you wish.

1	large baking potato	
1	tbsp. low-fat plain yogurt	15 mL
$\frac{1}{4}$	cup low-fat cheese, grated	50 mL
1	tbsp. green onion, thinly sliced	15 mL
$\frac{1}{2}$	tsp. jalapeno pepper, finely chopped	2 mL
1	tsp. fresh coriander, finely chopped	5 mL

Salt and freshly ground pepper to taste

Scrub the potato and prick it with a fork. Bake at 375°F/190°C for about 1 hour or until tender. Slice in half horizontally and scoop out the pulp, leaving some attached to the skin for support.

Mash the pulp in a bowl with the yogurt and cheese. Mix in the green onion, jalapeno pepper, coriander, salt, and pepper. Scoop the mixture into the potato shells. Bake on a baking sheet or in an ovenproof dish at 375°F/190°C for 20 minutes or until the cheese melts.

Mediterranean Baked Potato

Calories 345
Protein 12 g
Fat 10 g
Carbohydrate 55 g

Serves 1 as a main course.

A baked potato with a zing! Serve with a romaine or spinach salad.

1	large baking potato	
1	tbsp. low-fat plain yogurt	15 mL
3	tbsp. feta cheese	40 mL
1	tbsp. pimiento, chopped	15 mL
1	tsp. basil, finely chopped	5 mL

Salt and freshly ground pepper to taste

Scrub the potato and prick it with a fork. Bake at 375°F/190°C for about 1 hour or until tender. Slice in half horizontally and scoop out the pulp, leaving some attached to the skin for support.

Mash the pulp in a bowl with the yogurt and feta cheese. Mix in pimiento, basil, salt, and pepper. Scoop the mixture into the potato shells. Bake on a baking sheet or in an ovenproof dish at 375°F/190°C for 20 minutes or until the cheese melts.

Calories 30
Protein 1 g
Fat 3 g
Carbohydrate *1 g
(per tablespoon)

*Less than

Tofu Mayonnaise

Makes about 6 oz./175 g.

You'd never guess how little fat is in this untraditional but delightfully creamy mayo. And no eggs either.

5–6 oz. tofu (1 block), drained	150–175 g
2 tbsp. vegetable oil	25 mL
1 tbsp. virgin olive oil	15 mL
2 tbsp. cider vinegar	25 mL
1 tsp. Dijon mustard	5 mL
Salt and freshly ground pepper to taste	

Blend all ingredients in a food processor or blender until smooth. Refrigerate in an airtight container.

Calories 469
Protein 33 g
Fat 31 g
Carbohydrate 22 g
(entire recipe)

Oriental Spinach Dip

Makes about 2 cups/500 mL.

Your party guests will never know that this is a low-fat dip made with tofu. Ideal for dipping raw vegetable crudités or spreading on whole-grain toast rounds and crisp crackers. This recipe comes from Susan Joseph, who owns and operates her Slimcook cooking school in Bethesda, Maryland.

3	cups lightly packed fresh spinach, washed, dried, and with stems removed	750 mL
1	cup drained, mashed tofu	250 mL
$\frac{1}{2}$	English cucumber, peeled and seeded	
1	tbsp. sesame oil	15 mL
3	tbsp. lemon juice	45 mL
2	cloves garlic, minced	
$\frac{1}{2}$	cup low-fat plain yogurt	125 mL
$\frac{1}{4}$	cup finely chopped green onion	50 mL

Salt and freshly ground pepper to taste

Blend the first six ingredients in a food processor or blender until smooth, then transfer the mixture to a bowl. Stir in the yogurt and onions until blended. Season with salt and pepper.

Calories 215
Protein 18 g
Fat 11 g
Carbohydrate 16 g

Tofu Stir-Fry

Serves 4.

The tofu must be pressed (see below) before going into this tasty vegetarian stir-fry that is full of protein and other goodies.

2	cups drained tofu	500 mL
2	tsp. vegetable oil	10 mL
1	small onion, sliced	
1	clove garlic, minced	
1	cup sliced mushrooms	250 mL
1	medium zucchini, cut into thin julienne strips	
1	sweet red pepper, cut into thin julienne strips	
1	cup bamboo shoots, cut into thin julienne strips	250 mL
2	tsp. low-sodium soy sauce	10 mL
$\frac{1}{2}$	tsp. sesame oil	2 mL

Freshly ground pepper to taste

To press the tofu, cut the slabs into 2 or 3 slices. Place absorbent tea towels underneath and on top of the tofu slices. Place a cookie sheet or cutting board on top of the covered tofu. Place 2–4 1b./1–2 kg of weight on top (canned food works well) and leave for 20 minutes to 1 hour. Cut the tofu into small cubes.

Heat the oil in a wok until it is very hot. Sauté the onion, garlic, and mushrooms until the onions are soft. Add the zucchini, red pepper, and bamboo shoots and stir-fry for about 1 minute. Stir in the soy sauce and sesame oil. Then add the tofu, stirring gently or shaking the wok to mix the ingredients without breaking the tofu. Cook until the tofu is heated through. Add pepper to taste. Serve over rice or Chinese noodles.

Lemon Maple Tofu Cheesecake

Calories 336
Protein 16 g
Fat 18 g
Carbohydrate 33 g

Serves 12.

This is one of the most amazing facsimiles ever tasted. As good as regular cheesecake without the caloric side effects.

$1\frac{1}{2}$	cups walnut pieces	375 mL
$\frac{1}{2}$	cup rolled oats	125 mL
3	tbsp. soft margarine, melted	45 mL
3	tbsp. honey or maple syrup	45 mL
$1\frac{1}{2}$	lb. tofu, well drained	750 g
2	eggs	
Juice and grated rind of 1 lemon		
$\frac{1}{2}$	cup maple syrup	125 mL
1	tsp. grated fresh ginger root	5 mL
Pinch salt		

Icing

$\frac{1}{2}$	lb. tofu, drained	250 g
Rind of 1 lemon		
Juice of $\frac{1}{2}$ lemon		
2	tbsp. maple syrup	25 mL
1	cup blueberries, sliced strawberries, or raspberries	250 mL

Spread the walnut pieces on a cookie sheet in a single layer. Toast at 400°F/200°C for 5–7 minutes and cool. Reduce the oven temperature to 350°F/180°C.

Process the rolled oats in a food processor or blender using a few on-off turns. Add the toasted walnuts and process until just coarsely chopped. Transfer the mixture to a bowl and stir in the melted margarine and honey. Pat into an 8- or 9-inch/2- or 2.5-L springform pan. Bake at 350°F/180°C for 12 minutes. Cool.

Press the tofu (see page 227) for 30 minutes—no longer—and process in a food processor or blender until smooth. Add the eggs, lemon juice and rind, maple syrup, ginger root, and salt and process until smooth. Pour this mixture into the cooked crust and bake at 350°F/180°C for 50 minutes or until the cake has set. Let it cool in the pan.

Purée all the icing ingredients except the berries in a food processor or blender. Remove the rim of the springform pan and spread the icing on the cake. Arrange the berries on top of the icing.

11   Riding the Life Cycle

From babyhood to old age, the principles of good nutrition as outlined in this book have a common application.
But there are some special needs in the space of a lifetime that make some pretty particular demands on how
and what we eat.

The Mother-to-Be
The development of the fetus puts especially high nutrient
requirements on the mother because a baby's birth weight
and nutritional status depend on the mother's food intake
during pregnancy. Equally important, however, is her
state of health prior to becoming pregnant because in
many cases, the fetus has begun to develop before the
woman is even aware of her condition. (See folacin, page
8.) A pregnant woman's good health is particularly vital if
she suffers from nausea and vomiting, which can result in
a low nutrient intake during early pregnancy.

The nutritional demands of the teenage years require
that the pregnant teenager be particularly careful to meet
the growth requirements of both herself and her baby.

These days, a maternal weight gain of 25 to 30
pounds is thought to be optimum for the baby to be born
with a good birth weight and for a healthy placenta and
amniotic fluid to develop in the mother. It is not advisable
for the mother to restrict her weight gain because this can
result in insufficient nutrient intake and a small baby.

Some women who believe they are overweight think
that pregnancy is a time to watch their diet and perhaps
lose some body fat. However, the fetus needs a wealth
of nutrients to develop bones, muscles, and blood supply, and they must be supplied by the mother, so she
should not use pregnancy as a time to diet. One consola-
tion for the overweight pregnant woman is that her
weight gain may not be as high as that of a thin one.
How the mother-to-be gains weight is also important. A
good average pattern for weight gain is about five pounds
in the first 20 weeks of pregnancy and about one pound
a week until the birth.

If your eating habits before pregnancy were far from
ideal, then this is a good time to improve them. Not only
will it mean a healthier baby, but good parental eating

habits are also the best example for a growing child. After all, a mother who never eats fruit can hardly expect her child to buy that story about "an apple a day!"

Here are some substances that pregnant women should be wary of.

Caffeine
The effects of caffeine on the fetus are not completely known. What is known, however, is that it crosses the placenta to the fetus, so until more is known about its effects, moderation is recommended. An occasional caffeine-containing food is certainly all right. Regular doses of herbal teas may not be a good idea; their toxic effects have been documented, along with severe diarrhea and allergic reactions. More research is needed in this area.

Alcohol
Alcohol can cross the pregnant woman's placenta, and studies show that alcoholic mothers sometimes give birth to babies with deformities, mental retardation, or both. Women who consumed alcohol before they knew they were pregnant may be reassured by the fact that, although safe levels of alcohol consumption have not been determined, the occasional drink does not seem harmful to the fetus. But because there is no conclusive evidence of this, avoid alcohol if motherhood is in your immediate plans.

Smoking
Smoking during pregnancy can cause babies to be born with a lower birth weight; it also increases the risk of premature birth. Need I say more?

The Maternity Menu
The pregnant woman should eat the basic balanced diet recommended in this book—but with some extras.

Energy and caloric needs during pregnancy vary from one woman to another, but you should consume an average of 100 extra calories a day in the first three-month period and about 300 extra calories a day during the second and third. What these calories consist of is also important; they must contain the nutrient bonuses of iron, calcium, and folic acid.

Extra calcium is best consumed by boosting your intake of dairy products and other calcium-rich foods (see the chart on page 12).

The pregnant woman needs a lot of fluids because of increased blood volume and kidney function and will find herself thirstier than usual. Drinking more water and eating plenty of high-fibre cereals, vegetables, and fruits will help—they not only add fluid to the diet but also help prevent constipation, an unpleasant hazard of pregnancy.

North Americans are used to eating too many salty foods. And although the practice of restricting salt during pregnancy has lately been discontinued, the mother-to-be is advised to use salt in moderation for the same reasons that anyone else should (see the chart on pages 16–17).

Many pregnant women have cravings for foods that are low in nutrients but high in sugar or fat. Women who are regularly overcome by the overwhelming desire for a huge slice of banana cream pie or a bag of pretzels do, however, have some healthier options. The best way to deal with cravings (and giving in to them on occasion is not harmful) is to eat a number of mini-meals throughout the day. This will maintain your energy level and help reduce your cravings.

Eating mini-meals is also a good routine for pregnant women experiencing severe nausea. Small, frequent amounts of food—healthful snacks like a small bran muffin or some low-fat yogurt topped with blueberries and wheat germ—can prevent extreme hunger and seem to reduce that queasy feeling. Women who are nauseated first thing in the morning should keep some crackers beside the bed to eat on waking up and then wait a few minutes before getting out of bed. It is also advisable not to drink and eat at the same time if nausea is a problem.

Skipping breakfast is just as unhealthy for pregnant women as it is for other people and can lead to uncontrolled weight gain in some women.

The Mouths of Babes
Breast-feeding is, without a doubt, the best way to feed a newborn baby for nutritional, immunological, and psychological reasons.

Breast-feeding is beneficial nutritionally because a mother's milk is uniquely suited to her particular baby and has the wonderful quality of changing its composition to suit her baby's stages of development. For example, the milk of a mother whose baby has just been born has a different nutritional balance than the milk of a mother whose baby is four months old. Breast milk is the easiest food for a baby to digest and seems to protect the infant against iron deficiency. It also allows better absorption of fats than cow's milk does. In addition, it is difficult to overfeed a breast-fed infant, who will stop sucking on the breast once he or she is satiated; a bottle can be forced on a full baby more easily.

The immunological advantages of breast-feeding result from antibodies in the mother's milk that help the newborn fight germs. Colostrum is the first secretion to come from the nursing mother's breast. Being rich in antibodies, it is especially important because it ensures that the baby concentrates on growing without the obstacle of illness. A breast-fed baby is generally unlikely to catch any diseases that the nursing mother cannot catch. This fact is worth considering by the mother who plans to wean her baby and realizes that flu or cold season is not the ideal time!

In general, breast-fed babies have fewer gastrointestinal and respiratory infections than babies who are bottle-fed.

Breast-feeding is also a good idea if there is a family history of allergies. Babies whose parents have any kind of allergy can develop food or airborne allergies but are less likely to if they have a strong nutritional head start by being breast-fed. (Babies are never allergic to breast milk itself.) With maturity, infants are better able to handle the allergic load of new foods and the environment.

A baby can, on the other hand, have an allergic reaction to something the mother has eaten. The mother should then manipulate her diet to pinpoint the offending food. The mother of a bottle-fed baby, however, is faced with a more serious problem if she finds her baby is allergic to certain formulas, because she no longer has the option to begin to breast-feed.

One of the main benefits of breast-feeding is the psychological bond it promotes between baby and mother. It also seems to have a soothing effect on the baby that bottle-feeding does not.

Breast-feeding speeds up the process that returns the uterus to its pre-pregnancy size. It can also be a time-saver in the middle of the night by dispensing with that whole business of warming up bottles. And it makes travelling easier, because the nursing mother has no bottles or cans of formula to pack!

Nursing Know-How
Although breast-feeding might seem like a simple process, many women find it fraught with problems. Here are some important guidelines to help the milk flow freely.

The nursing mother produces milk, which stays in the breast ready for the infant. The amount of milk produced depends on how much the baby nurses. If the baby empties the breast, the mother produces more milk. If the mother's breasts are not emptied, milk production decreases.

At the beginning of a feeding, milk is produced extremely slowly as the baby sucks. The mother's body then releases a hormone called *oxytocin*, which causes her milk to flow more freely. This is called the *let-down*. If there is no let-down, the baby has to work hard for little result and will likely tire before the breast is emptied. The result is decreased milk production and more frequent feedings.

This brings us to the primary rule for nursing mothers—"Relax and get your rest!" Fatigue and nervousness can both prevent the let-down from occurring, a fact that might explain why a mother's supply of milk is sometimes diminished on coming home from hospital, when the demands of other children or of chores around the home add to the strain of being a new mother. This could be the beginning of a frustrating experience for all concerned. But nursing should be a priority at this time. For the first three to four weeks of breast-feeding, the nursing mother would do well to think of herself as a cow at pasture. Once the breast-feeding pattern is established, it is likely to continue without problems. A well-fed baby whose mother is calm and confident will sleep better at night, and so will the rest of the family—including mom!

How often does a baby need to breast-feed? This varies from child to child, but a breast-fed baby does eat more often than a bottle-fed one because mother's milk is more easily digested. Frequent feedings also help stimulate the breast supply.

Nutrition for the Nursing Mother
The ideal diet of the breast-feeding mother is similar to that of the pregnant woman, and because breast milk contains iron, she should continue to tuck into those iron-rich foods.

Her caloric needs depend on the amount of milk she produces, and some of them can be met by the breakdown of extra fat deposited during pregnancy. The nursing mother should lose weight gradually so that she does not jeopardize her milk supply, and the best way she can achieve this is with that old stand-by—a nutritious diet.

Quick weight loss is not advisable during breast-feeding for several reasons. A severe reducing diet not only lacks important nutrients, it also tires the nursing mother, whose taxing role at this time requires all kinds of extra energy and stamina. Another reason is the possible hazard of PCBs (polychlorinated biphenyls)—environmental pollutants found in some foods, air, and water. If the mother has been exposed to PCBs, they will have been stored in her adipose (fatty) tissue. When it breaks down during rapid weight loss, PCBs could be released into her breast milk. Although the chances of being seriously contaminated are rare (for example, by eating fish from polluted water), should you be concerned, get your breast milk tested.

Plenty of fluids are essential for the nursing mother's milk production, but they can also add up to a lot of calories. The mother who drinks three to four glasses of whole milk a day is ingesting 240 more calories a day, or 43,000 in six months, than the woman who drinks fat-free milk—that's more than 12 pounds in extra weight that the mother can likely do without! The woman who drinks 2 percent milk can add up an additional six pounds in the same six-month period. Juice is another liquid source of calories and should not be consumed in large doses if weight loss is to occur. Plenty of water, combined with fresh fruit for fibre, vitamins, and minerals, is a much better choice.

The new mom should also be careful not to miss out on meals because of her changed routine. If it is difficult to fit in regular meals between nursing, napping, and doing the odd chore around the house, then frequent small meals could be the answer. But above all, don't forget to eat, or you will run out of energy in no time!

The nursing mother should stay away from large amounts of alcohol because it can hinder the let-down reflex during breast-feeding and could affect her infant's health. Some people believe that small amounts, on the other hand, such as the occasional beer, may stimulate milk production. High consumption of caffeine by the nursing mom can not only make her too jumpy to nurse well, it can also make her baby restless and unable to sleep.

Smoking is thought to have a negative effect on both production and let-down of breast milk, not to mention any bad effects it might have on the infant. It is also wise for the woman who is breast-feeding to consult a physician or pharmacist before taking any drugs; they could be transferred to her milk and have adverse effects on her newborn child.

If the nursing mother decides to go back to work, she can continue breast-feeding two or three times a day. This could be first thing in the morning, on coming home from work, and then at bedtime. In order for this arrangement to work well, the breast-feeding pattern must be well established. During the day, the baby can be bottle-fed formula or stored breast milk. Breast milk that the mother has expressed can be stored for up to 48 hours in the fridge or frozen for a maximum of two months.

Formula Feeding—What to Choose
Commercially prepared formulas are the closest foods to breast milk available; they have a similar ratio of ingredients. There are two main types of formulas—those with a base of cow's milk and those with a base of soy. Even formulas with a base of cow's milk contain protein that is more like that of breast milk, and their fats are easier to digest than the fats in cow's milk. Both types of formula have added vitamins and minerals and supply all the necessary nutrients until the baby is four to six months old. Then the infant requires extra iron, which can be given in the form of an iron-fortified formula, an iron supplement, or iron-enriched infant cereals.

If there is a family history of allergies and your infant has been showing signs of them, it is not advisable to switch from a cow's milk formula to the soy-based version, because soy products are also allergenic. Speak to your physician about what less allergenic products are available.

Be careful to feed your infant formula according to instructions. Different products require different concentrations, and giving a baby a formula full strength when it should be diluted could cause dehydration.

If possible, feed your baby formula until the age of 12 months. Cow's milk is hard for an infant to digest, and cases of internal bleeding have been documented. When cow's milk is introduced, it should be whole milk, at least until the age of two, because it provides the fat required for healthy development.

Food, Glorious Food

It is not advisable to give babies solid food before the age of four to six months. Even if your baby is hungrier and needs to be fed more often for a week or two, as often happens at around three months when there is a growth spurt, resist the temptation to offer solid foods. Not only will the infant exhibit the *extrusion reflex* (sticking out of the tongue) during the first few months of life, making him or her spit out solid food, but breast milk and formula also contain all the necessary nutrients in perfect balance during this stage of development.

When you introduce solids, don't be in a hurry to offer all kinds of different foods at once. Start with one or two new items at a time to ensure that your baby does not have intolerances or allergies. In order to do this, serve foods individually, not in mixtures. Start new foods a little at a time over three to four days so you can observe any problems. Some signs of intolerance are obvious, but because an infant cannot tell you that he or she has stomachache, this might be manifested by sleeplessness or crying. Watch for patterns when trying to pinpoint such problems.

It is wiser to feed babies infant cereals than adult varieties. Some adult cereals like cream of wheat are fortified with iron; others are not. All infant cereals, however, are fortified with important vitamins and minerals, especially iron, and should be fed to babies up to one year old.

Homemade or Store Bought?

There is often little nutritional difference between homemade and store-bought baby food. It is, however, cheaper to make your own baby food and a good idea as long as you are careful to maximize nutrients. Commercial baby food is made with ingredients of peak nutritional quality, so they are a better choice in some cases.

Use fresh ingredients, and cook foods in ways that minimize loss of vitamins and minerals (see Chapter 5). Then purée and freeze them in ice cube trays for single serving portions. As your baby develops teeth, you can chop food to a coarser texture. Don't add sugar or salt to your baby's food, and when feeding your baby dishes eaten by the rest of the family, avoid strong spices; he or she may not like the taste.

When you buy commercial baby food, read the labels. A "beef dinner" could be quite different from beef alone and could be extended with cereal, making it lower in protein. Similarly, plain and simple fruits are a better choice than an infant "dessert." In general, avoid foods containing more than a trace of salt and sugar, whether they are homemade or not.

It is also best not to feed your baby homemade spinach or carrots before the age of six months because of the nitrate levels in these foods. Commercial processing removes nitrates. Because of the danger of botulism, honey is not recommended as a food for babies less than one year old. Nor is it wise to feed allergenic foods like wheat, cow's milk, eggs, fish, nuts, or chocolate to a baby with allergy-prone parents. Another no-no is putting your baby to bed with a bottle: the sugar in juice and the lactose in milk can cause cavities.

Childhood: Laying the Foundation

It is during childhood that a lifetime's eating habits are formed.

These habits are crucial to developing strong bodies and minds that can help prevent disease, so starting children on the path to healthful eating is a must. To ensure this, adults must first set the example and then involve the child in their own nutrition. Letting children make some decisions about what foods they eat, having them help plan meals, especially their school lunches, and even including them in some of the cooking are great ways to do this.

Children need to eat the same kinds of foods as adults, but in different amounts. How much depends on their stage of development as well as activity levels. The biggest growth spurt happens in the first year of life, and this explains why a child's appetite may become smaller at the start of the second year. This is a time to offer small portions of food and let your child eat as much as he or she wants.

A parent must keep in mind that a child's appetite varies from day to day and from season to season. The key is to offer a variety of foods and not to be discouraged if a new food is rejected. Don't offer a new food when your child is tired or not feeling well, and serve new foods in small amounts. If an unfamiliar vegetable, for example, is met with outright rejection, try serving it later in a more attractive disguise, such as puréed in a soup containing alphabet noodles. If a child refuses the meal at hand, it is not a good idea to offer substitutes.

Bargaining with children can be another way to teach them to accept a variety of nutritious foods. If, for example, a child usually refuses whole-grain bread, make an arrangement whereby you agree to alternately buy white and whole-wheat loaves to use in sandwiches for school. The child will feel that he or she is part of the decision-making process and will likely develop a taste for whole-grain breads at the same time.

Sometimes outside influences, such as television commercials that tempt children with surprise gifts tucked into the packages of yet another new, sugary breakfast cereal, can be a real problem. When a food of questionable nutritional quality is cleverly advertised this way, it is hard to convince a child that it is not a desirable food to eat. Stick to your guns and refuse to buy it without appearing too moralistic, and use the opportunity to teach your child not to believe everything he or she sees on TV. Complain to the television station or food company about the misuse of persuasive advertising as a way to try and change it.

Snacking is extremely important for children because they tend to eat small meals, so try to make snacks as nutritious as possible. Don't go to the extreme of never allowing a potato chip or candy to pass your child's lips—this could create a greater desire for such "forbidden fruit."

Try to avoid giving sugary snacks to kids; they cause cavities when plaque on their teeth combines with the sugar to form acids. Every time sugar is eaten, these acids stay in the mouth for 20 minutes, wreaking havoc. Sticky, chewy, sugary foods are the worst for this, and they include dried fruit as well as many kinds of candy.

Best snacking foods are fresh fruits and vegetables along with their juices, nuts and seeds, whole-grain crackers and cereals, and popcorn, especially when they are eaten with milk, plain yogurt, or low-fat cheese. Nuts, seeds, and popcorn, though, should not be given to children under three years of age because of the risk of choking. Cutting down on the fat and sugar in cake and cookie recipes is another good idea. Calling muffins cupcakes and baking them in fancy paper cups is a nifty way to make healthful eating fun.

Here are more ideas for easy, nutritious snacks that children can help prepare: peanut butter logs made of sliced bananas smeared with peanut butter; banana popsicles made by dipping whole bananas in orange juice and nuts and freezing them; seasoned popcorn made by sprinkling home-popped corn with grated cheese; fruit kebabs made by placing whole or chunks of fresh fruit on wooden skewers and then dipping them in low-fat yogurt blended with fresh fruit, vanilla, or a little honey. As for the ever-popular cookie, see the great recipes on pages 254 to 257.

Obesity, the most glaring nutritional problem in today's society, must be prevented during childhood. By applying the principles of this book along with an understanding that small people need small portions, even a child with a genetic tendency to be overweight can be helped to avoid obesity.

Studies have shown that in many cases, overweight children do not consume more calories than lean children; they just burn fewer calories by being less active. Nagging such children about being overweight only causes a bad self-image and could cause them to seek solace in food. A more productive approach is to encourage children to be physically active by involving them in family sports, outings, etc. Dieting during childhood is definitely out—this is a time when young people need plenty of nutrients for growth. It is better for the overweight child to grow while remaining at the same weight; the child therefore becomes leaner without compromising growth.

The Assertive Adolescent
During their teens—a time of growth and development when nutrient requirements increase substantially—many young people, especially girls, unfortunately do not pay much attention to nutrition. This is a point in life when young people need more calcium because of a growth in skeleton size.

At a time when there is so much concern over how to eliminate osteoporosis in women, we should be looking to the age when we can really prevent the problem from occurring at all. The emphasis should be on calcium intake during the adolescent years. This is the time of life when the calcium is being laid down in the bones. Worrying more about taking in calcium during the later years is much like bolting the barn door after the cows are gone. As well, most adolescent girls consume too little iron for their bodies' needs.

Teenage boys generally fare somewhat better in this regard than girls. Although they may not pay any more attention to nutrition, they are likely to get more nutrients simply by eating larger amounts of food.

A time of increasing independence, this can also be a period during which teens learn to make food choices that are often different from their parents'. It is now that the habit of skipping breakfast frequently begins—one that leads to low energy levels during the school day. A big breakfast and sizable lunch not only increase mental alertness during school but also help control the overeating that is common when teenagers arrive home and raid the cookie jar.

The teens are a time when it is easy to gain weight. After sitting all day in school, a walk or planned aerobic activity before going home are good ways to provide energy for homework and speed up the metabolic rate.

School lunches are another hazard for this age group, because they are often not nutritious enough. Parents and their children can put pressure on schools to make cafeteria food more nutritious and to add low-fat milk and fresh fruit to the pop and potato chip selection in vending machines. The latter is usually a surprisingly popular move with teenagers, who often pick a nutritious fastfood alternative when given the choice.

Teen Temptations

For girls, the teens are a time when growth spurts and a developing body can make them feel they are getting fat. In fact, it is normal for some weight gain to precede a growth spurt. However, girls often turn to fad dieting, and the resulting lack of nutrients can stop growth from taking place. At a time when a girl's self-image might be somewhat low, it is best for parents not to harp on her weight, but to discourage fad diets and be caring advisors, not dictators.

If a girl's weight begins to act like a yo-yo at this age, her concern about being overweight can get worse, and bulimia or anorexia nervosa could result. Both conditions are characterized by excessive dieting and obsessive exercising.

Bulimia and anorexia nervosa are both increasingly common diseases, and 90 percent of those afflicted are female. An anorexic, although emaciated, believes that she is overweight. Her fanatical dieting can cause loss of periods, lowered heart rate and metabolism, loss of hair, and electrolyte imbalance. In the most serious cases, she starves to death. Even if the anorexic stops her dieting, health problems can show up years later. Because of hormonal changes, the calcium status of an anorexic is similar to that of the post-menopausal woman.

Bulimia is characterized by binge eating followed by self-induced vomiting and the use of laxatives. Because these practices do not rid the body of many calories, body fat does not change drastically, and the person does not usually lose weight. Any weight loss that does occur is caused by loss of water and can result in dehydration. Electrolyte imbalance can also follow. Bulimics also commonly experience bloating, constipation, and the wearing away of dental enamel.

Because of the pressures to be thin and beautiful that our society exerts on women, they are more likely to succumb to the diet demons than teenage boys. This is, however, an age when boys might be tempted to build up their muscles with protein powders and expensive supplements. They would do better to concentrate on eating a balanced diet while exercising their muscles by means of training, which is much more effective and inexpensive!

Baby Boomers

Those people who are pushing or past 40 know only too well that this is a time when the body refuses to take abuse lying down!

Suddenly you find yourself getting older and feeling it. Your body is starting to speak up loud and clear when you mistreat it by overeating, drinking to excess, or not getting enough sleep. For the first time, perhaps, you cannot eat whatever you want without it showing on your stomach or hips. And overnight you, who used to be able to drink two cups of coffee before going to bed, realize it was that after-dinner cappuccino that kept you awake till 3 A.M.!

Skipping meals because your day is too full will not help matters. This is an age when eating correctly and exercising begin to be an absolute must to keep you feeling vital and stop your weight from creeping up. It's a time of reckoning, but also a time when preventive action is usually not too late.

Menopause—A Time of Change

For women, the time leading up to and including menopause is a time of transition. As levels of hormones such as estrogen diminish, special consideration must be given to lifestyle issues.

Waist management can become more difficult. Excess weight that used to appear on the hips and buttocks may suddenly find its way to the midsection. Being apple-shaped rather than the previous pear shape can increase the risk of disease. (See Waist Not, page 273.)

As women progress through menopause, they lose some of their protection against heart disease. A major contributor to the increased risk of cardiovascular disease is a drop in the protective HDL-cholesterol levels. Extra thought and action must now be directed towards boosting these levels. (See Heart of the Matter page 21.)

Bone health is another concern. Osteoporosis has been estimated to affect one in four women after menopause because of diminishing estrogen levels. Often, calcium intake is the only issue on the minds of those concerned (see page 162). Popping a calcium supplement may seem like the simple solution, but weight-bearing exercise, cigarette smoking, and alcohol and caffeine intake all affect the likelihood of developing osteoporosis.

The Golden Years

Youth may be wasted on the young, but there is no reason why age should not be accompanied by wisdom in the important matter of eating well. After all, the older one gets, the more crucial it is to maintain energy levels and a feeling of physical well-being.

Many elderly people consider themselves past the age when eating a nutritious diet is a top priority. They're more concerned about what they should *not* eat for medical reasons than they are about taking a positive attitude about what foods would be good for them. This is unfortunate because, along with pregnancy and breast-feeding, the senior years are a time when nutrition is more important than at any other stage of adulthood.

Certainly the metabolic rate slows down with increasing age, so that elderly people need fewer calories to maintain their weight. Less physical activity adds to this reduced need for calories. But the requirement for nutrients is in no way reduced, so packing these nutrients into a smaller quantity of food is the name of the game.

Many elderly folk have psychological reasons for lapsing into the "tea and toast" syndrome or other unhealthful eating habits. Lack of motivation to cook for onself after a lifetime of eating with a family or spouse or feelings of loneliness and isolation at this stage of life can lead to a lack of appetite. Many women complain that after years of cooking for a family and finding it a chore, they don't feel like preparing food. Whatever the reason, not having the will or the energy to think about meals could lead to malnourishment and all that goes with it.

Seek out a friend or group of friends to get together at mealtimes to solve the aversion to eating alone. Pot-luck meals are a good way of sharing the work and the cost of cooking as well as making mealtime a pleasant, social event. Picnicking outdoors in warm weather is also a good idea; the fresh air can be a terrific stimulant to conversation as well as appetite.

If you are forced to eat alone against your wishes, try reading a book, listening to the radio, or watching a favourite program on TV while you eat. This can help take your mind off the fact that you are alone. Set a proper place for yourself, perhaps pour a glass of wine to go with dinner, and even eat by candlelight—enjoy yourself!

Vitality – Keeping It

There are some physical conditions that often accompany aging that can be an obstacle to a nutritious diet. Here are some ideas on how to overcome them.

Osteoporosis, or loss of calcium from the bones, can occur in the jaw. This brings with it problems with teeth and difficulty chewing certain foods—raw fruits and vegetables, some meats, and whole grains, to name a few. A simple cure could be to ensure that your dentures fit well. If you still have a problem, roast, boil, or stew meats and then slice them thinly, cook vegetables in soups, and eat ripe, stewed, or canned fruit; these are all good ways to prepare nutrition-packed foods for easy chewing.

It is particularly important at this age to consume an adequate amount of protein. If the "tea and toast" routine becomes a substitute for proper meals, the muscles can begin to waste away. A lack of iron in the diet often makes an elderly person, whose meals should include some iron-rich foods, tired and listless. (See the discussion of iron in Chapter 1.)

To combat the increase in blood pressure that often accompanies the aging process, many elderly people follow sodium-restricted diets. But aging is also usually accompanied by reduced sense of taste and smell, so the lack of salt can render food almost tasteless.

Medication is another factor that can interfere with an elderly person's eating habits. Diuretics, for example, create an increased need for potassium-rich foods (again, see Chapter 1). And a drug like tetracycline should not be taken with dairy products. If you are taking medication, consult your physician or pharmacist about whether the drug should be taken with, before, or after meals and whether you should be avoiding or increasing certain foods while on the medication.

It is easy for people in this age group to become overweight because of their lower metabolic rates and decreased activity levels. You can combat this tendency by cutting down on foods that are high in empty calories and increasing activity wherever possible (more on this in Chapter 12).

If a physician has advised you to follow a special diet and you are having difficulty doing so, ask to be referred to a dietitian.

Shopping Tips for Seniors
Many of the food shopping pointers that we gave for singles in Chapter 10 also apply to seniors. Here are some more.

- An "emergency" shelf is an excellent idea in case there actually is an emergency. Perhaps you are unable to shop for food because of bad weather; the person who usually gives you a ride to the supermarket can't make it; or someone drops by unexpectedly. Foods on this shelf should include dairy products like skim milk powder, evaporated low-fat milk, UHT milk, and perhaps some instant pudding mix. Canned meat and fish, baked beans, dried legumes such as kidney beans, and peanut butter are protein stand-bys. Crackers, noodles, whole-grain cereals, and muffin or biscuit mixes are carbohydrate foods that keep well. Canned fruit and vegetables, canned juices and soups, as well as dried fruit complete the picture.

- A shopping list based on a careful reading of weekly specials advertised in the newspaper can be a big help. Evaluate whether an item on special is worth a detour. If you're saving only a small amount, it might not be worth the extra cost in transportation.

- Read labels on food packages to assess value for money as well as nutritional content of ingredients. In order to do this easily, don't forget to take your glasses when you are food shopping if you have eyesight problems.

- Shop with a friend and divide things up if sizes are too large. For example, milk is cheaper in the large plastic bags than in single cartons.

Stove Top Tuna Casserole

Calories 215
Protein 23 g
Fat 5 g
Carbohydrate 19 g

Serves 2–3.

A fast, low-fat version of an old reliable that kids will love.

1	tbsp. soft margarine	15 mL
2	tbsp. finely chopped onion	25 mL
2	tbsp. all-purpose flour	25 mL
$\frac{1}{8}$	tsp. freshly ground pepper	.5 mL
1	cup skim milk	250 mL
1	can (6.5 oz./184 g) water-packed tuna	
1	cup frozen mixed vegetables or peas and carrots	250 mL
$\frac{1}{2}$	cup low-fat plain yogurt	125 mL
$\frac{1}{2}$	tsp. grated lemon rind (optional)	2 mL

Cooked noodles, rice, or whole-wheat toast

Melt the margarine in a medium-sized saucepan. Add the onion and cook over medium heat until soft. Stir in the flour and pepper and cook, stirring, for about 1 minute. Gradually add milk and continue cooking, stirring constantly, until the sauce is smooth and thickened, 3–4 minutes. Add tuna and vegetables, cover, and cook 2–3 minutes, until vegetables are done. Stir in the yogurt. Serve over hot cooked noodles or rice or with whole-wheat toast.

Macaroni and Cheese with Spinach

Calories 444
Protein 24 g
Fat 15 g
Carbohydrate 52 g

Serves 4.

Kids will never guess that this is low in fat! A wonderfully healthful version of an old favourite.

2	tbsp. soft margarine	25 mL
1	small onion, finely chopped	
1	clove garlic, minced	
3	tbsp. all-purpose flour	45 mL
$2\frac{1}{2}$	cups skim milk	625 mL
Pinch cayenne pepper		
$\frac{1}{2}$	tsp. nutmeg	2 mL
Salt and freshly ground pepper to taste		
1	cup grated low-fat cheese	250 mL
2	cups elbow macaroni, cooked and drained	500 mL
1	10-oz./284-g package fresh spinach, cooked, well drained, and chopped	
$\frac{1}{2}$	cup freshly grated Parmesan cheese	125 mL

Melt the margarine in a medium-sized saucepan. Add the onion and garlic and cook over medium heat until soft. Stir in the flour and cook, stirring, for about 1 minute. Whisk in the milk, stirring until the sauce is smooth and thickened. Season with cayenne, nutmeg, salt, and pepper. Stir in the cheese and cook until it melts.

Place half the macaroni in a medium-sized ovenproof dish. Top with a layer of spinach. Spoon half the sauce over the spinach. Top with the remaining macaroni and sauce. Sprinkle with Parmesan. Bake at 350°F/180°C for about 20 minutes or until golden brown on top.

Pita Chips

Each recipe serves 4–6.

Try these crispy pita chips instead of the commercial variety. They're much lower in fat and sodium, but tops in flavour. Opt for the whole-wheat kind to increase your fibre intake.

Calories	76
Protein	2 g
Fat	3 g
Carbohydrate	11 g

Pesto Chips

2	pitas	
1	tbsp. virgin olive oil	15 mL
2	tsp. pesto (see page 102)	10 mL

Sprinkle of freshly grated Parmesan cheese for garnish

Cut each pita in half to make two circles. Then cut each circle into 8 triangles. Mix other ingredients and brush onto triangles. Place on baking sheet and bake in a preheated 200°F/95°C oven for 20–30 minutes. Serve with additional spread or as cocktail crackers.

Calories	86
Protein	3 g
Fat	3 g
Carbohydrate	11 g

Cheesy Chips

2	pitas	
1	tbsp. virgin olive oil	15 mL
3	tbsp. freshly grated Parmesan cheese	45 mL

Salt and freshly ground pepper to taste

Follow method for Pesto Chips.

Calories	75
Protein	2 g
Fat	3 g
Carbohydrate	11 g

Mediterranean Chips

2	pitas	
1	tbsp. virgin olive oil	15 mL
1	tsp. fresh parsley, finely chopped	5 mL
1	tsp. ground rosemary	5 mL

Follow method for Pesto Chips.

Pita Tuna Melts

Serves 3.

An old favourite with a twist.

3	whole-wheat pitas	
1	can (6.5 oz./184 g) water-packed tuna, drained and flaked	
$\frac{1}{4}$	cup celery, chopped	50 mL
2	tbsp. green onion, finely chopped	25 mL
2	tbsp. light mayonnaise	25 mL
$\frac{1}{2}$	cup grated part-skim mozzarella cheese	125 mL
9	tomato slices	

Freshly ground pepper

Combine tuna, celery, green onion, and light mayonnaise in a bowl. Cut top off each pita and open pocket. Carefully layer tuna mixture, cheese, and tomato slices inside. (Enlarge opening if necessary.) Wrap pitas in aluminum foil and bake at 375°F/190°C for 10–15 minutes or until cheese is melted and pita is crisp.

Bagel Thins

Each recipe serves 3–4.

Crunch your way through all these versions. For even more variety, use several kinds of bagels.

Plain Thins

2	bagels	
1	tbsp. vegetable oil	15 mL

Salt and freshly ground pepper to taste

Thinly slice each bagel into 6 rounds; set aside. Mix other ingredients; brush onto rounds. Place rounds on a baking sheet and bake in a preheated 200°F/95°C oven for 45 minutes or until bagel thins are crisp.

Garlic Thins

Calories 122
Protein 3 g
Fat 4 g
Carbohydrate 18 g

2	bagels	
1	tbsp. virgin olive oil	15 mL
1	clove garlic, minced	

Follow method for Plain Thins.

Cheesy Thins

Calories 136
Protein 4 g
Fat 4 g
Carbohydrate 18 g

2	bagels	
1	tbsp. virgin olive oil	15 mL
3	tbsp. freshly grated Parmesan cheese	45 mL

Follow method for Plain Thins.

Italian Thins

Calories 122
Protein 3 g
Fat 4 g
Carbohydrate 18 g

2	bagels	
1	tbsp. virgin olive oil	15 mL
1	tsp. fresh parsley, finely chopped	5 mL
1	clove garlic, minced	
1	tsp. ground rosemary	5 mL

Follow method for Plain Thins.

Cajun Thins

Calories 120
Protein 3 g
Fat 4 g
Carbohydrate 18 g

2	bagels	
1	tbsp. vegetable oil	15 mL
1	tsp. chili powder	5 mL
$\frac{1}{2}$	tsp. cayenne (optional)	2 mL
1	clove garlic, minced (optional)	

Pinch salt and pepper

Follow method for Plain Thins, but mix dry ingredients separately. (For spicier thins, add the cayenne and garlic.) Brush bagel rounds with oil, then lightly sprinkle on the seasonings.

Seasoned Popcorn

Seasoned popcorn has become a big business today. Make your own at home and spare yourself the salt, the fat, and the dollars.

Each recipe serves 4.

<table>
<tr><td>Calories 85</td></tr>
<tr><td>Protein 2 g</td></tr>
<tr><td>Fat 4 g</td></tr>
<tr><td>Carbohydrate 12 g</td></tr>
</table>

Mexican Popcorn

8	cups air-popped popcorn	2 L
1	tbsp. soft margarine, melted	15 mL
1–2 tsp.	chili powder	5–10 mL
$\frac{1}{2}$ tsp.	garlic powder	2 mL
$\frac{1}{2}$ tsp.	dried thyme	2 mL

Combine margarine and seasonings, stirring well, then drizzle mixture over the popped corn. (For added zip, increase the spices.) Toss gently to cool. Store in an airtight container.

<table>
<tr><td>Calories 108</td></tr>
<tr><td>Protein 4 g</td></tr>
<tr><td>Fat 5 g</td></tr>
<tr><td>Carbohydrate 12 g</td></tr>
</table>

Parmesan and Herb Popcorn

8	cups air-popped popcorn	2 L
1	tbsp. soft margarine, melted	15 mL
$\frac{1}{4}$	cup freshly grated Parmesan cheese	50 mL
1	tsp. dried oregano	5 mL
$\frac{1}{2}$	tsp. garlic powder	2 mL

Prepare as above, mixing Parmesan with the seasonings. Store in an airtight container.

<table>
<tr><td>Calories 154</td></tr>
<tr><td>Protein 3 g</td></tr>
<tr><td>Fat 4 g</td></tr>
<tr><td>Carbohydrate 30 g</td></tr>
</table>

Fruity Cinnamon Popcorn

8	cups air-popped popcorn	2 L
1	tbsp. soft margarine, melted	15 mL
$\frac{1}{2}$	tsp. ground cinnamon	2 mL
1	cup chopped dried mixed fruit (apples, apricots, dates, prunes, and raisins)	250 mL

Prepare as above, then add chopped fruit and toss again. Store in an airtight container.

Calories	92
Protein	2 g
Fat	1 g
Carbohydrate	21 g

Honey Popcorn

8	cups air-popped popcorn	2 L
2	tbsp. liquid honey, heated	25 mL
$\frac{1}{4}$	tsp. ground cinnamon	1 mL
$\frac{1}{8}$	tsp. ground nutmeg	.5 mL

Pour honey and sprinkle spices over popcorn; stir well. Store in an airtight container. (Great for making popcorn balls.)

Calories	99
Protein	4 g
Fat	6 g
Carbohydrate	9 g

Tofu Nuggets

Makes about 15 balls.

A nutritious substitute for fried chicken that children of all ages will enjoy. Make a meal of them with a crisp tossed salad.

1	cup tofu, drained and pressed (see page 241)	250 mL
$\frac{1}{2}$	cup brown long-grain rice, cooked	125 mL
2	tbsp. low-sodium soy sauce	25 mL
$\frac{3}{4}$	cup ground almonds	175 mL
$\frac{1}{4}$	cup wheat germ	50 mL
$\frac{3}{4}$	cup sesame seeds	175 mL

Place the tofu in a bowl and mash well. Blend half the cooked rice with the tofu in a food processor or blender until they form a thick paste. Transfer to a bowl and stir in the remaining rice, soy sauce, almonds, wheat germ, and $\frac{1}{4}$ cup/50 mL sesame seeds. Blend well.

Roll this mixture into 1-inch/2-cm balls. Roll each ball in the remaining $\frac{1}{2}$ cup/125 mL sesame seeds to coat. Bake on a lightly greased baking sheet at 350°F/180°C for about 45 minutes or until golden brown.

Calories 235
Protein 11 g
Fat 6 g
Carbohydrate 40 g

Tofu Fruit Pudding

Serves 2.

This is one of the tastiest ways to introduce tofu to children. It tastes better than any commercial pudding mix and is, of course, much more healthful. This recipe combines the protein of tofu with the fibre, vitamins, and minerals of fresh fruit.

$\frac{3}{4}$	cup drained, mashed tofu	175 mL
$\frac{3}{4}$	cup sliced fresh, ripe, tender fruit	175 mL
	(banana, peach, nectarine, or mango)	
1	tsp. honey	5 mL
1–2 tsp. lemon juice		5–10 mL

To remove the excess moisture from the tofu, wrap it in a clean tea towel and squeeze gently. Blend the tofu with the remaining ingredients in a food processor or blender until smooth. Pour into individual serving dishes and chill.

Note: If using banana, serve at once, or the pudding will turn brown.

Chewy Squares

Makes 12–16.

Crunchy, chewy, and healthful at the same time, these have a yummy peanut butter flavour plus a fibre-full cookie base. Carob chips can be used for caffeine- or chocolate-sensitive individuals.

¼	cup wheat germ	50 mL
3	cups rolled oats	750 mL
⅓	cup soft margarine	75 mL
¼	cup honey	50 mL
½	tsp. vanilla	2 mL
¼	cup raisins	50 mL
Topping	½ cup carob or chocolate chips	125 mL
	⅓ cup chunky peanut butter	75 mL

Combine the wheat germ and rolled oats in a medium-sized bowl. Melt the margarine together with the honey and vanilla in a small saucepan and mix well. Pour into the rolled-oat mixture and mix well. Stir in the raisins. Pat into an 8-inch/2-L square baking pan. Bake at 400°F/ 200°C for 10–15 minutes. Cool completely.

Melt the carob or chocolate chips in a small, heavy saucepan. Stir in the peanut butter until blended. Spread this mixture over the cooled crust. Cool, then cut into squares.

Calories	94
Protein	2 g
Fat	5 g
Carbohydrate	13 g

Great Granola Bars

Makes 12–16.

These are a must as part of anyone's brown-bag lunch and the perfect between-meal snack. A granola bar that's as nutritious as it's cooked up to be!

$\frac{1}{4}$	cup soft margarine, melted	50 mL
2	tbsp. brown sugar	25 mL
$\frac{1}{2}$	tsp. vanilla	2 mL
1	egg	
$2\frac{1}{2}$	cups homemade granola (see page 193)	625 mL

Combine the margarine and sugar in a medium-sized bowl and blend well. Add the vanilla and egg and beat until smooth. Stir in the granola. Pat the mixture into a lightly oiled 8-inch/2-L square baking pan. Bake at 400°F/ 200°C for about 15 minutes or until golden brown. Cool completely before cutting into bars.

Calories 100
Protein 1 g
Fat 5 g
Carbohydrate 12 g

Nutty Oatmeal Cookies

Makes about 3 dozen.

These cookies are so tasty, they could turn anyone into a monster! But go easy on them because they are fairly high in fat and sugar. This recipe uses a food processor, but you can also make them by hand.

$\frac{1}{2}$	cup soft margarine	125 mL
$\frac{1}{3}$	cup vegetable oil	75 mL
$\frac{3}{4}$	cup lightly packed brown sugar	175 mL
1	tsp. vanilla	5 mL
$\frac{1}{4}$	cup boiling water	50 mL
$1\frac{3}{4}$	cups whole-wheat flour	425 mL
$\frac{1}{2}$	tsp. salt	2 mL
1	tsp. baking soda	5 mL
2	cups rolled oats	500 mL
$\frac{1}{2}$	cup chopped walnuts	125 mL

Process the margarine, oil, sugar, and vanilla in a food processor or blender until well blended. Add the boiling water and process until blended. Add the flour, salt, baking soda, and rolled oats and process with several on-off turns until they are mixed.

Transfer the mixture to a bowl and stir in the walnuts. Shape into 1-inch/2-cm balls. Place on a lightly greased or paper-lined cookie sheet and flatten completely with a floured fork. Bake at 325°F/160°C for about 18 minutes or until golden brown.

Oatmeal Chocolate Chip Cookies

Calories 124
Protein 2 g
Fat 6 g
Carbohydrate 17 g

Makes about 4 dozen.

Fibre and flavour all in one delectable package! All kids seem to love chocolate chip cookies, so give them one that's more nutritious.

$\frac{2}{3}$	cup soft margarine	150 mL
$\frac{1}{2}$	cup granulated sugar	125 mL
$\frac{1}{2}$	cup lightly packed brown sugar	125 mL
2	eggs	
$1\frac{1}{2}$	cups whole-wheat flour	375 mL
1	tsp. baking soda	5 mL
$\frac{1}{2}$	tsp. salt	2 mL
3	cups rolled oats	750 mL
1	cup chopped walnuts	250 mL
$\frac{1}{2}$	cup chocolate chips	125 mL

Cream together the margarine and sugars until light and creamy. Beat in the eggs one at a time.

Mix together the flour, baking soda, and salt in a medium-sized bowl, then stir them into the creamed mixture. Stir in the rolled oats, walnuts, and chocolate chips and mix well. Drop the dough in spoonfuls onto a lightly oiled or paper-lined cookie sheet. Bake at 350°F/180°C for 10–12 minutes or until golden brown.

Calories 65
Protein 1 g
Fat 4 g
Carbohydrate 8 g

Double Oat Cookies

Makes about $4\frac{1}{2}$ dozen.

The perfect after-school cookie.

$\frac{3}{4}$	cup soft margarine	175 mL
1	cup brown sugar, loosely packed	250 mL
1	large egg	
1	tsp. vanilla extract	5 mL
$\frac{1}{2}$	cup whole-wheat flour	125 mL
$1\frac{1}{2}$	cups rolled oats	375 mL
1	cup oat bran	250 mL
1	tsp. baking soda	5 mL
$\frac{1}{8}$	tsp. salt	.5 mL
$\frac{1}{2}$	cup chopped pecans	125 mL
$\frac{1}{2}$	cup raisins	125 mL

Cream together the margarine and sugar until light and creamy. Beat in the egg and vanilla.

Combine the flour, rolled oats, oat bran, baking soda, and salt in a separate bowl. Stir into the creamed mixture and mix well. Stir in the pecans and raisins. Drop the dough in teaspoonfuls onto a lightly oiled or paper-lined cookie sheet. Flatten slightly with a floured fork. Bake at 350°F/180°C for 10–12 minutes or until golden brown. After taking cookies out of oven, wait one minute before removing cookies from the pan.

Calories 64
Protein 2 g
Fat 4 g
Carbohydrate 7 g

Peanut Butter Cookies

Makes about 3 dozen.

The best ever, these are a high-fibre version of an old favourite.

$\frac{1}{3}$	cup soft margarine	75 mL
$\frac{1}{2}$	cup natural peanut butter	125 mL
$\frac{1}{3}$	cup granulated sugar	75 mL
$\frac{1}{3}$	cup lightly packed brown sugar	75 mL
1	egg	
1	tsp. vanilla	5 mL
$\frac{1}{2}$	cup natural bran	125 mL
$\frac{1}{2}$	cup all-purpose flour	125 mL
1	tsp. baking soda	5 mL
Pinch salt		
$\frac{1}{3}$	cup blanched, unsalted, chopped peanuts	75 mL

Cream together the margarine, peanut butter, and sugars in a large bowl until smooth and fluffy. Blend in the egg and vanilla.

Combine the bran, flour, baking soda, and salt in a separate bowl. Stir into the peanut butter mixture and mix well. Stir in the peanuts. Shape the dough into 1-inch/2-cm balls on an ungreased cookie sheet and flatten with a floured fork. Bake at 350°F/180°C for 10–12 minutes or until golden brown.

12   The Diet Dilemma

Let's wipe the weight control slate clean.

First, let's dispel all thoughts of what is usually called dieting—that mind-numbing process of self-denial that can obsessively govern each movement of fork to mouth day after day, month upon month, year in and year out. Next, let's see what weight control really means. The good news is that although there is no magic formula for losing weight, the subject is much less complicated than the diet gurus would have us think.

Weight control is simply a matter of making the right food choices, feeling good physically and mentally, and developing realistic attitudes about our bodies and how they are fuelled.

The Body Beautiful – A Changing Standard
What does being overweight really mean?

We have only to look at a Rubens painting or photos of that curvaceous sex goddess Marilyn Monroe to realize that standards of body weight have changed over the years. In North America today, ideal looks are unfortunately epitomized by bony fashion models so thin and lacking in curves that they seem almost emaciated. No wonder anorexia and bulimia are two diseases of our age.

One of the reasons for our obsession with weight is a misconception of how the body is made up. Contrary to popular belief, our bodies do not consist mainly of fat. Lean body mass, or muscle, bones, water, and other substances all make up our body weight. Tables showing what we "should" weigh that do not take into account physical variations like body frame and muscle mass should therefore be used only as guidelines—nothing more.

Health and Welfare Canada's Guidelines For Healthy Weight uses a formula, called Body Mass Index, (BMI) to evaluate the potential for health risks as a result of being either overweight or underweight.

Using the BMI (a ratio of height to weight), a range of healthy weights has been established rather than an ideal weight or number. As a result, the "healthy weight" method for assessing body weight makes allowances for the different body shapes that make up our society. Check the Body Mass Index chart on page 274–75 to see what your BMI reading is.

If your BMI is below 20 and you're at a natural weight, then there may not be a health risk for you. But if you're at this level and are perpetually dieting to maintain your weight, then there is a message here for you. A few added pounds and sensible eating might be in order.

If your BMI is within the acceptable range and you feel that you're a little overweight, then the answer may be "eating right" along with a little extra physical activity.

Although there are numerous people dieting to lose those extra 5 pounds, we must not dismiss the dangers of being legitimately overweight. Those with a reading of more than 27 fall into this category. Such people tend to die younger than people of average weight, especially if they were fat at an early age. In addition, the consequences of being overweight often take years to surface as disease. Heart disease, hypertension, diabetes, and degenerative arthritis are all prevalent in our society and tend to strike overweight people progressively over a matter of years. These people are also at risk of developing certain cancers, including cancer of the colon, endometrium, and breast, all of which seem to be linked with diets high in fat.

Waist Not, Want Not
The next step in assessing whether you're at risk is to measure your waist-hip ratio. Divide your waist measurement by your hip measurement to see how your body fat is distributed. Where you store that spare tire may be a good indicator of whether or not it's likely to cause health problems.

If you're a male, your ratio should be less than one, that is, your waist should be the same or smaller than your hips. For females, who naturally have considerably larger hips, a positive reading is 0.8. Studies show that if you're overweight and pear-shaped as opposed to apple-shaped, you're less likely to run into problems because of your excess weight. Men are much more apt to develop those "love handles" around the waist, making them more apple-shaped.

As you can see by the examples of two males and two females (see page 275), male #2 is much larger around the waist than male #1. Statistics of disease risk show that he's much more likely to experience health problems as a result of his body shape.

BODY MASS INDEX

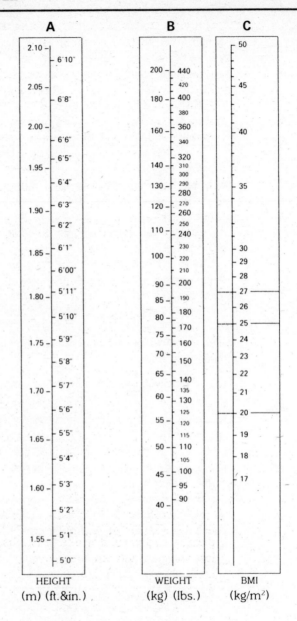

A	B	C
HEIGHT	WEIGHT	BMI
(m) (ft.&in.)	(kg) (lbs.)	(kg/m²)

How to find your BMI:
1) mark an X at your height on line A,
2) mark an X at your weight on line B,
3) take a ruler and join the two Xs, and
4) extend the line to line C to find your BMI.

Zone A	Zone B	Zone C	Zone D
BMI	BMI	BMI	BMI
less than 20	between 20 and 25	between 25 and 27	more than 27
May be associated with health problems for some people	Good weight for most people	May lead to health problems in some people	Increasing risk of developing health problems

generally acceptable range

These same statistics show that female #2 with the same waist-hip ratio as male #1 is at higher risk than female #1.

Male #1	Waist: 34 inches/86 cm
	Hip: 35 inches/90 cm
	Waist-Hip Ratio: 0.97
Male #2	Waist: 40 inches/102 cm
	Hip: 35 inches/90 cm
	Waist-Hip ratio: 1.14
Female #1	Waist: 26 inches/66 cm
	Hip: 36 inches/91 cm
	Waist-Hip ratio: 0.72
Female #2	Waist: 34 inches/86 cm
	Hip: 35 inches/90 cm
	Waist-Hip Ratio: 0.97

Don't Be a Yo-Yo

"Yo-yo" diets on which weight is quickly shed and then just as quickly regained, have become a trend over the past few decades and also carry serious risks. People who lose and gain large amounts of weight are likely to develop medical problems such as gallstones, not to mention the nutritional hazards that such diets usually entail.

These diets may also be one of the reasons why North American women are unusually prone to osteoporosis. A North Dakota study found that when women reduced their weight, they lost bone mass, even when exercising regularly and consuming sufficient amounts of calcium during the weight-loss regimen. Repeated bouts of dieting may certainly take their toll on bone health.

Why certain people become overweight is a complex question that is the subject of extensive research and much debate. What seems clear amid the controversy is that genetic factors and environment both play a part.

If a child has one overweight parent, the likelihood of the child being overweight is 50 percent. If both parents are overweight, the likelihood jumps to 70 percent. In a family whose weekend ritual is going for walks, the chances of offspring being overweight are lower than in one whose favoured activity is eating out! Developing healthy attitudes toward food as a family and encouraging physical activity help prevent weight problems, particularly if there is a genetic predisposition to amass body fat.

Another problem is the scale. It is certainly a helpful tool in determining body weight, but it does not accurately measure changes in body fat. A person's weight often depends on fluctuations in bodily fluids. If you drank 16 ounces of water and then stepped on the scale, you would weigh one pound more—a gain of fluid, not fat. Body fluids and electrolytes can easily affect your weight if you are on a weight-loss program. The best way to determine weight is to step on the same scale in the same place wearing the same weight of clothes once a week.

Animal Instincts

To discover the ideal eating plan that will keep us at an optimum weight, each of us must get back to basics. This means rediscovering the animal in us. Animals eat when they're hungry and stop eating when they have had enough, provided, of course, that they have an adequate source of food. When it's time to hibernate, they put on fat.

Human beings, whose bodies have the same ability to regulate weight and appetite as animals, carry with them a complicating factor that can cause problems, namely, the mind. The human mind can override the body's basic need for food with cerebral notions such as dining out to celebrate, nibbling on hors d'oeuvres at a cocktail party, or downing a package of chocolate chip cookies to quell pre-exam nerves! In fact, our habit of using food as a means to socialize or solve a psychological problem has made sustenance its secondary function. The result is the nutritional mess in which we find ourselves today.

But all is not lost. We can return to a more animal-like approach to eating that allows us to listen to our bodies with sensitivity and feed ourselves with the care and nurturing we all deserve. But first, we have to rediscover the animal regulation of appetite in order to know when we are hungry and when we are full.

If you don't eat when your body is hungry, you will not know when it is full. Responses to this vary from "I know when I'm hungry—for sure not in the morning" to "Whether I'm full depends on the meal, the company, how I'm feeling, and what my day's been like." In a nutshell, most people believe they cannot change their eating patterns, even though these patterns are based on habit and the power of the mind rather than on the body's physical need for food.

The main task when tackling weight control, therefore, is to develop eating habits that are in harmony with your body's need for food. First, you must learn to eat when you are hungry and not eat when you are full. Next, you must establish an eating pattern and stick to it. The result will be a nutritious way of eating that is easy to maintain and does not obsess you as most ways of dieting do.

It's all a matter of listening to our bodies' cues. The reason that fad diets don't work is that nearly all of them run counter to our bodies' need for food. This sets up a battleground on which our bodies fight the regimen being forced on them and explains why most people on such diets stick with them for only a short time.

The body has another mechanism that must be considered when discussing weight loss. This is its desire to maintain the status quo. The healthy body wants to stay at the weight it is, overweight or not. In fact, it is a sign of illness to lose weight easily with no appetite changes. Because of this, hunger that results from an attempt to lose weight is actually a positive sign—a sign of good health.

Perpetual dieters, whose days are dominated by feelings of hunger, are eventually unable to cope, quit the diet, and often seek solace from their frustration by eating even more than before they began their diet. In these cases, dieting can actually be a cause of gaining weight!

On a healthy weight-loss program, however, you should eat often and stave off hunger. You will be hungry before meals and satisfied afterward. If you are eating properly, you will be hungry after a meal only at a time when your weight is dropping—a sure sign of success!

For most people, the first week of a weight-loss program is the time the hungries really hit and the biggest weight loss happens. For others, the drop in weight and accompanying hunger occur only after two weeks of a change in eating habits. It is thus important to realize that weight loss varies from person to person and from week to week and that the long-term shedding of pounds during healthy weight loss averages out. It is also crucial to develop a positive attitude to hunger when you are losing weight and to realize that it is a happy sign of impending weight loss—not a cue to throw in the tea towel!

Fast or Feast
What is a proper weight loss?

A healthy rate at which to shed weight is an average of two pounds a week. This is small compared to the amounts advocated by some diets, but still substantial, especially if you visualize the equivalent two pounds of butter or lard!

Keep in mind that the goal of losing weight is to shed fat, not just to weigh less. The quick weight loss that results from crash dieting is often loss of water combined with lean body mass and fat—a loss that returns almost as fast as it disappeared. Fat takes time to accumulate and time to lose, and there are no miracles that can make it otherwise. People who state that they can gain and lose weight in the blink of an eye are kidding themselves that this is loss of fat. And those who tout diets that will help you do this may be kidding themselves as well as hoodwinking you!

The Energy Equation
Body fat is nature's way of storing excess energy, or calories. An increase in body fat causes an increase in body weight. How much fat we store is a matter of how the energy equation balances out:

Energy intake equals energy expenditure: fat stores are stable.

Energy intake is greater than energy expenditure: fat stores increase.

Energy intake is less than energy expenditure: fat stores decrease.

This is what these equations mean. One pound of body fat is equal to 3,500 calories. In order to gain or lose one pound of body fat a week, the body must have an excess or deficit of an average of 500 calories per day.

AVERAGE ENERGY REQUIREMENTS OF INDIVIDUALS

Sex	Weight	Calories per Day
Male	150 lb./68 kg	2,450
	160 lb./73 kg	2,600
	170 lb./77 kg	2,800
	180 lb./82 kg	2,950
	190 lb./86 kg	3,100
	200 lb./91 kg	3,300
	225 lb./102 kg	3,700
	250 lb./114 kg	4,100
Female	100 lb./45 kg	1,450
	110 lb./50 kg	1,600
	120 lb./54 kg	1,750
	130 lb./59 kg	1,900
	140 lb./64 kg	2,050
	150 lb./68 kg	2,200
	160 lb./73 kg	2,350
	170 lb./77 kg	2,500
	180 lb./82 kg	2,600
	190 lb./86 kg	2,750
	200 lb./91 kg	2,900
	225 lb./102 kg	3,272

Note: The above are averages based on ages 25 to 49. Energy needs of younger individuals are greater, whereas those of older individuals are slightly lower.

To gain or lose two pounds a week requires an excess or deficit of 1,000 calories per day, or 7,000 calories a week. Therefore, an excess or deficit of 100 calories a day would mean a gain or loss of 36,500 calories, or 10 pounds, over a period of one year. In order to determine your caloric needs, you must consider your present weight and activity levels.

A person who weighs more than 200 pounds can lose weight with a much higher intake of calories than someone who weighs 130 pounds. Chances are, too, that the 200-pound person will stick to the higher calorie intake better than to a severe reducing diet that could doom him or her to failure.

A good reducing program must include all the daily nutrient requirements while cutting down on calories. This requires a minimum of 1,200 calories a day. If nutrients are lacking, weight loss will go hand in hand with fatigue, feelings of malaise, and a lacklustre, sickly appearance—not great when your aim is to look as good as you feel! Crash diets that cause these symptoms create dips in energy levels, and often cause the dieter to give up the regimen. A nutritious weight-loss program, however, has the opposite effect and makes the dieter feel and look healthy while he or she gradually sheds weight.

There are exceptions to the 1,200-calorie-per-day rule of thumb. One is if the dieter has an orthopedic problem in the back or joints and must lose some weight before he or she can become more active. A vitamin or mineral supplement would likely be advised to accompany such a low calorie intake.

Each person's daily energy requirement or calorie intake also depends on his or her basal metabolic rate and activity levels (see chart on page 279).

Today's lifestyle has caused a dramatic shift in the energy equation. All manner of devices, from the automobile to the electric clothes dryer, have made our way of life more sedentary than it was in the past, and we must adjust our activity levels accordingly (see Chapter 9 for a discussion of the benefits of exercise).

Compounding this problem is the body's reaction to a person's effort to lose weight. When a person embarks on a weight-loss program, the body shifts into a survival mode that turns into a real battle of the bulge! First, the body calls on its hunger troops to maintain the status quo, thinking that it is fighting for survival. When the hunger continues, the body thinks it has to struggle against starvation. Its next tactic is to decrease its metabolic rate to conserve energy in the form of calories. At this point, the dieter has a simple choice: either cut down even more on calories, or increase the body's metabolic rate by exercise. The latter choice is certainly preferable.

Here is how exercise can change the energy balance in the dieter's favour. By decreasing your food intake by 500 calories a day, you would lose one pound a week. By increasing the energy you expend by exercising regularly, you could add another 500 calories to your daily expenditure. Exercise not only burns calories but also gives you a feeling of well-being, firms up your muscles, and is a terrific way to combat stress (again, see Chapter 9)—whether you're dieting or not!

More Than Calories Count

Many people believe that all there is to losing weight is adding up the number of calories they consume in a day and then cutting down. In fact, the energy equation is more complex than this. Energy taken in can affect energy burned in several ways, and considerable research is being done on this relationship of food intake to the metabolic rate.

Food has a heating, or thermal, effect on the body. When you eat, you increase your metabolism to some extent. Thus, if you ate six small meals a day, your metabolic rate would be faster than if you ate larger amounts two or three times a day. In fact, the very act of eating breakfast revs up your body's engine and increases your metabolic rate. This effect lasts for a short while, and then it's time to eat again. As with everything, though, don't take this idea too far and consume too many calories in a futile effort to make your body's metabolic rate go over the top.

The ideal energy intake should be spread over three meals a day plus a couple of snacks. By eating more often, you can sneak in a little more food and still lose weight. The kinds of food you eat can also affect the metabolic rate. One study found that a meal that was high in carbohydrate raised the metabolic rates of overweight people higher than a meal containing a comparable number of calories, but made up mostly of fats.

All this points to the pitfalls of counting calories as the sole way of controlling weight.

Someone who only counts calories might save up his or her calorie quota for one meal and thus miss out on the thermal effect of eating often. By rating foods just according to calories, foods high in fat can be consumed instead of carbohydrates with the same calorie count, causing the dieter to lose out on an increase in metabolic rate. What is more, counting calories with no thought to nutrients, particularly carbohydrate, protein, and fat, can lead to a severe drop in energy.

This plummeting energy level can result in cravings—often for all the wrong foods, like the sugary Danish that is the breakfast skipper's answer to hunger pangs. Eating nutrient-dense foods at frequent intervals is a better way to diet than relying on calorie counts alone. Remember also that eating correctly early in the day becomes preventive eating when it controls the intake later in the day (there's more on breakfast in Chapter 8).

Eating a large evening meal is another pitfall of the dieter who relies on counting calories. Instead, eating a big meal in the morning and tapering off consumption toward day's end is a much better method. By eating a smaller evening meal and forgoing those midnight snacks, your body will begin to be hungrier in the morning, which is what you want.

Another minefield for calorie counters is the "I'll be good today" or "I'll be really good tomorrow" school of thought. People who are wracked by guilt if they eat a chocolate bar or piece of cake are likely to give up their weight-loss program completely and are headed down the perpetual dieters' path to failure. This is why rigid diets that promote self-denial and guilt are self-defeating.

Yet another weakness of calorie counting as a way of losing weight is that it keeps you out of touch with that most important of mechanisms—regulation of appetite. A meal pattern that paces your food intake regularly throughout the day with built-in calorie controls, however, will help your body relearn the animal ability to recognize hunger and satiety. This means eating small quantities of food every three to four hours and cutting down, if necessary, at the evening meal when your body needs food least.

Mind Games — The Importance of Motivation
No matter how sound your weight-loss program is, however, it will not work if you do not have motivation.

Trying to lose weight without being motivated can be more detrimental than not trying at all. When hunger strikes the unmotivated dieter—a good sign that weight is being lost—he or she tends to eat more. Failure to stick to the diet leads to frustration and a tendency to simply give up. There goes the diet, and up goes the weight! Such a person would do well to figure out why he or she is not motivated and, if possible, reverse the situation.

For many people, motivation is difficult when they are faced with a task that seems so overwhelming and a goal that seems so far away. One solution is to make short-term goals. Try planning for a two-week stint, which could mean losing four pounds, and then renegotiating for two weeks more.

Some people lose motivation after they have lost a substantial amount of weight because they cannot face the hunger that would be caused by losing more. They should stop dieting at this point, concentrate on trying to maintain their weight loss, and then find a way to get motivated if they need to lose more. If losing more weight is critical for health reasons, their best recourse is to seek the help of a qualified professional.

Today's obsession with thinness can cause another problem—dieting by people who have no reason to and whose goals are unrealistic. These efforts are doomed to failure and can be risky to people's health, especially that of teenage girls. Those with normal weight who diet in fear of gaining are equally misguided and should learn the art of healthful eating.

Set the Record Straight

The best way to start losing weight is to write down everything you eat *before* you eat it so you can assess exactly what aspects of your eating habits need to be changed. This can be an extremely helpful, if sometimes painful, revelation of where your eating problems lie and what habits should be changed. It is also a good idea to keep this food record during the period you are trying to lose weight. By analyzing it once a week, you will gain many insights into what foods you missed as well as what foods you could have done without. Keep it in a handy spot, and put it on a convenient size of paper so you can carry it with you easily.

In particular, this record will pinpoint "danger" foods that you consume in excess—much to your body's dismay. These could be salty items like potato chips, which seem to have an addictive quality that has you eating the whole package when you intended only to munch a couple. Realizing which foods cause such snack attacks will

DAILY FOOD RECORD

Time	Food*	Amount	Place	Am I Hungry? (Yes/No)

* Include type of preparation, for example, fried, baked, or broiled.

help you plan your strategy, which might be to avoid salty munchies altogether or to grab a few and to start eating them only once the package is safe and sound inside a cupboard!

What you learn from your food record can also help you understand why certain eating habits die hard. An adult who returns home to the family nest where overeating is a way of life can easily slip back into the old routine. Stress can also cause old habits to reappear. Once life is back to normal or the person is back home, however, it takes special concentration to get back into that healthful way of eating.

A food record can also reveal how moods or physical condition influence the way you eat. Feeling tired, for example, is the cue for many people to open the fridge. Try taking a cat nap or doing a little exercise instead. If holidays are your time to sample different foods, this might not be the time to lose weight, but rather to maintain it. Finding other ways to fill your holiday time is also a good idea.

Above all, use your food record to make positive changes in your eating habits. Once you have noted how problems or habits influence what you eat, don't be negative about your ability to change. Work at one area at a time in order to make permanent changes. One good way is to go meal by meal, perhaps working on breakfast first, then moving on to lunch, and so on. Soon you will have a whole new set of eating habits that, like the pieces of a jigsaw puzzle, fall happily into place.

Diet Downfalls

One unfortunate sign of our times is the way nutrition has become for many people a moral issue with all the evangelical trappings of a new religion. So fanatical are its adherents that eating a whole chocolate bar or devouring several scoops of ice cream are labelled major transgressions for which one must surely pay!

This attitude has no place in the down-to-earth matter of healthful eating. Anyone who tries to unlearn certain eating habits and replace them with new ones is bound to make mistakes. There is absolutely no place here for perfectionism, criticism, blame, or guilt.

Changing many small aspects of your behaviour and weathering the setbacks are all part of the weight-loss learning process. Alter one aspect at a time, and you will end up with a new, improved set.

Make It a Ten!

One nifty trick for overcoming dieter's guilt is to approach a delicious-looking food that you know is not nutritious with the following game plan. Take one bite and rate it from one to ten. Finish eating it only if it scores a top-notch ten out of ten. You will be surprised how many chocolate cakes do not live up to their gorgeous looks! You will also discover a discriminating palate you may not have known you had.

A positive attitude is the key to making any change, whether the problem is food or anything else. A negative attitude ensures failure.

An example of this is the person who eats the wrong kinds of food at parties with the rationalization, "I've always overeaten at parties and it's a bad habit, but there's nothing I can do about it." A positive approach would be to try some new strategies such as eating regularly on the day of the party and having a snack before leaving home so as not to arrive starving. Another trick is not to eat while you are engaged in stimulating conversation. If you do, you won't fully appreciate the food's taste and probably won't notice if it is laden with fat.

Learn from each experience. Discover which ways of eating work for you and which do not. The good experiences will encourage you to make more changes.

Diet Works
If you need the structure of a reducing diet to lose weight, you must assess its safety, reliability, and prognosis for helping you make long-term changes.

This is not an easy task, because fad diets that feed on the public's desire for slimness are an ever-growing breed. Beware of diets promising miracles, claiming that you will shed pounds effortlessly either by eating food in intricate combinations, by avoiding milk, or by consuming only fruit for breakfast. If a diet makes claims that are too good to be true, then its claims are exactly that!

Diets that give day-to-day menus are not a good idea either. The most efficient, lasting way to lose weight is learning to make choices and gaining control of your eating pattern, not giving it up. What matters in the end is the freedom to decide what foods to eat when *you* decide to eat them, not when someone else's menu plan decides you should.

Joining a weight-loss group is helpful to some people for the benefits of peer pressure. Before you join, assess the group's common sense and let good nutrition principles be your guide. Again, beware of get-thin-quick fads and scams.

Detecting Demon Diets
Here are some pointers to help you avoid fad diets. Watch out for these danger signs in a diet if:

- It advocates unusual eating patterns in an enthusiastic, often messianic fashion.

- It promotes a particular food or combination of foods as having special virtues. Such foods take on an aura of "super" or "wonder" foods.

- It eliminates certain nutritious foods from the diet, claiming that they are harmful.

- It relies on the testimony of individuals rather than on scientific study and makes false claims that are often difficult to spot because they are couched in scientific terminology.

- It is endorsed by pseudo-professionals and takes on a cult-like quality.

The results of diets that fill this bill are plain and simple: losing weight temporarily and regaining weight rapidly.

Loss Leaders

Here are some guidelines for choosing a good weight-loss program. Once you have made sure the program complies with these guidelines, embark on it only after you have discussed your choice with your physician.

- It follows the principles of the four food groups and meets the body's needs for nutrients rather than relying on supplements. It also advocates a sensible balance of protein to fat to carbohydrate.

- It advocates an adequate intake of calories. A diet of less than 1,000 calories a day should be followed only under a doctor or dietitian's supervision and only in rare instances.

- It assesses individual eating habits and nutrient requirements and takes the dieter's likes, dislikes, and lifestyle into consideration.

- There are few if any forbidden foods.

- It allows healthful snacks and emphasizes controlling portions.

- Its weight-loss claims are reasonable, that is, an average of one to two pounds a week.

- It attempts to change undesirable eating habits in order to initiate and then maintain weight loss on a long-term basis.

- It recommends exercise.

- It does not advocate special foods or treatments like hormone injections.

Staying Power
Once you have lost the amount of weight you wanted, maintaining your new body weight can be tricky. So here are some tips to help you:

- Beware of keeping a constant vigil over everything you eat. This is likely to result in a routine whereby you find yourself dieting from Monday to Friday and eating non-stop from Friday evening to Sunday night. This pattern is doomed to failure.

- Find a meal pattern that allows you to relax your vigil without causing you to gain weight. The best way to do this is to increase your intake by small amounts throughout the day and monitor your resulting hunger. If you find that dinner is your hungry time, eat a little extra at lunch and add an afternoon snack. This will help you establish an eating pattern in tune with your body's appetite that maintains a good weight.

- Keep tabs on your weight by weighing yourself once a week. If your weight inches up a pound or two, cut back on unnecessary treats. If your weight goes up four or five pounds, then you need to follow a more stringent plan for several weeks. Plan meals that keep fat at a minimum, and keep tabs on your hunger as a good sign of weight loss. The importance of preventing your weight from climbing more than five pounds above the ideal level cannot be overemphasized.

Winning the Losing Game
The best way to keep your weight where you want it is to eat right.

Eating right allows your body to regulate your weight so you won't be dieting for the rest of your life. You may have to lose a few pounds from time to time, but you won't be an obsessive dieter watching every mouthful. Once eating right becomes second nature, you and your body will become a harmonious team, choosing nutritious foods in the right amounts.

Follow the principles outlined in this book, and battling the bulge will be a struggle that is just plain history!

13   Food Fantasy

How easy things would be if there were a wonder food that could meet all our nutritional needs in one fell swoop. However, this kind of wishful thinking belongs in the wonderful world of fantasy, along with the princess and the pea and Love Potion No. 9!

The search for miracle foods that would relieve us of the often mundane responsibility of seeking out the right things to eat is understandable, but misguided. Here are some common fallacies and their accompanying facts.

Fallacy   Honey is a better choice of sweetening agent than white sugar because it is nutritionally superior.

Fact   Both honey and white sugar are simple sugars, of which the average North American eats too much. Honey does contain some vitamins and minerals, but in negligible amounts. A person would have to eat 50 tablespoons of honey, for example, to get the same amount of calcium as he or she would get from one ounce of cheddar or two-thirds of a cup of milk!

There are also some hazards associated with honey. It should not be fed to infants under one year of age because of the slight risk of botulism poisoning. Although extremely rare, such poisoning can occur if honey is a carrier of clostridium botulinum spores. These spores are not dangerous to adults but can cause constipation, progressive weakness, and ultimately respiratory arrest in infants. Corn syrup, which can also be a carrier of these spores, is not recommended to infants under one year for the same reasons. Research is currently being directed at a possible connection between Sudden Infant Death Syndrome and botulism poisoning in infants.

Honey's one nutritional advantage over sugar is that it is slightly sweeter and can thus be used in recipes in smaller amounts and for fewer calories.

Fallacy   Lecithin is a wonder product that can retard senility, aid in weight loss, and lower blood cholesterol.

Fact   Lecithin is a compound produced by the body and is therefore not an essential nutrient. It is found in many of the foods we eat, for example, eggs, meat, wheat, and legumes, and is used by the body to maintain cell structure.

Lecithin is useful in therapeutic doses to treat certain neurological disorders such as Huntingdon's disease and the senile dementia that occurs with Alzheimer's disease, where the body is deficient in *acetylcholine*, a substance the body manufactures from lecithin. This does not mean, however, that taking lecithin is beneficial to people without an acetylcholine deficiency.

Research has not yet proved that lecithin helps lower blood cholesterol substantially, whereas it has been shown that cholesterol is lowered by consumption of polyunsaturated fats and soluble fibres like oat bran.

Taking lecithin supplements as part of a weight-loss diet has only a placebo effect. They are ineffectual in a physical sense, but could give the dieter the incentive to stick to a low-calorie eating plan and lose weight. As with all placebos, however, lecithin is no substitute for will-power and common sense.

Fallacy   Bee pollen can act as an appetite suppressant to aid weight loss and can promote weight gain, prevent premature aging, aid in mental retardation, remedy bowel problems, increase energy levels, and help treat allergies.

Fact   The list of wonders attributed to bee pollen—the tiny seeds carried by bees from the flower to the hive—is as long as it is mind-boggling! However, the preceding and other purported merits of bee pollen have not been documented in scientific literature. What have been documented are cases of people who have had an allergic reaction to the bee pollen they took as a treatment for allergies!

Fallacy   Special dietary regimes and nutritional aids such as caffeine, bee pollen, vitamins, and minerals can give you the "racer's edge" in athletic competition.

Fact   First, one cannot discount the psychological edge that may be produced by the belief that a particular meal is the answer. It is not unusual for an athlete to try to reproduce the setting of a winning event by eating the identical precompetition meal time after time.

Caffeine is taken by many athletes prior to competition to enhance their performance, but in certain cases its ingestion may actually be a hindrance. Its effect depends on the amount consumed as well as the individual's body weight and caffeine sensitivity. Taking caffeine prior to an endurance event has been reported to allow an individual to exercise somewhat more intensely than he or she otherwise would. Caffeine may alter the perception of effort. In one study by exercise physiologist David Costill, participants were tested on a treadmill with and without caffeine taken prior to testing. The participants worked harder and performed better after consuming caffeine, yet they felt the effort they put forth was the same in both tests.

But consuming caffeine before an athletic event can have its drawbacks. Caffeine can lead to anxiety in sensitive individuals, and a nervous athlete may not perform as well. It can also have a dehydrating effect, which may impair performance. An acceptable caffeine intake for one person may be too great for another. The best way to find your tolerance is to try it in moderation while training, but not on the day of an important contest. Keep in mind, though, that high caffeine intakes have been associated with other health risks (see pages 179–82).

Bee pollen has had numerous wonders attributed to it, including increased athletic performance, all unsubstantiated.

As for vitamin and mineral supplements, it appears that for the well-nourished athlete a vitamin and mineral supplement is ineffective in enhancing performance. A study reported by L.M. Weight in February 1988 found that three months of multivitamin and mineral supplementation did not have any beneficial effect on the competitive male runners in the study. This finding has been corroborated by numerous other studies.

But in certain instances more attention should be paid to the vitamin and mineral status. An athlete who suffers from vitamin or mineral deficiencies will not perform at the height of his or her ability. For example, wrestlers who are trying to make their weight may turn to quick weight-loss diets. If these diets are repeated or prolonged, they may take their toll on the intake of certain essential nutrients. Individual tastes can also steer one in the wrong direction. Many athletes have shunned red meat in their pursuit of a low-fat diet. Their sources of iron in the diet may not be adequate, resulting in anemia. Because of the role of iron in the production of hemoglobin, which is necessary for oxygen transport by the blood, iron deficiency can lead to fatigue and specifically a reduction of aerobic capacity. Long-distance runners and female athletes generally seem also to be at risk and may be in need of iron supplementation. A diet rich in iron from alternate sources could avert this problem.

The effect of massive doses of vitamins and minerals on athletic performance has not been well-documented to date owing to the concern over possible ill effects that such testing may cause.

An athlete's goal is to be well-trained, but should he or she not be nutritionally conditioned too? There is no evidence to indicate that the racer's edge can be found in a tablet. Top-notch nutrition can separate the champion from the runner-up — and that is certainly easier to swallow!

Fallacy	Eating products made with oats and oat bran is a way of ensuring a lower blood cholesterol level.
Fact	Oat bran is just one of many foods that has cast a spell on North Americans, and while many believe it's the ultimate weapon in our fight against heart disease, soluble fibres are only a component of a heart-healthy diet.

As well, the amount and type of other ingredients besides oat bran should be looked at when buying an oat bran product. For example, check the amount of oat bran in a cereal boasting this product, and check whether or not the product contains saturated tropical oils.

Fallacy	Unbuttered popcorn is a better snack to have than potato chips.
Fact	Plain popcorn is virtually fat-free but some popcorn products are another matter. For example, natural-flavoured microwave popcorn can contain up to 56 percent fat while potato chips, a well-known high-fat snack, tallies in at a close 60 percent. Don't be fooled by the claim that a package contains air-popped popcorn. Read the labels to see how much fat is used in the preparation. One popular cheese popcorn, which is air-popped, contains as much fat and sodium as potato chips.

Accompanying the fat, in many cases, is its frequent

partner, salt. Popping your kernels in an air-popper or with a minimal amount of oil, and then adding your own toppings (see recipes on pages 264–65), is an easy way to save on fat and sodium.

Fallacy   Foods containing stearic acid, such as beef and chocolate, are actually good for your cholesterol.

Fact   Stearic acid is a saturated fat that lowered blood cholesterol when fed as a sole fat in a formula used in laboratory experiments. In the real world, however, it is found in the company of other saturated fats (e.g., palmitic acid), which are potent cholesterol raisers. When you read about various laboratory studies in the popular press, remember that we eat foods, not formulas. In some cases, research material cannot be directly applied to what we eat. These studies give researchers direction in which to look for answers.

Fallacy   Hair analysis can diagnose everything from heavy metal toxicity to nutritional deficiencies, headaches, and sallow skin.

Fact   Hair analysis may be a valuable diagnostic tool in the future because of the ease of obtaining and storing samples. The problem to date, however, has been that methods of analysis and interpretation have not been standardized. In addition, there are many factors that can affect the results of hair analysis. Trace minerals found in hair are affected by hair treatments (shampoo, colouring, conditioners, etc.) as well as environmental factors like air pollution and chlorinated water from a swimming pool.
    Until the results and interpretations of hair analysis have been standardized to reflect excesses or deficiencies, be wary of anyone who uses it as a test on you!

Fallacy   High-colonic enemas are helpful in ridding the body of toxins.

Fact   High-colonic enemas are the irrigation of the bowel with large amounts (more than 15 gallons) of water mixed with various herbs and enzymes. They are administered by some chiropractors, naturopaths, and self-styled "nutrition professionals," who claim that they wash toxins out of the body. The healthy way to maintain regular bowel movements and to rid one's body of waste products most efficiently is to eat a balanced diet that is high in fibre and water. High-colonic enemas are a risky procedure that could cause electrolyte and fluid imbalance as well as infection or even perforation of the bowel.

Fallacy   Herbs are a safe, natural way to treat ailments and are superior to pharmaceutical drugs.

Fact   Medication prescribed by a doctor, unlike a herbal remedy, is carefully tested for dosage and long-term effects before it is allowed on the market. Herbs, however, are readily available in unrestricted amounts and have not been reliably tested for dosage or long-term effects.

With all the concern these days about the caffeine contained in tea and coffee, many people are switching to herbal teas without being aware of their hazards. Allergic reactions to herbal teas are quite common; for example, drinking camomile tea, a member of the ragweed family, could adversely affect a person who suffers from hayfever.

Some herbal teas have even stranger properties. Coca leaf tea, for example, is a herbal tea packaged in Peru. Its ingredients are listed as "decocainized coca leaves," but random sampling in the United States has shown that these leaves do indeed contain some cocaine. In fact, most of the cocaine is released by simple infusion when the leaves are made into tea. Although two cups of coca leaf tea a day contain less cocaine than one intranasal dose and do not cause any serious side effects, cocaine ingested this way shows up in a urine test. It also causes mild stimulation, mood elevation, and increased heart rate.

In general, when drinking herbal teas as an alternative beverage, treat them the same way you would any others that contain caffeine—drink them in moderation and alternate them with other liquids.

Other herbs are taken as laxatives. Aloe vera, which causes intestinal cramping, could be dangerous to pregnant women because of its action on the abdominal muscles. Like other herbs that are purported to cure constipation, aloe vera is no substitute for a healthy diet in promoting regular bowel movements. If a laxative is absolutely necessary to cure constipation, then a pharmaceutical version that acts as a stimulant to the bowel is a wiser choice than a herbal one that does exactly the same thing, simply because the pharmaceutical version has been more thoroughly tested.

"Diet" teas—herbal products sold as aids for weight loss—simply act as laxatives, frequently causing cramps and diarrhea. They carry the added risk of water loss and dehydration. Drinking them is hardly a desirable way to lose weight and no different from the unhealthy practice of using an over-the-counter laxative to slim down!

When you cook with herbs, there is no danger as long as you use them in moderation. However, a Health and Welfare Canada committee researching the effects of all manner of herbs, from oregano to saffron, warns that some herbs eaten in large amounts can have toxic effects. Some herbs simply should not be consumed. For example, the *British Medical Journal* has told the story of a man who had been diagnosed as having digoxin toxicity, with the symptoms of headache, nausea, loss of appetite, and heart block. It was discovered that for many years, he had been concocting and drinking a special herbal tea containing foxglove. Equally dangerous are white poppy seeds and castor beans. Herbs that may be harmful to a fetus when consumed in abnormal amounts during pregnancy include parsley oil and oregano.

Fallacy   We all need a certain amount of refined sugar in our diets.

Fact   The body cannot differentiate between the simple sugars contained in fruit, vegetables, and milk and the sugars contained in refined products such as table sugar. It seems obvious then that we should opt for foods like fruits and vegetables that combine sugar with vitamins and minerals rather than choosing the refined sugar in a chocolate bar that consists almost entirely of empty calories. Remember that to identify the amount of sugar in a product, check the label for sucrose, fructose, glucose, dextrose, and maltose. Ingredients are listed in descending order of amount, so the closer a sugar is to the beginning of the list, the greater the amount.

Fallacy   Certain pills or aids such as amphetamines, thyroid extracts, bulk producers, diuretics, and injections of substances like human chorionic gonadotropin (HCG) are helpful in weight reduction.

Fact	Amphetamines act as stimulants and thereby cause a decrease in appetite. Their unfavourable side effects include nervousness, irritability, insomnia, and possible addiction. Thyroid extracts increase the metabolic rate and thus cause people to burn more calories—but not without negative side effects such as heart palpitations and hyperactivity.

Bulk producers do reduce appetite by causing a "full" sensation. What they don't do is help a person learn new, more healthful eating habits. If they are high in insoluble fibres and the person's diet is already low in certain trace minerals, they can lower the absorption of certain nutrients. Diuretics cause water loss, not fat loss. It is only temporary and can have side effects such as depletion of certain minerals, in particular potassium.

Injections of human chorionic gonadotropin, a sex hormone, are of no proven benefit when it comes to weight loss. It is rather the accompanying low-calorie diet, along with the psychological effects of daily visits to the therapist for injections, that cause any weight reduction. The exorbitant fees usually charged are added reason for the patient to believe that this diet really works! The hazards of these injections are the use of accompanying diuretics and a low-calorie diet lacking in nutrients.

Fallacy	Eating a little mouldy food won't hurt you. After all, penicillin comes from mouldy cheese.

Fact	Moulds are fungi that grow on a variety of vegetable and animal matter, especially under warm, moist conditions.

Recent research has shown that mouldy food can be extremely dangerous because of the toxins—called *mycotoxins*—that some moulds produce. Mycotoxins have been found to cause cancer in animal tests. They seep in and around the mould and cannot therefore simply be scraped off along with it. Some mycotoxins can survive in food for a long time, and some are not even destroyed by heat during cooking.

Here are some tips on avoiding the risk of mycotoxins on mouldy food. Don't buy foods with a musty odour or produce with bruises on the skin or signs of rot around the stems. Avoid nuts that are discoloured, and store nuts in a cool, dry place.

Avoid exposing cheese to air unnecessarily after use. It can become contaminated, and mould can grow days later, even in the fridge. If hard cheese develops a patch of mould, you can salvage the cheese by cutting the mould away to a depth of 1 inch (2.5 cm). Discard liquid or semi-solid foods like jam or maple syrup if you find mould on them. Discard wrappings that have been in contact with mouldy foods to prevent cross-contamination. The rule of thumb is: When in doubt, throw it out!

Fallacy   Sulphites used to preserve food are harmless.

Fact   Sulphites are chemicals used to preserve packaged foods and to retain the crisp texture and prevent the browning of fresh produce. They are used extensively to keep salad bars looking bright and perky and preserve potatoes prepared for commercial use. Sulphites are also used in the production of wine and beer.

Most people, it seems, are not sensitive to the effects of sulphites. There is a small segment of the population, however, that has such an adverse physical reaction to them that their use must be examined. Reactions include hives, stomach upset, shortness of breath, severe wheezing, and in extreme cases, even death. People at risk are frequently asthmatic.

Sulphites are listed among ingredients on packaged foods and are contained in the following additives: potassium bisulphite, potassium metabisulphite, sodium bisulphite, sodium metabisulphite, sodium sulphite, sodium dithionite, and sulphurous acid.

Because sulphites are often used in bulk foods for which there is no ingredient list, here is a list of foods in which they are often used: fresh and dried fruits and vegetables; alcoholic and fruit beverages; pastries and baked goods; jams, jellies, pickles, and relishes; mustards; molasses; frozen fish; and processed tomato products such as spaghetti sauce and tomato paste.

If you suspect that you are sensitive to sulphites, start looking for sources in your diet. Ask whether foods in a restaurant have been treated with sulphites, although you may or may not get an answer—it is often the suppliers who use them, a fact the management may not be aware of. It is a good idea, however, to let the restaurant know why you are avoiding a food that might contain sulphites in order to help increase awareness of the problem. Avoiding sulphite-containing processed foods will also help deter food companies from using them. And reporting any adverse reaction to foods containing sulphites to the appropriate government agency will also speed up efforts to determine the extent of public sensitivity.

Fallacy   "Natural" foods are better for you.

Fact   The word *natural* has become a catch-all and is often used by food companies eager to jump on the nutritional bandwagon. These companies are well aware of the increasing concern among consumers about the meaning of ingredient lists on the foods they buy. Worried about chemical additives as well as the nutritional content of packaged foods, the food-buying public is understandably drawn to foods that are as close to their natural states as possible.

But here's the hitch. There are no rules governing the use of the word *natural*, nothing that says that it must mean "unadulterated" or "minus food additives." As a result, it can mean almost anything. *Natural* can be just an adjective describing the noun it precedes. For example, "natural apple flavour" can be one of the ingredients in a dessert that is chock-full of additives. One thing the word *natural* does usually mean is a few cents added to the price of the food it's in. This is another case of "Food buyer beware!"

In general, it is best to opt for the fresh product whenever possible. However, all of us must eat processed foods in certain instances to attain a balanced diet, so we should choose nutritious foods that additives increase our use of. For example, the lecithin added to whole-milk powder helps it dissolve in water, and the sequestering agent used in canned lima beans helps to retain their colour. On the other hand, it's not essential to buy a salad dressing to which emulsifiers have been added so you won't have to shake it before use—a little elbow grease is a better solution than unnecessary additives. If you have a choice, for example, of canned cherries with or without added colouring, go for the unadulterated version. Exercise your power as a consumer. The more demand there is for processed foods free of additives, the more such foods will be produced.

Let's not forget that dismissing processed foods altogether is another case of throwing the baby out with the bath water. Processing adds to the variety of foods available to us—and variety and its cohort, moderation, are keys to healthful eating.

Fallacy	Eating plenty of grapefruit helps you lose weight.
Fact	Contrary to popular belief, grapefruit does not burn or melt fat! Even unsweetened grapefruit contains a fair amount of calories because of its sugar content. Its main virtue is a good dose of vitamins and minerals. Grapefruit, like the hot water and lemon juice recommended on some diets, has no magical powers to cause weight loss and must be included in a total calorie count like any other food.

Fallacy	Lead poisoning is passé.. Modern technology has eliminated the problem.
Fact	Anemia, memory loss, lack of concentration, and behavioural changes may all be a result of exposure to lead. The real risks of long-term exposure, though, to low levels of lead hasn't been determined yet, but one thing is for sure—the less the better. For most of us, much of the lead we're exposed to comes from our food. There are some simple ways to minimize the lead you consume.

First, the water you drink. Use only cold water for drinking and food preparation. Lead from pipes can leach into hot water more easily than cold. Run the cold water for a few minutes if the tap hasn't been used for several hours.

Canned foods can also be a source of lead, depending on where the food was canned. The canning industry in Canada no longer uses lead solder, so Canadians cans aren't a risk. But cans from other countries may contain lead, so it's wise to store them for no longer than one year. After opening, remove the food and store leftovers in other containers rather than an opened can.

The dishes you serve your food on may also be a source of lead. Lead-glazed pottery should be used for decoration, not for serving. Chances are that souvenir piece of pottery you picked up in a foreign country has a lead glaze. (See p. 185 for more on lead)

When you determine how much lead is toxic, you need to look at how much is absorbed. Adults generally absorb only about 10 percent of lead consumed while infants and young children absorb about 50 percent. You'll also absorb more if your intake of calcium and phosphorus are low. So as you can see, kids with poor diets can be much more at risk.

Fallacy	All barbecued food is bad for you.
Fact	How food is barbecued may affect the apparent carcinogenic effects of this cooking method. When fat drips onto a wood or charcoal fire, benzopyrene forms. This is a carcinogen that can get into the food through the smoke or flames. Smoked foods, such as meat and fish, can also contain benzopyrene. To minimize the risk of benzopyrene getting into your food when you are barbecuing, cook food slowly over a raised grill or wrap it in foil before cooking to avoid contact with the offending agents.

Fallacy	"Light" foods are lower in calories and a better nutritional choice.
Fact	Legislation governing the use of the word *light* is so vague that it can mean almost anything. Foods described this way can be legitimately fat-reduced, like certain salad dressings, or can actually be high in fat and sugar, like some "light" muffins that are actually cupcakes! A "light" pudding can be low in sugar and fat, but is certainly not once it has been baked into a pastry crust. This is another case of reading the label and "Food buyer beware": "light" may be describing the taste, colour, or texture of the food product, not the number of calories.

Fallacy	Natural calcium supplements, like bone meal and dolomite are superior to food sources of calcium because they contain the right magnesium-calcium balance for maximum calcium absorption.
Fact	First, valid scientific research has not shown that a specific magnesium-calcium balance affects calcium absorption. Second, bone meal and dolomite contain, along with calcium, toxic metals such as arsenic, cadmium, mercury, and lead. These substances could be dangerous to small children and pregnant women, who absorb them more readily, or to anyone who consumes them in excess.

The best way to consume adequate calcium is in food, but if you need a supplement, look for the amount of elemental calcium on the label. The amount of calcium in a supplement depends on the type of calcium. Calcium carbonate, for example, is 40 percent calcium, whereas calcium gluconate is only 9 percent. |

Fallacy	Foods labelled "Cholesterol Free" are a good choice for those on a heart-healthy diet.
Fact	These foods may be low in cholesterol, but they could be loaded with fat and not always healthy fat. True, they're not high in saturated fat; however, they could contain appreciable amounts of trans fatty acids (see p. 28).

(see p. 28)

Fallacy	Hypoglycemia is a very common condition.
Fact	Hypoglycemia is not a common medical condition, but some of the symptoms experienced by hypoglycemics may be common.

Hypoglycemia is a disease in which too much insulin is released into the bloodstream. This causes low blood sugar. Low blood sugar can also occur after an absence of food in the body or when too much sugar is eaten alone. As the blood sugar drops to low levels, symptoms such as headache, irritability, and nausea can progress to blackouts. The less severe symptoms can be experienced by people with poor eating habits, who could be mistakenly diagnosed as hypoglycemic. Going for hours on end without eating can cause many of the symptoms of hypoglycemia without the disease.

If you think you are hypoglycemic, see a physician. An improvement in eating habits can help alleviate symptoms for people who have the disease and for those who have not been eating properly.

The Bottom Line

Much as we might like to have total control over our bodies, this is not possible. Many diseases are the result of complex variables, which cannot be connected with what we eat or any other aspect of daily life that is within our control.

There are, nonetheless, many things we do to our bodies that clearly affect our health. Here are some of the ways we can adapt our lifestyles to the body's advantage:

- Maintain a healthy body weight.

- Decrease the amount of fat in our diets.

- Increase our intake of dietary fibre.

- Moderate our intake of sugar, caffeine, alcohol, and salt.

- Increase our exercise or activity levels.

- Eat small, balanced meals more often.

Simple as these guidelines are, however, there are many complexities in the whole matter of nutrition that we must keep in mind. With the continual barrage of scientific information that comes our way about the latest finding on this or that nutrient, it is easy to become confused. This is why we must be aware of the crucial ingredients in the recipe for a healthy diet—namely, moderation and balance.

The more we fool around with nutrients, the more we can disturb their balance. A nutrient may not be toxic by itself, but too much of it could disturb the balance of certain others. An example is the iron-zinc-copper balancing act. If you take too much iron in supplement form, you could upset your body's zinc status. Overdo the amount of zinc you ingest, as some food faddists recommend, and you could lower your HDL cholesterol levels and set the amount of copper in your body off kilter. The same applies to vitamin C.

And so the list continues.

What is the solution? Given that eating certain foods can contribute to better health and even help prevent disease, what is the ideal eating plan?

The answer is sweet and simple. Vary your diet,

while incorporating the nutrition guidelines listed above. I trust that this book will also help demystify what sometimes seems like a mind-boggling task.

Make changes gradually. The more changes you need to make, the longer the process will take. Plan to overhaul your eating habits meal by meal, habit by habit. One good method is to start at the beginning of the day with breakfast. Move on to lunch through the morning snack, then to the afternoon snack. Finally, work on that evening meal.

And if you need outside help, a dietitian can give terrific insights—not to mention moral support. Above all, learn to be in harmony with your body. Once you and it are a team, you'll have it made!

Appendixes

Food	Measure	Weight (g)	Water (%)	Energy (Kcal)	Protein (g)	Carbohydrate (g)	Fat (g)	SFA*
Milk, Cheese, Cream, Related Products — Cheese								
Cheese, blue		45	42	159	10	1	13	8
Cheese, brick		45	41	167	10	1	13	8
Cheese, camembert		45	52	135	9	tr	11	7
Cheese, cheddar		45	37	181	11	tr	15	9
Cheese, cheddar, grated	15 mL	7	37	28	2	tr	2	1
Cheese, cottage, creamed, 4.5% B.F.	250 mL	222	79	229	28	6	10	6
Cheese, cottage, 2% B.F.	250 mL	239	79	214	33	9	5	3
Cheese, cottage, dry curd, 0.4% B.F.	250 mL	153	80	129	26	3	tr	tr
Cheese, cream	15 mL	15	54	52	1	tr	5	3
Cheese, feta		45	53	123	7	2	10	7
Cheese, gouda		45	41	164	11	1	13	8
Cheese, gruyere		45	33	186	13	tr	15	9
Cheese, mozzarella, made with partly skimmed milk		45	52	118	11	1	7	5
Cheese, mozzarella		45	52	132	9	1	10	6
Cheese, muenster		45	42	166	11	tr	14	9
Cheese, parmesan, grated	15 mL	5	18	23	2	tr	2	tr
Cheese, provolone		45	41	158	12	tr	12	8
Cheese, ricotta, made with partly skimmed milk		45	74	62	5	2	4	2
Cheese, ricotta, made with whole milk		45	72	78	5	1	6	4
Cheese, swiss		45	37	169	13	2	12	8
Cheese: processed spread, cheddar	15 mL	15	48	44	2	1	3	2
Cheese: processed spread, made with skim milk	15 mL	15	—	29	4	2	tr	0
Cheese: processed food cheddar, cold pack		45	43	149	9	4	11	7

* Saturated fatty acids

PUFA* (g)	Cholesterol (mg)	Calcium (mg)	Iron (mg)	Sodium (mg)	Potassium (mg)	Vitamin A (RE)	Thiamin (mg)	Riboflavin (mg)	Niacin (NE)	Folate (mcg)	Vitamin C (mg)	Dietary Fibre (g)
tr	34	237	.1	628	115	103	.01	.17	2.8	16	0	—
tr	42	303	.2	252	61	136	tr	.16	2.5	9	0	—
tr	32	174	.1	379	84	113	.01	.22	2.6	28	0	—
tr	47	325	.3	279	44	136	.01	.17	2.4	8	0	—
tr	7	50	tr	43	7	21	tr	.03	.4	1	0	—
tr	33	133	.3	899	187	107	.05	.36	5.4	27	0	—
tr	20	164	.4	970	230	48	.06	.44	6.4	31	0	—
tr	10	49	.4	20	50	12	.04	.22	5.1	23	0	—
tr	16	12	.2	44	18	66	tr	.03	.2	2	0	—
tr	41	229	.3	519	29	60	.07	.39	2.0	15	0	—
tr	52	321	.1	376	55	80	.01	.15	2.7	10	0	—
tr	50	455	tr	151	36	135	.03	.13	3.2	5	0	—
tr	27	305	.1	217	39	82	tr	.14	2.7	4	0	—
tr	37	242	tr	175	31	113	tr	.11	2.2	3	0	—
tr	43	323	.2	282	60	142	tr	.14	2.5	5	0	—
tr	4	69	tr	93	5	9	tr	.02	.5	tr	0	—
tr	31	340	.2	394	62	119	tr	.14	2.7	5	0	—
tr	14	122	.2	56	56	51	tr	.08	1.0	6	0	—
tr	23	93	.2	38	47	60	tr	.09	1.0	5	0	—
tr	41	432	tr	117	50	114	.01	.16	3.0	3	0	—
tr	8	84	tr	244	36	28	tr	.07	.6	1	0	—
0	—	—	—	296	61	—	—	—	.9	—	0	—
tr	29	224	.4	435	163	91	.01	.20	2.2	2	0	—

* Polyunsaturated fatty acids

Food	Measure	Weight (g)	Water (%)	Energy (Kcal)	Protein (g)	Carbohydrate (g)	Fat (g)	SFA (g)
Cheese: processed, cheddar		45	39	169	10	tr	14	9
Cheese: processed, cheddar, made with skim milk		45	—	86	11	4	3	—
Cheese: processed, swiss		45	42	150	11	tr	11	7
Milk, Cheese, Cream, Related Products — Cream								
Cream, cereal (half & half), 12% B.F.	250 mL	256	80	344	8	11	31	19
Cream, cereal (half & half), 12% B.F.	15mL	15	80	20	tr	tr	2	1
Cream, sour, 14% B.F.	250 mL	253	74	475	8	11	46	28
Cream, sour, 14% B.F.	15 mL	15	74	28	tr	tr	3	2
Cream, table (coffee), 18% B.F.	250 mL	253	75	467	7	10	46	28
Cream, table (coffee), 18% B.F.	15 mL	15	75	28	tr	tr	3	2
Cream, whipped topping pressurized	15 mL	4	61	10	tr	tr	tr	tr
Cream, whipping, 35% B.F.	250 mL	251	60	822	5	7	88	55
Cream, whipping, 35% B.F.	15 mL	15	60	49	tr	tr	5	3
Milk, Cheese, Cream, Related Products — Frozen Desserts								
Ice cream, vanilla, hard, rich, 16% B.F.	125 mL	78	59	184	2	17	12	8
Ice cream, vanilla, hard, 10% B.F.	125 mL	70	61	142	3	17	8	5
Ice milk, vanilla soft serve	125 mL	92	69	129	4	20	4	2
Sherbet, orange	125 mL	102	66	143	1	31	2	1
Milk, Cheese, Cream, Related Products — Imitation Cream Products								
Coffee whitener, (nondairy), liquid, frozen	15 mL	15	77	20	tr	2	1	1
Coffee whitener, (nondairy), powdered	5 mL	2	2	11	tr	1	tr	tr
Dessert topping, (nondairy), powdered + whole milk	15 mL	5	67	9	tr	tr	tr	tr
Dessert topping, (nondairy), semisolid (frozen)	15 mL	5	50	16	tr	1	1	1

PUFA (g)	Cholesterol (mg)	Calcium (mg)	Iron (mg)	Sodium (mg)	Potassium (mg)	Vitamin A (RE)	Thiamin (mg)	Riboflavin (mg)	Niacin (NE)	Folate (mcg)	Vitamin C (mg)	Dietary Fibre (g)
tr	42	277	.2	644	73	131	.01	.16	2.5	4	0	—
—	—	253	.1	693	133	47	.02	.19	1.2	—	0	—
tr	38	347	.3	617	97	103	tr	.12	2.7	3	0	—
1	99	267	.2	105	331	286	.09	.38	2.0	5	2	—
tr	6	16	tr	6	19	17	tr	.02	.1	tr	tr	—
2	106	283	.2	123	352	424	.09	.38	2.0	28	2	—
tr	6	17	tr	7	21	25	tr	.02	.1	2	tr	—
2	155	247	.1	102	312	429	.08	.37	1.8	5	2	—
tr	9	15	tr	6	19	25	tr	.02	.1	tr	tr	—
tr	3	4	tr	5	6	8	tr	tr	tr	tr	0	—
3	322	166	tr	90	206	953	.06	.29	1.3	10	1	—
tr	19	10	tr	5	12	57	tr	.02	tr	tr	tr	—
tr	46	80	tr	57	116	115	.02	.15	.6	1	tr	—
tr	31	92	tr	61	135	70	.03	.17	.7	1	tr	—
tr	13	124	.1	73	186	37	.05	.24	.9	2	tr	—
tr	7	55	.2	47	105	20	.02	.05	.3	7	2	—
0	0	1	tr	12	29	1	.00	.00	tr	0	0	—
0	0	tr	tr	4	16	tr	.00	tr	tr	0	0	—
tr	tr	5	tr	3	8	2	tr	tr	tr	tr	tr	—
tr	0	tr	tr	1	tr	4	.00	.00	tr	0	0	—

Food	Measure	Weight (g)	Water (%)	Energy (Kcal)	Protein (g)	Carbohydrate (g)	Fat (g)	SFA (g)
Dessert topping, (nondairy), whipped, pressurized	15 mL	4	60	11	tr	tr	tr	tr
Milk, Cheese, Cream, Related Products — Milk Beverages								
Eggnog, commercial	250 mL	268	74	361	10	36	20	12
Milk, chocolate, partly skimmed, 2% B.F.	250 mL	264	84	189	8	27	5	3
Milk, hot cocoa, made with whole milk	250 mL	264	82	230	10	27	10	6
Milk, malted, made with whole milk	250 mL	280	81	250	11	28	11	6
Milk, shake, chocolate thick, commercial type	250 mL	211	72	250	6	45	6	4
Milk, shake, vanilla, thick, commercial type	250 mL	207	74	231	8	37	6	4
Milk, Cheese, Cream, Related Products — Milk Desserts								
Pudding mix, low calorie, prepared with skim milk	125 mL	137	78	137	4	27	3	tr
Pudding, canned, chocolate	125 mL	132	68	191	3	28	10	9
Pudding, canned, vanilla	125 mL	132	69	205	2	31	9	9
Pudding, cornstarch, cooked	125 mL	137	70	170	5	31	4	2
Pudding, cornstarch, instant + whole milk	125 mL	137	69	171	4	33	3	2
Pudding, custard, baked	125 mL	140	77	161	8	16	8	4
Pudding, rice with raisins	125 mL	140	66	204	5	37	4	2
Pudding, tapioca (minute)	125 mL	87	72	117	4	15	4	2
Milk, Cheese, Cream, Related Products — Milk Fluids								
Milk, buttermilk	250 mL	259	90	105	9	12	2	1
Milk, goat, whole	250 mL	258	87	178	9	11	11	7
Milk, human, whole, mature	250 mL	260	88	181	3	18	11	5
Milk, partly skimmed, 2% B.F.	250 mL	258	89	128	9	12	5	3
Milk, skim	250 mL	259	91	90	9	13	tr	tr
Milk, soybean, fluid	250 mL	258	92	85	9	6	4	0
Milk, whole, 3.3% B.F.	250 mL	258	88	159	8	12	9	5

PUFA (g)	Cholesterol (mg)	Calcium (mg)	Iron (mg)	Sodium (mg)	Potassium (mg)	Vitamin A (RE)	Thiamin (mg)	Riboflavin (mg)	Niacin (NE)	Folate (mcg)	Vitamin C (mg)	Dietary Fibre (g)
tr	0	tr	tr	2	tr	2	.00	.00	tr	0	0	—
tr	157	348	.5	146	443	214	.09	.51	2.7	2	4	—
tr	18	300	.6	159	446	150	.10	.43	2.3	13	2	—
tr	35	315	.8	130	507	90	.11	.46	2.6	13	3	—
tr	39	367	.3	228	559	98	.22	.57	3.9	23	2	—
tr	22	279	.7	234	473	44	.10	.47	1.8	10	0	—
tr	24	302	.2	197	378	58	.06	.40	2.2	14	0	—
tr	2	197	.7	190	194	21	.04	.21	.1	8	tr	—
tr	tr	69	1.1	265	236	29	.04	.16	1.1	—	tr	—
tr	tr	73	.2	284	144	tr	.03	.11	.9	—	tr	—
tr	16	140	.4	177	186	53	.03	.21	1.0	4	tr	—
tr	15	197	.7	170	177	53	.04	.21	.9	4	1	—
tr	147	157	.6	111	204	147	.06	.27	1.5	10	tr	—
tr	15	137	.6	99	248	46	.04	.20	1.2	7	0	—
tr	84	91	.3	136	117	76	.04	.16	.9	5	tr	—
tr	9	301	.1	272	392	21	.09	.40	1.7	13	3	—
tr	29	344	.1	128	527	144	.12	.36	2.6	2	3	—
1	36	84	tr	44	133	166	.04	.09	1.2	14	13	—
tr	19	314	.1	129	398	147	.10	.43	2.2	13	2	—
tr	5	320	.1	133	429	158	.09	.36	2.3	13	3	—
0	0	54	2.1	0	506	10	.21	.08	2.1	8	0	—
tr	35	308	.1	126	391	80	.10	.42	2.2	13	2	—

Food	Measure	Weight (g)	Water (%)	Energy (Kcal)	Protein (g)	Carbohydrate (g)	Fat (g)	SFA (g)
Milk, Cheese, Cream, Related Products — Milk Processed								
Milk, condensed, sweetened, canned	250 mL	323	27	1036	26	176	28	18
Milk, dry, skim, powder, instantized	25G->250 mL	25	91	90	9	13	tr	tr
Milk, dry, whole	15 mL	8	2	40	2	3	2	1
Milk, evaporated, whole, 7.6% B.F. undiluted	250 mL	266	74	357	18	27	20	12
Milk, evaporated, 2% B.F. undiluted	250 mL	268	78	246	20	30	5	3
Milk, evaporated, skim 0.2% B.F. undiluted	250 mL	270	79	210	20	31	tr	tr
Milk, Cheese, Cream, Related Products — Yogurt								
Yogurt, coffee and vanilla varieties, 1.25% B.F.		125	79	107	6	17	2	1
Yogurt, frozen, fruit, 6.3% B.F.	125 mL	125	—	148	4	23	5	—
Yogurt, fruit flavour, 1.4% B.F.		125	74	131	6	23	2	1
Yogurt, plain, 1.5% B.F.		125	85	79	7	9	2	1
Eggs								
Egg, large, fried in butter	1 egg	46	72	83	5	tr	6	2
Egg, large, raw/cooked in shell, without shell	1 egg	50	75	79	6	tr	6	2
Egg, large, scrambled, + milk + butter	1 egg	64	76	95	6	1	7	3
Egg, white, large, raw or cooked in shell	1 white	33	88	16	3	tr	tr	0
Egg, yolk, large, raw/cooked in shell	1 yolk	17	49	63	3	tr	6	2
Egg: substitute, frozen (yolk replaced)	egg = 60 mL	61	73	97	7	2	7	1
Meat, Poultry, Fish, Shellfish, Related Products — Assorted Meat Products								
Bologna, beef and pork	SL 11DMX.2	22	54	70	3	tr	6	2
Bologna, turkey	SL 11DMX.2	22	65	44	3	tr	3	1
Ham, luncheon meat, sliced, packaged	SL11X11X.2	27	65	49	5	tr	3	tr

PUFA (g)	Cholesterol (mg)	Calcium (mg)	Iron (mg)	Sodium (mg)	Potassium (mg)	Vitamin A (RE)	Thiamin (mg)	Riboflavin (mg)	Niacin (NE)	Folate (mcg)	Vitamin C (mg)	Dietary Fibre (g)
1	109	916	.6	410	1200	262	.29	1.34	6.7	36	8	—
tr	5	308	tr	137	426	178	.10	.44	2.3	12	1	—
tr	8	73	tr	30	106	22	.02	.10	.5	3	tr	—
tr	78	694	.5	281	806	144	.13	.84	4.8	21	44	—
tr	21	738	.6	296	851	314	.12	.84	5.1	23	44	—
tr	10	782	.8	311	895	316	.12	.83	5.3	23	44	—
tr	6	214	tr	82	274	16	.05	.25	.7	13	tr	—
—	—	145	—	63	199	—	.03	.27	.2	—	4	—
tr	7	211	tr	81	270	19	.05	.25	.7	13	tr	—
tr	8	228	.1	88	292	20	.06	.27	.8	14	1	—
tr	246	26	.9	144	58	83	.03	.13	1.5	22	0	—
tr	274	28	1.0	69	65	78	.04	.15	1.6	33	0	—
tr	248	47	.9	155	85	89	.04	.16	1.6	22	tr	—
0	0	4	tr	50	45	0	tr	.09	.9	5	0	—
tr	272	26	.9	8	15	94	.04	.07	.7	26	0	—
4	1	44	1.2	122	130	82	.07	.24	1.8	10	tr	—
tr	12	3	.3	224	40	0	.04	.03	1.0	1	5	—
tr	22	18	.3	193	44	0	.01	.04	1.2	2	0	—
tr	15	2	.3	356	90	0	.23	.07	2.4	tr	8	—

Food	Measure	Weight (g)	Water (%)	Energy (Kcal)	Protein (g)	Carbohydrate (g)	Fat (g)	SFA (g)
Liverwurst	15 mL	15	52	49	2	tr	4	2
Salami, cooked, beef and pork	SL 11DMX.2	22	60	55	3	tr	4	2
Salami, cooked, turkey	SL 11DMX.2	22	66	43	4	tr	3	tr
Salami, dry type	SL 4.5DMX.3	6	35	25	1	tr	2	tr
Sausages, beef & pork, cooked, 16 per 500 g package	1 sausage	15	45	59	2	tr	5	2
Sausages, pork, cooked 16 per 500 g package	1 sausage	15	45	55	3	tr	5	2
Wieners, beef and pork 12 per 450 g package	1 weiner	37	54	118	4	tr	11	4
Wieners, chicken, 12 per 450 g package	1 wiener	37	58	95	5	3	7	2
Wieners, turkey, 12 per 450 g package	1 wiener	37	63	84	5	tr	7	2
Meat, Poultry, Fish, Shellfish, Related Products — Beef								
Beef, corned, brisket, cooked		90	60	226	16	tr	17	6
Beef, corned, canned	4 slices	84	58	210	23	0	13	5
Beef, corned, hash with potatoes	250 mL	232	67	420	20	25	26	13
Beef, ground, lean, broiled, medium	1 8DMX1.5	88	59	212	23	0	13	5
Beef, ground, regular, broiled, medium	1 8DMX1.5	88	54	254	21	0	18	7
Beef, roast, blade, lean and fat, braised	2 11X6X0.6	88	49	286	25	0	20	8
Beef, roast, blade, lean only, braised	2 11X6X0.6	88	55	229	28	0	12	5
Halibut, broiled with butter or margarine	PC 12X7X1	92	67	157	23	0	6	4
Herring, smoked, kippered	11X4X0.6	55	61	116	12	0	7	1
Lobster, canned	150 mL	92	77	87	17	tr	1	0
Mackerel, canned, solids and liquid	150 mL	95	66	174	18	0	11	3
Oysters, raw, meat only	9 small	90	85	59	8	3	2	tr

PUFA (g)	Cholesterol (mg)	Calcium (mg)	Iron (mg)	Sodium (mg)	Potassium (mg)	Vitamin A (RE)	Thiamin (mg)	Riboflavin (mg)	Niacin (NE)	Folate (mcg)	Vitamin C (mg)	Dietary Fibre (g)
tr	24	4	1.0	129	26	1245	.04	.16	1.0	5	0	—
tr	14	3	.6	234	44	0	.05	.08	1.2	tr	3	—
tr	18	4	.4	221	54	0	.01	.04	1.4	tr	0	—
tr	5	tr	tr	112	23	0	.04	.02	.5	tr	2	—
tr	11	2	.2	121	28	0	.05	.02	.8	tr	0	—
tr	12	5	.2	194	54	0	.11	.04	1.1	tr	tr	—
1	19	4	.4	414	62	0	.07	.04	1.5	1	10	—
1	37	35	.7	507	31	14	.02	.04	1.8	1	0	—
2	40	39	.7	528	66	0	.02	.07	2.2	3	0	—
tr	88	7	1.7	1021	131	—	.02	.15	5.2	—	0	—
tr	72	—	1.7	845	114	0	.02	.12	5.5	—	1	—
tr	77	30	4.6	1253	464	0	.02	.21	8.6	30	0	—
tr	74	6	2.1	62	275	—	.05	.24	9.1	8	0	—
tr	79	10	2.1	73	257	—	.03	.17	9.4	8	0	—
tr	91	13	2.6	43	240	—	.06	.21	6.3	4	0	—
tr	93	16	3.1	51	287	—	.07	.25	7.5	5	0	—
tr	55	15	.7	123	483	188	.05	.06	11.9	11	0	—
1	60	36	.8	3427	86	5	.01	.15	4.1	9	0	—
0	78	60	.7	193	166	0	.09	.06	4.5	16	0	—
—	89	176	2.0	70	399	123	.06	.20	8.9	12	0	—
tr	45	85	5.0	66	109	84	.13	.16	3.6	—	27	—

Food	Measure	Weight (g)	Water (%)	Energy (Kcal)	Protein (g)	Carbohydrate (g)	Fat (g)	SFA (g)
Perch, ocean, frozen, breaded, fried, reheated	PC 17X5X1	93	43	297	18	15	18	5
Salmon, canned, solids and liquid	150 mL	95	64	193	21	0	12	2
Salmon, fresh, broiled or baked with butter or margarine	PC 12X7X1	92	63	167	25	0	7	2
Sardines, canned in oil, solids only	7 medium	84	62	171	20	0	9	2
Scallops, steamed	7 scallops	90	73	101	21	3	1	0
Shrimp, canned solids	28 medium	90	70	104	22	tr	tr	tr
Shrimp, french fried, batter dipped	11 large	88	57	198	18	9	10	3
Sole, baked with lemon juice, without added fat	1 fillet	90	78	85	18	tr	1	tr
Trout, lake, broiled or baked	PC 17X5X1	93	71	201	21	tr	13	6
Tuna, canned in oil, drained solids	125 mL	85	61	167	24	0	7	2
Tuna, canned in water, drained solids	125 mL	85	63	135	30	0	1	tr
Whitefish, baked, stuffed	PC 12X7X1	92	63	198	14	5	13	4

Meat, Poultry, Fish, Shellfish, Related Products — Lamb

Food	Measure	Weight (g)	Water (%)	Energy (Kcal)	Protein (g)	Carbohydrate (g)	Fat (g)	SFA (g)
Lamb, leg, roasted, lean and fat	2SL 11X6X.6	87	54	243	22	0	16	9
Lamb, leg, roasted, lean only	2SL 11X6X.6	87	62	162	25	0	6	3
Lamb, loin chop, broiled, lean and fat	198G RAW	118	47	424	26	0	35	19
Lamb, loin chop, broiled, lean only	198G RAW	87	62	164	25	0	7	4
Lamb, shoulder, roasted, lean and fat	3SL 7X6X.6	83	50	281	18	0	23	13
Lamb, shoulder, roasted, lean only	3SL 7X6X.6	83	61	170	22	0	8	5

Meat, Poultry, Fish, Shellfish, Related Products — Organ and Glandular Meats

Food	Measure	Weight (g)	Water (%)	Energy (Kcal)	Protein (g)	Carbohydrate (g)	Fat (g)	SFA (g)
Heart, beef, simmered	150 mL pc	92	64	161	26	tr	5	2
Kidney, beef, simmered	150 mL pc	89	69	128	23	tr	3	tr

PUFA (g)	Cholesterol (mg)	Calcium (mg)	Iron (mg)	Sodium (mg)	Potassium (mg)	Vitamin A (RE)	Thiamin (mg)	Riboflavin (mg)	Niacin (NE)	Folate (mcg)	Vitamin C (mg)	Dietary Fibre (g)
54	31	1.2	142	264	0	.09	.10	4.9	8	0	—	
35	146	.9	70	399	67	.03	.15	10.8	25	0	—	
43	117	1.1	107	408	44	.15	.06	13.6	24	0	—	
118	367	2.4	691	496	55	.03	.17	8.2	13	0	—	
48	104	2.7	239	428	27	.09	.05	5.0	15	0	—	
135	104	2.8	126	110	16	tr	.03	5.6	18	0	—	
132	63	1.8	164	202	0	.04	.07	5.7	17	0	—	
62	14	.3	107	303	11	.05	.09	5.1	—	1	—	
58	47	4.7	85	272	89	.11	.25	5.4	12	3	—	
55	7	1.6	680	256	20	.04	.10	14.6	13	0	—	
48	17	.6	468	255	32	.03	.10	16.9	—	0	—	
40	33	.5	179	268	552	.10	.10	4.7	12	0	—	
85	10	1.5	54	247	0	.13	.24	8.8	2	0	—	
87	11	1.9	61	280	0	.14	.26	10.0	2	0	—	
116	11	1.5	64	291	0	.14	.27	10.7	2	0	—	
87	10	1.7	60	275	0	.13	.24	9.8	2	0	—	
81	8	1.0	44	202	0	.11	.19	7.2	6	0	—	
83	10	1.6	55	249	0	.13	.23	8.8	6	0	—	
178	6	6.9	58	2	0	.13	1.42	8.7	2	1	—	
344	15	6.5	119	159	332	.17	3.61	10.5	87	tr	—	

Food	Measure	Weight (g)	Water (%)	Energy (Kcal)	Protein (g)	Carbohydrate (g)	Fat (g)	SFA (g)
Kidney, pork, braised	150 mL pc	89	69	134	23	0	4	1
Liver, calves, fried	3SL 8X6X.6	95	51	248	28	4	13	3
Liver, chicken, simmered	5 livers	100	68	157	24	tr	5	2
Liver, pork, braised	1 16X6X1	86	64	142	22	3	4	1
Meat, Poultry, Fish, Shellfish, Related Products — Pork, Cured								
Bacon, back, sliced, grilled	1 slice	23	62	43	6	tr	2	tr
Bacon, side, pan-fried crisp	2 slices	13	13	75	4	tr	6	2
Ham, roasted, lean only	2SL11X6X.6	87	68	128	19	tr	5	2
Ham, roasted, lean and fat	2SL11X6X.6	87	58	211	19	0	15	5
Meat, Poultry, Fish, Shellfish, Related Products — Pork, Fresh								
Pork, loin, centre cut chop, lean and fat, broiled	1 chop	87	50	275	24	0	19	7
Pork, loin, centre cut chop, lean only, broiled	1 chop	72	57	166	23	0	8	3
Pork, shoulder, whole, roasted, lean and fat	3SL 8X6X.6	86	52	280	19	0	22	8
Pork, shoulder, whole, roasted, lean only	3SL 8X6X.6	86	59	210	22	0	13	4
Pork, spareribs, braised, lean and fat	2 medium	70	40	278	20	0	21	8
Meat, Poultry, Fish, Shellfish, Related Products — Poultry								
Chicken, broiler/fryer breast, meat only, roasted	1/2	86	65	142	27	0	3	tr
Chicken, broiler/fryer breast, meat + skin + batter, fried	1/2	140	52	364	35	13	18	5
Chicken, broiler/fryer breast, meat + skin, roasted	1/2	98	62	193	29	0	8	2
Chicken broiler/fryer drumstick, meat only, roasted	2	88	67	151	25	0	5	1
Chicken, canned, boned with broth	100 mL	87	69	144	19	0	7	2
Turkey roll, light and dark meat	2 slices	57	70	85	10	1	4	1
Turkey, all classes, dark meat only, roasted	2 slices	86	63	161	25	0	6	2

PUFA (g)	Cholesterol (mg)	Calcium (mg)	Iron (mg)	Sodium (mg)	Potassium (mg)	Vitamin A (RE)	Thiamin (mg)	Riboflavin (mg)	Niacin (NE)	Folate (mcg)	Vitamin C (mg)	Dietary Fibre (g)
tr	427	12	4.7	71	127	69	.35	1.41	10.0	36	9	—
tr	416	12	13.5	112	430	9320	.23	3.96	20.8	190	35	—
tr	631	14	8.5	51	140	4913	.15	1.75	10.2	770	16	—
tr	305	9	15.4	42	129	4643	.22	1.89	12.5	140	20	—
tr	13	2	.2	356	90	0	.19	.05	2.5	tr	5	—
tr	11	2	.2	207	63	0	.09	.04	1.6	tr	4	—
tr	45	6	.7	1319	323	0	.81	.20	8.5	3	0	—
2	54	6	.8	1033	249	0	.52	.19	7.4	3	0	—
2	84	3	.7	61	312	3	.87	.24	9.5	4	tr	—
tr	71	4	.7	56	302	1	.83	.22	9.2	4	tr	—
3	83	6	1.1	58	261	2	.46	.27	7.5	3	tr	—
2	83	7	1.3	65	303	2	.50	.31	8.6	4	tr	—
2	85	33	1.3	65	224	2	.29	.27	8.4	3	0	—
tr	73	13	.9	64	220	5	.06	.10	17.0	3	0	—
4	119	28	1.8	385	281	28	.16	.20	21.4	8	0	—
2	82	14	1.0	70	240	26	.07	.12	18.0	4	0	—
1	82	11	1.1	84	216	16	.07	.21	10.2	8	0	—
2	54	12	1.4	438	120	30	.01	.11	9.0	3	2	—
1	31	18	.8	334	154	0	.05	.16	4.6	3	0	—
2	73	28	2.0	68	249	0	.05	.21	7.8	8	0	—

Food	Measure	Weight (g)	Water (%)	Energy (Kcal)	Protein (g)	Carbohydrate (g)	Fat (g)	SFA (g)
Turkey, all classes, light meat only, roasted	2 slices	86	66	135	26	0	3	tr

Meat, Poultry, Fish, Shellfish, Related Products — Veal

Food	Measure	Weight (g)	Water (%)	Energy (Kcal)	Protein (g)	Carbohydrate (g)	Fat (g)	SFA (g)
Veal, loin, cutlet or chop, broiled	1 PC 7X6X2	92	59	215	24	0	12	6
Veal, round with rump, broiled	2SL 11X6X.6	87	60	188	24	0	10	5

Lentils, Nuts and Seeds — Dry Beans

Food	Measure	Weight (g)	Water (%)	Energy (Kcal)	Protein (g)	Carbohydrate (g)	Fat (g)	SFA (g)
Beans, common white, cooked, drained	250 mL	195	69	230	15	41	1	tr
Beans, lima, dry, cooked, drained	250 mL	201	64	277	16	51	1	tr
Beans, red kidney, cooked, drained	250 mL	195	69	230	15	42	tr	tr
Chickpeas (garbanzos), boiled, drained	250 mL	172	60	285	16	47	4	tr
Lentils, cooked, drained	250 mL	211	72	224	16	41	1	tr
Soybeans, mature seeds cooked, drained	250 mL	190	71	247	21	21	11	2
Tofu	PC 7X6X2	89	85	63	7	2	4	tr

Lentils, Nuts and Seeds — Dry Peas

Food	Measure	Weight (g)	Water (%)	Energy (Kcal)	Protein (g)	Carbohydrate (g)	Fat (g)	SFA (g)
Peas, split, cooked	250 mL	211	70	243	17	44	tr	tr

Lentils, Nuts and Seeds — Nuts

Food	Measure	Weight (g)	Water (%)	Energy (Kcal)	Protein (g)	Carbohydrate (g)	Fat (g)	SFA (g)
Almonds, shelled, whole	125 mL	75	4	442	15	15	39	4
Brazil nuts, raw	125 mL	74	3	485	11	9	49	12
Cashew nuts, roasted	125 mL	69	4	397	11	20	33	7
Coconut, dried, sweetened, shredded	125 mL	49	13	245	1	23	17	15
Nuts, mixed, dry roasted, with peanuts	125 mL	72	2	428	12	18	37	5
Nuts, mixed, dry roasted, with peanuts, salt added	125 mL	72	2	428	12	18	37	5
Nuts, mixed, oil roasted with peanuts, salt added	125 mL	75	2	463	13	16	42	7
Peanut butter	15 mL	16	1	95	5	3	8	1

PUFA (g)	Cholesterol (mg)	Calcium (mg)	Iron (mg)	Sodium (mg)	Potassium (mg)	Vitamin A (RE)	Thiamin (mg)	Riboflavin (mg)	Niacin (NE)	Folate (mcg)	Vitamin C (mg)	Dietary Fibre (g)
tr	59	16	1.2	55	262	0	.05	.11	10.8	5	0	—
tr	93	10	2.9	60	272	0	.06	.23	9.4	5	0	—
tr	88	10	2.8	58	264	0	.06	.22	9.0	5	0	—
tr	0	98	5.3	14	811	0	.27	.14	4.1	89	0	12.3
tr	0	58	6.2	4	1230	0	.26	.12	4.4	91	0	10.9
tr	0	74	4.7	6	663	1	.22	.12	4.2	91	0	15.4
2	0	84	5.2	12	501	tr	.19	.10	3.9	—	0	—
tr	0	53	4.4	27	525	4	.15	.13	4.3	71	0	7.8
6	0	139	5.1	4	1026	6	.40	.17	5.0	117	0	—
2	0	80	1.7	6	37	0	.05	.03	1.3	—	0	—
tr	0	23	3.6	27	625	8	.32	.19	5.0	23	0	9.9
8	0	200	2.7	8	549	0	1.6	.58	7.0	44	tr	5.4
8	0	130	2.5	1	444	0	.74	.09	4.4	3	tr	—
6	0	28	2.8	12	366	0	.29	.12	4.1	47	0	—
tr	0	7	.9	128	165	0	.02	.01	.5	4	tr	—
8	0	50	2.7	9	430	tr	.14	.14	6.6	36	tr	—
8	0	50	2.7	482	430	tr	.14	.14	6.6	36	tr	—
0	0	81	2.4	489	436	2	.37	.17	6.9	62	tr	—
2	0	5	.3	3	110	0	.02	.02	3.1	13	0	—

Food	Measure	Weight (g)	Water (%)	Energy (Kcal)	Protein (g)	Carbohydrate (g)	Fat (g)	SFA (g)
Peanut butter, salt added	15 mL	16	1	95	5	3	8	1
Peanuts, oil roasted	125 mL	77	2	447	21	14	38	5
Peanuts, oil roasted, salt added	125 mL	77	2	447	21	14	38	5
Pecans, halves	125 mL	57	5	380	4	10	39	3
Pistachio nuts, dry roasted, salt added	125 mL	68	2	412	10	19	36	5
Walnuts, english, chopped	15 mL	6	4	39	tr	1	4	tr
Walnuts, english, halves	125 mL	53	4	340	8	10	33	3
Lentils, Nuts and Seeds — Seeds								
Pumpkin and squash, seed kernels, dry	125 mL	73	7	395	18	13	33	6
Sesame butter (tahini) from unroasted kernels	15 mL	14	3	85	3	3	8	1
Sesame seeds, dry	125 mL	79	5	465	21	7	43	6
Sunflower seed kernels, dry	125 mL	76	5	433	17	14	38	4
Vegetables, Related Products								
Alfalfa seeds, sprouted with seed, raw	250 mL	35	91	10	1	1	tr	tr
Asparagus, boiled, drained spears	4 1CM DM	60	92	15	2	3	tr	tr
Asparagus, canned, drained pieces	250 mL	256	94	49	5	6	2	tr
Bamboo shoots, canned, drained solids	250 mL	138	94	26	2	4	tr	tr
Bean sprouts, mung, boiled, drained	250 mL	131	93	28	3	5	tr	tr
Beans, lima, boiled, drained	250 mL	180	67	221	12	43	tr	tr
Beans, snap, green/yellow/ italian, boiled, drained	250 mL	132	89	46	2	10	tr	tr
Beans, snap, green/yellow/ italian, canned, drained	250 mL	144	93	29	2	6	tr	tr
Beets, canned, sliced, drained	250 mL	180	91	56	2	13	tr	tr
Beets, diced or sliced boiled, drained	250 mL	180	91	56	2	12	tr	tr
Beets, greens, boiled, drained	250 mL	152	89	41	4	8	tr	tr

UFA (g)	Cholesterol (mg)	Calcium (mg)	Iron (mg)	Sodium (mg)	Potassium (mg)	Vitamin A (RE)	Thiamin (mg)	Riboflavin (mg)	Niacin (NE)	Folate (mcg)	Vitamin C (mg)	Dietary Fibre (g)
0	5	.3	75	110	0	.02	.02	3.1	13	0	—	
0	66	1.5	12	541	0	.23	.08	15.6	81	0	6.2	
0	66	1.5	333	541	0	.23	.08	15.6	81	0	6.2	
0	21	1.2	tr	223	7	.48	.07	2.4	22	1	—	
0	48	2.2	530	650	16	.29	.17	3.3	40	5	—	
0	6	.1	tr	30	tr	.02	tr	.3	4	tr	—	
0	50	1.3	5	266	6	.20	.08	2.2	35	2	—	
0	31	10.9	13	589	28	.15	.23	6.5	42	1	—	
—	20	.9	tr	64	tr	.22	.02	1.7	14	0	—	
0	103	6.2	32	322	6	.57	.07	9.9	76	0	—	
0	88	5.1	2	524	4	1.74	.19	7.8	173	1	—	
0	11	.3	2	28	6	.03	.04	.4	13	3	.8	
0	14	.4	2	186	50	.06	.07	.9	59	16	.9	
0	41	4.7	998	440	136	.16	.26	3.3	245	47	3.8	
0	11	.4	10	110	1	.04	.04	.6	4	2	3.6	
0	16	.9	13	132	1	.07	.13	1.7	38	15	1.4	
0	58	4.4	31	1026	67	.25	.17	4.5	47	18	9.5	
0	61	1.7	4	395	88	.10	.13	1.3	44	13	3.4	
0	37	1.3	361	157	50	.02	.08	.6	46	7	3.7	
0	27	3.3	493	266	2	.02	.07	.6	54	7	—	
0	20	1.1	88	562	2	.06	.03	.9	96	10	—	
0	173	2.9	366	1382	775	.18	.44	1.8	22	38	—	

Food	Measure	Weight (g)	Water (%)	Energy (Kcal)	Protein (g)	Carbohydrate (g)	Fat (g)	SFA (
Broccoli, frozen, chopped, boiled, drained	250 mL	194	91	54	6	10	tr	tr
Broccoli, raw	1 spear	151	91	42	5	8	tr	tr
Brussels sprouts, boiled drained	250 m L 7-8	165	87	64	4	14	tr	tr
Cabbage, red, shredded raw	250 mL	74	92	20	1	5	tr	tr
Cabbage, shredded, raw	250 mL	74	93	18	tr	4	tr	tr
Carrots, boiled, drained	250 mL SL	165	87	74	2	17	tr	tr
Carrots, canned, drained	250 mL SL	154	93	35	tr	9	tr	tr
Carrots, frozen, boiled, drained	250 mL SL	154	90	55	2	13	tr	tr
Carrots, raw	1 19X2.9DM	72	88	31	tr	7	tr	tr
Cauliflower, boiled, drained	250 mL	131	93	31	2	6	tr	tr
Cauliflower, raw	250 mL	106	92	25	2	5	tr	tr
Celery, diced, raw	250 mL	127	95	20	tr	5	tr	tr
Celery, outer stalk, raw	19 cm long	40	95	6	tr	1	tr	tr
Chard, swiss, boiled, drained	250 mL	185	93	37	3	8	tr	0
Coleslaw (cabbage salad)	250 mL	127	82	88	2	16	3	tr
Corn, sweet, boiled, drained kernels	1 ear	77	70	83	3	19	tr	tr
Corn, sweet, canned cream style	250 mL	270	79	194	5	49	1	tr
Corn, sweet, canned, kernels, drained	250 mL	173	77	140	5	32	2	tr
Cucumber, raw	250 mL SL	111	96	14	tr	3	tr	tr
Eggplant, cubed, boiled, drained	250 mL	101	92	28	tr	7	tr	tr
Fiddlehead greens, frozen, cooked	250 mL	150	93	30	4	5	tr	–
Lettuce, iceberg, raw	1 leaf	20	96	3	tr	tr	tr	tr
Mushrooms, canned, pieces, drained	250 mL	165	91	40	3	8	tr	tr
Mushrooms, pieces, raw	250 mL	74	92	19	2	3	tr	tr
Olives, black	5 large	20	80	26	tr	tr	3	tr
Olives, green	5 medium	20	78	23	tr	tr	3	tr

PUFA (g)	Cholesterol (mg)	Calcium (mg)	Iron (mg)	Sodium (mg)	Potassium (mg)	Vitamin A (RE)	Thiamin (mg)	Riboflavin (mg)	Niacin (NE)	Folate (mcg)	Vitamin C (mg)	Dietary Fibre (g)
0	99	1.2	47	349	367	.11	.16	1.9	109	78	5.4	
0	72	1.3	41	491	233	.10	.18	1.7	107	141	4.2	
0	59	2.0	35	523	119	.18	.13	1.8	99	102	5.0	
0	38	.4	8	152	3	.04	.02	.4	15	42	1.5	
0	35	.4	13	182	10	.04	.02	.4	42	35	1.5	
0	51	1.0	109	375	4051	.06	.09	1.2	23	4	5.0	
0	39	1.0	371	276	2121	.03	.05	1.0	14	4	4.6	
0	43	.7	91	243	2726	.04	.06	1.0	17	4	4.6	
0	19	.4	25	233	2025	.07	.04	.8	10	7	2.2	
0	35	.6	8	423	1	.08	.07	1.3	67	73	2.2	
0	31	.6	16	376	2	.08	.06	1.1	70	76	1.8	
0	46	.6	112	361	17	.04	.04	.6	11	8	1.9	
0	14	.2	35	114	5	.01	.01	.2	4	3	.6	
0	107	4.2	331	1016	581	.06	.16	1.2	16	33	—	
10	57	.7	29	230	104	.08	.08	.7	34	42	—	
0	2	.5	13	192	17	.17	.06	1.5	36	5	2.2	
0	8	1.0	770	362	27	.07	.14	3.1	121	12	7.6	
0	9	1.5	559	337	28	.06	.14	2.6	84	15	4.8	
0	16	.3	2	165	6	.03	.02	.4	15	5	.9	
0	6	.4	3	250	6	.08	.02	.7	15	1	—	
0	8	1.2	2	332	—	.00	.38	—	—	14	—	
0	4	.1	2	32	7	tr	tr	tr	11	tr	.3	
0	18	1.3	701	213	0	.14	.04	3.8	20	0	4.1	
0	4	.9	3	274	0	.08	.33	3.6	16	3	1.9	
0	17	.3	163	7	1	.00	.00	.0	—	0	—	
0	12	.3	480	11	6	.00	.00	.0	—	0	—	

Food	Measure	Weight (g)	Water (%)	Energy (Kcal)	Protein (g)	Carbohydrate (g)	Fat (g)	SFA
Onion rings (breaded), frozen, heated in oven	5	50	29	204	3	19	13	4
Onions, chopped, boiled drained	250 mL	222	92	62	2	14	tr	tr
Onions, chopped, raw	250 mL	169	91	57	2	12	tr	tr
Onions, spring, chopped, raw	15 mL	6	92	2	tr	tr	tr	tr
Parsley, chopped, raw	15 mL	4	88	1	tr	tr	tr	0
Parsnips, boiled, drained slices	250 mL	165	78	134	2	32	tr	tr
Peas, edible-podded (snow peas), raw	250 mL	153	89	64	4	12	tr	tr
Peas, green, boiled, drained	250 mL	169	78	142	9	26	tr	tr
Peas, green, canned, drained	250 mL	180	82	124	8	23	tr	tr
Peppers, hot, red, dried (chili) powder	15 mL	15	8	47	2	8	3	0
Peppers, sweet, green, raw	1 pepper	74	93	19	tr	4	tr	tr
Pickles, assorted, sweet	1 piece	10	69	12	tr	3	tr	0
Pickles, dill	1 4.5DMX10	136	93	15	tr	3	tr	0
Pickles, gherkins	PC 2DMX7	20	61	29	tr	7	tr	0
Pickles, relish, sweet	15 mL	9	63	12	tr	3	tr	0
Potato salad	250 mL	264	76	378	7	29	22	4
Potatoes, baked in skin, flesh and skin	1 12X6DM	206	71	225	5	52	tr	tr
Potatoes, baked in skin, flesh only	1 12X6DM	159	75	148	3	34	tr	tr
Potatoes, dehydrated flakes, prepared	250 mL	222	76	251	4	33	12	8
Potatoes, french fried cooked in deep fat	10 strips	50	38	158	2	20	8	3
Potatoes, french fried frozen, heated	10 strips	50	53	111	2	17	4	2
Potatoes, hashed brown home prepared	250 mL	165	75	252	4	12	23	9
Potatoes, mashed, milk and butter added	250 mL	222	76	235	4	37	9	2

PUFA (g)	Cholesterol (mg)	Calcium (mg)	Iron (mg)	Sodium (mg)	Potassium (mg)	Vitamin A (RE)	Thiamin (mg)	Riboflavin (mg)	Niacin (NE)	Folate (mcg)	Vitamin C (mg)	Dietary Fibre (g)
0	16	.8	188	65	12	.14	.07	2.4	7	tr	—	
0	60	.4	18	337	0	.09	.02	.7	28	13	2.9	
0	42	.6	3	262	0	.10	.02	.6	34	14	2.2	
0	4	.1	tr	15	30	tr	tr	tr	tr	3	—	
0	5	.2	2	21	21	tr	tr	tr	7	4	—	
0	61	1.0	17	606	0	.14	.08	1.6	96	21	5.8	
0	66	3.2	6	306	21	.23	.12	1.6	64	92	2.9	
0	46	2.6	5	458	101	.44	.25	4.5	107	24	7.6	
0	36	1.7	394	311	139	.22	.14	2.2	80	17	8.1	
0	42	2.1	152	287	524	.05	.12	1.3	—	10	—	
0	4	.9	2	144	39	.06	.04	.5	13	95	1.0	
0	2	.2	53	20	tr	.00	tr	.0	—	tr	—	
0	35	1.4	1942	272	14	.00	.03	.0	—	8	—	
0	2	.2	142	40	2	.00	tr	.0	—	1	—	
0	2	tr	64	18	tr	.00	tr	.0	—	tr	—	
180	50	1.7	1397	671	87	.20	.16	4.2	18	26	—	
0	21	2.8	16	861	0	.22	.07	4.6	23	27	3.5	
0	8	.6	8	622	0	.17	.03	3.0	14	20	1.6	
31	109	.5	737	517	47	.25	.11	2.2	16	22	—	
7	10	.4	108	366	0	.09	.01	2.1	15	5	—	
0	5	.7	16	229	0	.06	.02	1.5	8	5	.5	
0	13	1.3	40	530	0	.12	.03	4.2	13	9	1.7	
4	58	.6	655	642	44	.19	.09	3.5	18	14	2.2	

Food	Measure	Weight (g)	Water (%)	Energy (Kcal)	Protein (g)	Carbohydrate (g)	Fat (g)	SFA (g)
Potatoes, peeled before boiling	1 6-7cm DM	135	77	116	2	27	tr	tr
Potatoes, peeled after boiling	1 6-7cm DM	136	77	118	3	27	tr	tr
Potatoes, scalloped, dry mix, prepared	250 mL	259	79	241	5	33	11	7
Pumpkin, canned	250 mL	259	90	88	3	21	tr	tr
Radishes, raw, without tops	10	45	95	8	tr	2	tr	tr
Rutabagas, boiled, drained, cubed	250 mL	180	90	61	2	14	tr	tr
Rutabagas, raw, cubed	250 mL	148	90	53	2	12	tr	tr
Sauerkraut, canned, solids and liquid	250 mL	249	93	47	2	11	tr	tr
Spinach, boiled, drained	250 mL	190	91	44	6	7	tr	tr
Spinach, chopped, raw	250 mL	59	92	13	2	2	tr	tr
Squash, summer, zucchini, boiled, drained	250 mL SL	190	95	30	1	7	tr	tr
Squash, winter, butternut, frozen, boiled	250 mL	254	88	99	3	26	tr	tr
Squash, winter, hubbard, boiled, mashed	250 mL	249	91	75	4	16	tr	tr
Squash, winter, baked, cubes	250 mL	217	89	85	2	19	1	tr
Sweet potatoes, candied	PC 7X5DM	112	67	153	tr	31	4	2
Sweet potatoes, baked, peeled after baking	5DMX13 raw	114	73	117	2	28	tr	tr
Tomato juice, canned or bottled	250 mL	258	94	44	2	11	tr	tr
Tomato puree, canned	50 mL	53	87	22	tr	5	tr	tr
Tomato sauce, canned	50 mL	52	89	16	tr	4	tr	tr
Tomatoes, canned, stewed	250 mL	269	91	70	3	17	tr	tr
Tomatoes, canned, whole	250 mL	254	94	51	2	11	tr	tr
Tomatoes, raw	1 medium	123	123	23	1	5	tr	tr
Turnips, boiled, drained, mashed	250 mL	243	94	44	2	12	tr	tr
Turnips, raw, cubed	250 mL	137	92	37	1	9	tr	tr
Vegetable juice cocktail, canned	250 mL	256	94	49	2	12	tr	tr

PUFA (g)	Cholesterol (mg)	Calcium (mg)	Iron (mg)	Sodium (mg)	Potassium (mg)	Vitamin A (RE)	Thiamin (mg)	Riboflavin (mg)	Niacin (NE)	Folate (mcg)	Vitamin C (mg)	Dietary Fibre (g)
tr	0	11	.4	7	443	0	.13	.03	2.4	12	10	1.4
tr	0	7	.4	5	515	0	.14	.03	2.6	14	18	1.4
tr	—	93	1.0	883	526	54	.05	.15	3.7	25	9	—
tr	0	67	3.6	13	534	5714	.06	.14	1.5	32	11	—
tr	0	9	.1	11	104	tr	tr	.02	.2	12	10	—
tr	0	76	.8	32	517	0	.13	.07	1.5	28	39	4.0
tr	0	70	.8	30	499	0	.13	.06	1.4	30	37	3.3
r	0	75	3.7	1646	423	5	.05	.06	.8	59	37	—
tr	0	258	6.8	133	885	1556	.18	.45	2.2	277	19	4.4
tr	0	58	1.6	47	329	396	.05	.11	.8	115	17	2.4
r	0	25	.7	6	481	46	.08	.08	1.0	32	9	3.8
r	0	48	1.5	5	338	848	.13	.10	1.9	42	9	—
r	0	25	.7	12	533	998	.11	.07	1.7	24	16	—
r	0	30	.7	2	948	773	.18	.05	2.0	61	21	2.6
r	9	29	1.3	78	212	469	.02	.05	.6	13	8	2.7
r	0	32	.5	11	397	2487	.08	.15	1.1	26	28	2.7
r	0	23	1.5	931	568	144	.12	.08	2.0	51	47	—
r	0	8	.5	11	223	72	.04	.03	1.0	6	19	—
r	0	7	.4	315	193	51	.03	.03	.7	5	7	—
r	0	89	2.0	683	643	148	.12	.09	2.2	15	36	4.0
r	0	66	1.5	414	561	152	.11	.08	2.2	20	38	3.8
r	0	9	.6	10	255	139	.07	.06	.9	12	22	1.8
r	0	53	.5	122	328	0	.07	.06	1.0	22	28	5.3
r	0	41	.4	92	262	0	.06	.04	.8	20	29	3.0
r	0	28	1.1	934	494	300	.11	.07	2.2	54	71	—

Food	Measure	Weight (g)	Water (%)	Energy (Kcal)	Protein (g)	Carbohydrate (g)	Fat (g)	SFA (g)
Vegetables, mixed, canned, drained	250 mL	172	87	81	4	16	tr	tr
Vegetables, mixed, frozen, boiled, drained	250 mL	172	83	101	5	23	tr	tr
Fruits, Related Products — Fruits and Fruit Juices								
Apple juice, canned or bottled, + Vit C	250 mL	262	88	123	tr	31	tr	tr
Apple sauce, canned, sweetened	250 mL	269	80	204	tr	54	tr	tr
Apple sauce, canned, unsweetened	250 mL	258	88	111	tr	29	tr	tr
Apples, raw, with skin	1 7 CM DM	138	84	81	tr	21	tr	tr
Apricot nectar, canned + Vit C	250 mL	265	85	148	tr	38	tr	tr
Apricots, canned whole heavy syrup, no skin	250 mL	273	78	227	1	59	tr	tr
Apricots, dried, cooked without sugar	250 mL	264	76	224	3	58	tr	tr
Apricots, dried, uncooked	10 halves	35	31	83	1	22	tr	tr
Apricots, raw	1 whole	36	86	17	tr	4	tr	tr
Avocados, california, (winter), raw	1 whole	173	73	306	4	12	30	4
Avocados, florida (summer/autumn), raw	1 whole	230	80	258	4	20	20	4
Bananas, raw	1 22X3.6DM	114	74	105	1	27	tr	tr
Blackberries, raw	250 mL	152	86	79	1	19	tr	0
Blueberries, raw	250 mL	153	85	86	1	22	tr	0
Cantaloup, raw	1/2 13 DM	267	90	93	2	22	tr	0
Cherries, sour, red, canned, water pack	250 mL	258	90	93	2	23	tr	tr
Cherries, sweet, raw	250 mL	153	81	110	2	25	1	tr
Cranberries, whole, raw	250 mL	100	87	49	tr	13	tr	0
Cranberry juice, cocktail, bottled	250 mL	267	85	155	tr	40	tr	0
Cranberry sauce, canned, sweetened	250 mL	293	61	442	tr	114	tr	—
Dates, pitted, chopped	250 mL	188	23	517	4	138	tr	0

PUFA (g)	Cholesterol (mg)	Calcium (mg)	Iron (mg)	Sodium (mg)	Potassium (mg)	Vitamin A (RE)	Thiamin (mg)	Riboflavin (mg)	Niacin (NE)	Folate (mcg)	Vitamin C (mg)	Dietary Fibre (g)
0		46	1.8	256	501	2004	.08	.08	1.7	41	9	4.1
0		43	1.4	60	291	736	.12	.21	2.3	33	6	4.0
0		18	1.0	8	312	0	.06	.05	.3	tr	87	.8
0		11	.9	8	164	3	.04	.08	.6	2	5	3.8
0		8	.3	5	194	8	.03	.07	.6	2	3	3.6
0		10	.2	0	159	7	.02	.02	.2	4	8	3.5
0		19	1.0	8	302	350	.02	.04	.9	3	88	.8
0		25	1.2	30	366	339	.05	.06	1.5	5	8	—
0		42	4.4	8	1291	623	.02	.08	3.5	0	4	—
0		16	1.6	4	482	253	tr	.05	1.4	4	tr	2.8
0		5	.2	tr	107	94	.01	.01	.3	3	4	.6
0		19	2.0	21	1097	106	.19	.21	4.0	113	14	—
0		25	1.2	12	1122	140	.25	.28	5.1	123	18	—
0		7	.4	1	451	9	.05	.11	.8	22	10	2.4
0		49	.9	0	298	24	.05	.06	.8	52	32	6.9
0		9	.3	9	136	15	.07	.08	.6	10	20	4.1
0		29	.6	24	825	860	.10	.06	2.0	45	113	2.7
0		28	3.5	18	253	194	.04	.11	.8	21	5	—
0		23	.6	0	343	32	.08	.09	.9	6	11	1.8
0		7	.2	1	71	5	.03	.02	.2	2	14	—
0		8	.4	11	64	0	.01	.04	.1	tr	60	—
0		12	.6	85	76	6	.04	.06	.4	—	6	—
0		60	2.2	6	1226	9	.17	.19	5.7	24	0	14.3

Food	Measure	Weight (g)	Water (%)	Energy (Kcal)	Protein (g)	Carbohydrate (g)	Fat (g)	SFA (
Figs, dried, uncooked	1 fig	19	28	48	tr	12	tr	tr
Fruit cocktail, canned heavy syrup	250 mL	269	80	196	1	51	tr	tr
Fruit cocktail, canned juice pack	250 mL	262	87	121	1	31	tr	tr
Fruit cocktail, canned water pack	250 mL	259	91	83	1	22	tr	tr
Fruit salad, tropical, canned	250 mL	272	77	234	1	61	tr	—
Grapefruit juice, canned, sweetened	250 mL	264	87	121	2	29	tr	tr
Grapefruit juice, canned, unsweetened	250 mL	261	90	99	1	23	tr	tr
Grapefruit juice, fresh	250 mL	261	90	102	1	24	tr	tr
Grapefruit juice, frozen, unsweetened, diluted	250 mL	261	89	107	1	25	tr	tr
Grapefruit, canned, syrup pack	250 mL	268	84	161	2	41	tr	tr
Grapefruit, pink and red, raw	1/2 fruit	123	91	37	tr	9	tr	tr
Grapefruit, white, raw	1/2 fruit	118	90	39	tr	10	tr	tr
Grapes, canadian type (slip skin), raw	10 grapes	24	81	15	tr	4	tr	tr
Grapes, european type (adherant skin), raw	250 mL	169	81	120	1	30	tr	tr
Grapes, juice, canned or bottled	250 mL	267	84	163	1	40	tr	tr
Grapes, juice, frozen, sweetened, diluted, + Vitamin C	250 mL	264	87	135	tr	34	tr	tr
Honeydew melon, raw	1/10 fruit	129	90	45	tr	12	tr	0
Kiwifruit, raw	1 large	91	83	56	tr	14	tr	—
Lemon juice, canned or bottled, unsweetened	250 mL	258	92	54	1	17	tr	tr
Lemon juice, fresh	250 mL	258	91	65	tr	22	0	0
Lemon, raw, without peel	1 6 CM DM	84	89	24	tr	8	tr	tr
Lemonade, frozen concentrate, diluted	250 mL	262	89	115	tr	30	0	0
Lime juice, canned or bottled, unsweetened	250 mL	260	93	55	tr	17	tr	tr

UFA (g)	Cholesterol (mg)	Calcium (mg)	Iron (mg)	Sodium (mg)	Potassium (mg)	Vitamin A (RE)	Thiamin (mg)	Riboflavin (mg)	Niacin (NE)	Folate (mcg)	Vitamin C (mg)	Dietary Fibre (g)
0	27	.4	2	135	2	.01	.02	.2	1	tr	—	
0	16	.8	16	237	54	.05	.05	1.2	7	5	1.6	
0	21	.6	10	249	81	.03	.04	1.3	7	7	1.6	
0	13	.6	10	243	65	.04	.03	1.1	7	5	1.6	
0	35	1.4	5	356	35	.15	.12	1.7	—	48	—	
0	21	1.0	5	428	0	.11	.06	1.1	27	71	1.1	
0	18	.5	3	399	3	.11	.05	.9	27	76	1.0	
0	23	.5	3	423	3	.10	.05	.8	27	99	—	
0	21	.4	3	355	3	.11	.06	.8	9	88	—	
0	38	1.1	5	346	0	.10	.05	.7	23	57	—	
0	14	.1	0	159	32	.04	.03	.3	15	47	1.6	
0	14	tr	0	175	1	.04	.02	.4	12	39	1.5	
0	3	tr	tr	46	2	.02	.01	tr	tr	tr	.3	
0	19	.4	3	313	12	.16	.10	.6	7	18	2.2	
0	24	.6	8	352	3	.07	.10	1.0	7	tr	1.3	
0	11	.3	5	55	3	.04	.07	.4	3	40	tr	
0	8	tr	13	350	5	.10	.02	.9	39	32	—	
0	24	.4	5	302	16	.02	.05	.6	—	68	—	
0	28	.3	54	263	5	.11	.02	.7	26	64	—	
0	18	tr	3	320	5	.08	.03	.4	33	119	—	
0	22	.5	2	116	3	.03	.02	.3	9	45	—	
0	3	.0	0	42	—	.01	.02	.2	12	18	—	
0	31	.6	42	195	5	.09	tr	.5	21	17	—	

Food	Measure	Weight (g)	Water (%)	Energy (Kcal)	Protein (g)	Carbohydrate (g)	Fat (g)	SFA (g)
Lime juice, fresh	250 mL	260	90	70	1	23	tr	tr
Mangos, raw, peeled	1 fruit	176	82	114	tr	30	tr	tr
Nectarine, raw, peeled	1 6.4 DM	136	86	67	1	16	tr	0
Orange juice, canned	250 mL	263	89	110	2	26	tr	tr
Orange juice, fresh	250 mL	262	88	118	2	27	tr	tr
Orange juice, frozen concentrate, diluted	250 mL	263	88	118	2	28	tr	tr
Orange-grapefruit juice, canned	250 mL	261	89	112	2	27	tr	tr
Oranges, raw, peeled	1 6.7 DM	131	87	62	1	15	tr	tr
Papayas, raw, peeled	1 9DMX13	311	89	121	2	31	tr	tr
Peaches, canned halves/slices, + heavy syrup	250 mL	270	79	200	1	54	tr	tr
Peaches, canned halves/slices, juice pack	250 mL	262	87	115	2	30	tr	tr
Peaches, canned halves/slices, water pack	250 mL	258	93	62	1	16	tr	tr
Peaches, raw, pared whole	1 6.4CM DM	87	88	37	tr	10	tr	tr
Pears, canned halves/slices, + heavy syrup	250 mL	269	80	199	tr	52	tr	tr
Pears, canned halves, juice pack	250 mL	262	86	131	tr	34	tr	tr
Pears, raw, with skin	1 6.4DMX9	169	84	100	tr	26	tr	tr
Pineaple juice, canned, + Vitamin C	250 mL	264	86	148	tr	36	tr	tr
Pineapple, canned cubes, water pack	250 mL	260	91	83	1	22	tr	tr
Pineapple, canned, + heavy syrup, sliced	SL 8DMX0.8	64	79	50	tr	13	tr	tr
Pineapple, canned, + heavy syrup, crushed	250 mL	269	79	210	tr	54	tr	tr
Pineapple, raw, diced	250 mL	164	87	80	tr	20	tr	tr
Plums, purple, canned, + heavy syrup	250 mL	273	76	243	tr	63	tr	tr
Plums, raw	1 5.4CM DM	66	85	36	tr	9	tr	tr

PUFA (g)	Cholesterol (mg)	Calcium (mg)	Iron (mg)	Sodium (mg)	Potassium (mg)	Vitamin A (RE)	Thiamin (mg)	Riboflavin (mg)	Niacin (NE)	Folate (mcg)	Vitamin C (mg)	Dietary Fibre (g)
0	23	tr	3	283	3	.05	.03	.5	21	76	—	
0	18	.2	4	275	685	.10	.10	1.3	—	49	1.9	
0	7	.2	0	288	101	.02	.06	1.6	5	7	—	
0	21	1.2	5	460	47	.16	.07	.9	48	90	1.1	
0	29	.5	3	524	52	.24	.08	1.1	79	131	1.0	
0	24	.3	3	500	21	.21	.05	.6	115	102	—	
0	21	1.2	8	412	31	.15	.08	1.2	37	76	—	
0	52	.1	0	237	28	.11	.05	.6	40	70	2.6	
0	75	.3	9	799	625	.08	.10	1.5	—	192	2.8	
0	8	.7	16	248	89	.03	.07	1.7	9	8	1.4	
0	16	.7	10	335	100	.02	.05	1.6	9	9	1.2	
0	5	.8	8	255	137	.02	.05	1.4	9	7	1.3	
0	4	tr	0	171	47	.02	.04	.9	3	6	1.2	
0	13	.6	13	175	0	.03	.06	.7	3	3	4.8	
0	24	.8	10	252	3	.03	.03	.7	3	4	4.8	
0	19	.4	0	211	3	.03	.07	.3	12	7	4.7	
0	45	.7	3	354	0	.15	.06	.8	61	87	—	
0	39	1.0	3	330	5	.24	.07	1.0	12	20	—	
0	9	.2	tr	67	tr	.06	.02	.2	3	5	—	
0	38	1.0	3	280	3	.24	.07	1.0	12	20	—	
0	11	.6	2	185	3	.15	.06	.8	17	25	2.3	
0	25	2.3	52	248	71	.04	.10	1.0	7	1	—	
0	3	tr	0	114	21	.03	.06	.4	1	6	1.1	

Food	Measure		Weight (g)	Water (%)	Energy (Kcal)	Protein (g)	Carbohydrate (g)	Fat (g)	SFA (g)
Prune juice, canned or bottled	250 mL		270	81	192	2	47	tr	tr
Prunes, dried, uncooked	10 fruits		84	32	201	2	53	tr	tr
Prunes, dried, cooked, without added sugar	250 mL		224	70	240	3	63	tr	tr
Raisins, seedless	250 mL pkd		174	15	522	6	138	tr	tr
Raspberries, frozen, sweetened	250 mL		264	73	272	2	69	tr	tr
Raspberries, raw	250 mL		130	87	64	1	15	tr	tr
Rhubarb, frozen, cooked with added sugar	250 mL		254	68	295	tr	79	tr	0
Rhubarb, raw, diced	250 mL		129	94	27	1	6	tr	0
Strawberries, frozen, sweetened, sliced	250 mL		269	73	258	1	70	tr	tr
Strawberries, frozen, sweetened, whole	250 mL		269	78	210	1	56	tr	tr
Strawberries, frozen, unsweetened	250 mL		157	90	55	tr	14	tr	tr
Strawberries, raw, hulled	250 mL		157	92	47	tr	11	tr	tr
Tangerines (mandarins) fruit raw	6 DM		84	88	37	tr	9	tr	tr
Tangerines (mandarins) canned, light syrup pack	250 mL		266	83	162	1	43	tr	tr
Watermelon, raw	SL 25DMX2		368	92	118	2	26	2	0

Fruits, Related Products — Fruit Flavoured Drinks

Food	Measure		Weight (g)	Water (%)	Energy (Kcal)	Protein (g)	Carbohydrate (g)	Fat (g)	SFA (g)
Fruit flavoured drinks canned/bottled, + Vit C	250 mL		264	87	129	tr	33	0	0
Fruit flavoured drinks crystals + water + Vit C	250 mL		284	88	117	0	31	0	0

Bread, Cereals, Related Products — Biscuits and Crackers

Food	Measure		Weight (g)	Water (%)	Energy (Kcal)	Protein (g)	Carbohydrate (g)	Fat (g)	SFA (g)
Biscuits, baking power	1 5X3		28	27	103	2	13	5	1
Crackers, cheese	4	round	14	4	67	2	8	3	1
Crackers, graham	4	squares	28	6	108	2	21	3	tr
Crackers, saltines (soda)	4	squares	11	4	48	tr	8	1	tr
Crackers, snack type	1 round		3	3	15	tr	2	1	tr

PUFA (g)	Cholesterol (mg)	Calcium (mg)	Iron (mg)	Sodium (mg)	Potassium (mg)	Vitamin A (RE)	Thiamin (mg)	Riboflavin (mg)	Niacin (NE)	Folate (mcg)	Vitamin C (mg)	Dietary Fibre (g)
0		32	3.2	11	745	0	.04	.19	2.4	1	11	—
0		43	2.1	3	626	167	.07	.14	2.0	3	3	10.0
0		52	2.5	4	748	69	.05	.22	2.1	tr	6	—
0		85	3.6	21	1307	2	.27	.15	2.5	6	6	15.1
0		40	1.7	3	301	16	.05	.12	.9	69	44	13.5
0		29	.7	0	198	17	.04	.12	1.4	34	33	6.6
0		368	.5	3	244	18	.05	.06	.7	13	8	2.5
0		111	.3	5	372	13	.03	.04	.6	9	10	—
0		30	1.6	8	264	5	.04	.14	1.3	40	111	5.4
0		30	1.3	3	264	8	.04	.21	1.1	10	106	5.4
0		25	1.2	3	232	6	.04	.06	.9	26	65	3.1
0		22	.6	2	261	5	.03	.10	.5	28	89	3.1
0		12	tr	tr	132	77	.09	.02	.2	17	26	—
0		19	1.0	16	207	223	.14	.12	1.4	12	53	—
0		29	.6	7	427	136	.29	.07	1.2	8	35	1.1
0		13	.6	24	71	4	.05	.04	.7	tr	67	.3
0		78	.1	19	1	0	.00	.00	.0	0	60	.0
tr		34	.7	175	33	0	.08	.08	1.1	3	tr	—
4		47	.5	145	15	15	.06	.05	.8	2	0	—
0		11	1.0	188	108	0	.03	.17	1.3	5	0	—
0		2	.5	121	13	0	.05	.04	.7	2	0	—
0		3	.1	30	4	0	.01	.01	.2	—	0	—

Food	Measure	Weight (g)	Water (%)	Energy (Kcal)	Protein (g)	Carbohydrate (g)	Fat (g)	SFA (
Crackers, wheat thin	4	8	3	35	1	5	1	tr
Crackers, whole wheat wafers	2	8	4	35	1	5	2	tr
Bread, Cereals, Related Products — Breads, Rolls and Buns								
Bagels	1 9 CM DM	68	29	200	7	38	2	tr
Bread, cracked wheat	1 slice	25	35	66	2	13	tr	tr
Bread, french/vienna	1 slice	20	31	58	2	11	tr	tr
Bread, italian	1 slice	30	32	83	3	17	tr	0
Bread, melba toast	1 piece	4	—	16	tr	3	tr	—
Bread, mixed grain	1 slice	25	37	65	2	12	tr	tr
Bread, oatmeal	1 slice	25	37	65	2	12	1	tr
Bread, pita	1 16.5 DM	60	31	165	6	33	1	tr
Bread, raisin	1 slice	25	35	66	2	13	tr	tr
Bread, rye, dark, pumpernickel	1 slice	32	34	79	3	17	tr	tr
Bread, rye, light	1 slice	25	36	61	2	13	tr	tr
Bread, white	1 slice	28	36	76	2	14	tr	tr
Bread, white, calcium carbonate added to flour	1 slice	28	36	76	2	14	tr	tr
Bread, whole wheat (100% whole wheat)	1 slice	25	36	61	3	12	tr	tr
Bread, whole wheat (60% whole wheat)	1 slice	25	36	63	2	12	1	tr
Breadcrumbs, white bread, dry	250 mL	106	7	416	13	78	5	1
Buns, hamburger	1 bun	60	31	179	5	32	3	tr
Buns, hot dog	1 bun	50	31	149	4	27	3	tr
Croissants	1	57	22	235	5	27	12	4
English muffins	1	57	42	140	5	27	1	tr
Rolls, commercial, hard	1 round	50	25	156	5	30	2	tr
Tortillas, corn	1 tortilla	30	45	65	2	13	1	tr
Bread, Cereals, Related Products — Breakfast Cereals								
Cereal, bran flakes with raisins	200 mL	42	10	133	3	32	tr	—
Cereal, bran flakes, whole wheat	200 mL	40	5	139	4	32	tr	—

PUFA (g)	Cholesterol (mg)	Calcium (mg)	Iron (mg)	Sodium (mg)	Potassium (mg)	Vitamin A (RE)	Thiamin (mg)	Riboflavin (mg)	Niacin (NE)	Folate (mcg)	Vitamin C (mg)	Dietary Fibre (g)
tr	0	3	.3	69	17	0	.04	.03	.6	—	0	—
tr	0	3	.2	59	31	0	.02	.03	.6	—	0	—
tr	0	29	1.8	245	50	0	.26	.20	3.7	—	0	.7
tr	tr	22	.7	132	34	0	.09	.06	1.2	11	0	1.0
tr	tr	9	.6	116	18	0	.08	.05	1.0	7	0	.4
0	tr	5	.8	176	22	0	.12	.07	1.5	11	0	.3
—	—	5	.1	29	6	0	tr	.01	.1	1	0	—
tr	0	27	.8	106	56	0	.10	.10	1.5	—	0	.9
tr	0	15	.7	124	39	0	.12	.07	1.3	—	0	.6
tr	0	49	1.4	339	71	0	.27	.12	3.3	—	0	.5
tr	tr	18	.7	91	58	0	.10	.06	.9	9	0	.6
tr	tr	27	.9	182	145	0	.09	.07	1.1	7	0	1.0
tr	tr	19	.7	139	36	0	.08	.06	1.1	6	0	—
tr	tr	24	.8	142	29	0	.11	.07	1.4	10	0	.4
tr	tr	46	.8	142	29	0	.11	.07	1.4	10	0	.4
tr	tr	25	.8	132	68	0	.06	.03	1.2	14	0	1.4
0	1	23	.8	133	69	0	.07	.05	1.1	12	0	—
1	5	129	4.3	780	161	0	.37	.37	7.5	38	0	—
tr	4	44	1.7	304	57	0	.24	.15	2.9	21	0	—
tr	3	37	1.4	253	48	0	.20	.12	2.4	18	0	—
1	13	20	2.1	452	68	13	.17	.13	2.2	—	0	—
tr	0	96	1.7	378	331	0	.26	.19	3.1	—	0	—
tr	2	24	1.4	313	49	0	.20	.12	2.6	18	0	—
tr	0	42	.6	1	43	8	.05	.03	.8	—	0	—
—	0	18	5.6	284	221	0	.84	.00	3.1	25	0	3.7
—	0	1	5.3	291	175	4	.80	.04	2.7	24	0	3.9

Food	Measure	Weight (g)	Water (%)	Energy (Kcal)	Protein (g)	Carbohydrate (g)	Fat (g)	SFA (g)
Cereal, bran, all bran	125 mL	45	4	113	5	34	tr	—
Cereal, bran, bran buds	125 mL	44	3	122	5	34	tr	—
Cereal, bran, 100%	125 mL	35	3	90	4	29	tr	tr
Cereal, corn bran	200 mL	30	2	118	2	26	1	—
Cereal, corn flakes, plain	200 mL	19	4	70	1	16	tr	—
Cereal, corn flakes, sugar coated (frosted flakes)	200 mL	30	3	114	1	27	tr	—
Cereal, corn + oats, Cap'N Crunch	250 mL	39	2	154	2	31	2	2
Cereal, corn + wheat + oats, Froot Loops	200 mL	24	3	93	1	21	tr	—
Cereal, corn, puffed, presweetened, Sugar Corn Pops	250 mL	30	4	114	1	27	tr	—
Cereal, granola, homemade	125 mL	64	3	312	8	35	17	3
Cereal, oatmeal, regular/quick cooking, cooked	125 mL	124	85	77	3	13	1	tr
Cereal, oatmeal, regular/quick cooking, dry	125 mL	43	9	165	7	29	3	tr
Cereal, oatmeal, ready to serve, dry	1 pouch	32	9	120	4	21	2	tr
Cereal, oats + marshmallows, Lucky Charms	250 mL	34	3	134	2	29	tr	tr
Cereal, oats + puffed Cheerios	250 mL	24	7	92	3	17	2	tr
Cereal, oats + puffed, presweetened, Alpha-Bits	250 mL	30	2	118	2	26	tr	—
Cereal, red river, cooked	125 mL	125	—	82	3	16	tr	—
Cereal, rice flakes	200 mL	27	5	103	2	24	tr	—
Cereal, rice krispies	250 mL	30	4	112	2	25	tr	—
Cereal, rice + wheat, Special K	250 mL	22	4	82	4	16	tr	—
Cereal, rice, puffed	250 mL	15	2	59	tr	14	tr	—
Cereal, wheat, flakes, Grapenuts	200 mL	27	6	97	3	22	tr	—
Cereal, wheat, flakes, Wheaties	200 mL	24	5	86	3	20	tr	tr

PUFA (g)	Cholesterol (mg)	Calcium (mg)	Iron (mg)	Sodium (mg)	Potassium (mg)	Vitamin A (RE)	Thiamin (mg)	Riboflavin (mg)	Niacin (NE)	Folate (mcg)	Vitamin C (mg)	Dietary Fibre (g)
—	0	38	6.0	410	475	0	.90	.09	7.7	43	0	13.2
—	0	36	5.9	221	400	0	.88	.09	6.6	38	0	10.7
tr	0	27	4.7	—	437	0	.70	.13	8.9	25	0	9.9
—	0	23	4.0	259	66	0	.60	.01	1.8	18	0	6.1
—	0	tr	2.5	185	21	0	.38	tr	1.2	11	0	tr
—	0	tr	4.0	171	23	0	.60	tr	1.7	18	0	.1
tr	0	6	5.2	289	39	0	.78	.01	2.1	23	0	.6
—	0	2	3.2	98	28	0	.48	tr	1.4	14	0	.3
—	0	2	4.0	122	23	0	.60	—	1.7	18	0	.2
9	0	40	2.5	6	321	2	.38	.16	2.7	52	tr	—
tr	0	10	.8	1	69	2	.14	.03	.9	5	0	1.1
1	0	22	1.8	2	151	4	.31	.06	1.9	14	0	2.6
—	0	17	4.5	323	113	3	.70	.05	8.0	10	tr	1.5
tr	0	0	4.5	163	61	0	—	.03	2.2	20	0	.6
tr	0	28	3.2	214	86	0	.02	.02	1.9	14	0	.8
—	0	tr	4.0	12	47	2	.60	.05	1.9	18	0	.5
—	0	—	.4	7	—	0	.04	tr	1.1	13	0	2.4
—	0	8	3.6	—	—	0	.54	.02	1.6	16	0	.0
—	0	4	4.0	312	37	0	.60	tr	1.8	18	0	.1
—	tr	9	2.9	190	35	0	.44	—	1.9	13	0	.2
—	0	1	tr	1	17	0	tr	.01	.5	1	0	tr
—	0	tr	3.6	128	85	1	.54	.02	2.1	16	0	1.7
tr	0	0	3.2	187	97	0	.48	.00	2.0	14	0	1.7

Food	Measure	Weight (g)	Water (%)	Energy (Kcal)	Protein (g)	Carbohydrate (g)	Fat (g)	SFA (g)
Cereal, wheat, puffed	250 mL	13	2	50	2	10	tr	—
Cereal, wheat, puffed, presweetened, Sugar Crisp	250 mL	35	4	132	3	30	tr	—
Cereal, wheat, to be cooked, enriched, cooked	125 mL	133	87	68	2	15	tr	—
Cereal, wheat, whole, Shredded Wheat	1 biscuit	25	6	95	3	21	tr	—
Cereal, wheat, whole, Shreddies	200 mL	44	5	169	4	37	tr	—

Bread, Cereals, Related Products — Cakes

Food	Measure	Weight (g)	Water (%)	Energy (Kcal)	Protein (g)	Carbohydrate (g)	Fat (g)	SFA (g)
Cake from mix, angelfood	1/12 25 DM	76	34	197	4	45	tr	0
Cake from mix, cupcakes	1 7 cm DM	33	26	116	2	18	4	1
Cake from mix, gingerbread	1/9 21X21	63	37	174	2	32	4	1
Cake from mix, coffee cake	1/6 cake	72	30	232	5	38	7	2
Cake from mix, devil's food + icing	1/16 23 DM	69	24	234	3	40	8	3
Cake from mix, white layer + chocolate icing	1/16 23 DM	71	21	249	3	45	8	3
Cake, home recipe, boston cream pie	1/12 20 DM	69	35	208	3	34	6	2
Cake, home recipe, carrot + cream cheese frosting	1/8 cake	60	23	241	2	30	13	3
Cake, home recipe, fruitcake, dark	SL 4X7. 5X2	60	18	227	3	36	9	2
Cake, home recipe, pound cake	SL 9X8X1	30	17	142	2	14	9	2
Cake, home recipe, sponge	1/12 22DM	44	32	131	3	24	3	tr
Came, home recipe, white + boiled white icing	PC 8X8X5	114	23	401	4	70	12	3
Cake, home recipe, white, plain	PC 8X8X5	85	25	313	4	48	12	3
Cake, home recipe, yellow layer + chocolate icing	1/16 23 DM	75	21	274	3	45	10	3

PUFA (g)	Cholesterol (mg)	Calcium (mg)	Iron (mg)	Sodium (mg)	Potassium (mg)	Vitamin A (RE)	Thiamin (mg)	Riboflavin (mg)	Niacin (NE)	Folate (mcg)	Vitamin C (mg)	Dietary Fibre (g)
—	0	3	.5	tr	46	0	.01	.03	1.2	3	0	.6
—	0	1	.8	40	65	tr	.70	.06	2.4	21	0	.8
—	0	3	8.0	1	23	0	.01	.01	.5	4	0	.4
—	0	10	.8	2	85	0	.07	.07	2.0	10	0	2.4
—	0	16	5.9	—	—	0	.88	.07	2.9	26	0	3.2
0	0	72	.5	111	46	0	.05	.11	1.3	5	0	—
tr	20	53	.6	149	28	15	.06	.07	.8	3	tr	—
tr	tr	57	1.2	192	173	0	.10	.11	1.2	4	tr	—
2	47	44	1.2	310	79	32	.14	.15	2.1	—	tr	—
1	33	41	1.4	181	90	31	.07	.10	1.2	4	tr	—
1	1	70	.9	161	82	13	.09	.11	1.3	3	tr	—
1	59	46	.9	128	61	43	.09	.10	1.5	6	tr	—
4	46	28	.8	175	67	10	.07	.08	1.0	—	tr	—
2	27	43	1.7	95	298	22	.10	.10	1.2	7	tr	—
2	44	6	.5	33	18	25	.05	.05	.7	3	0	—
tr	108	13	.9	73	38	59	.06	.09	1.0	6	0	—
2	56	56	1.3	299	73	44	.14	.16	1.9	8	tr	—
2	56	55	1.3	258	68	44	.14	.16	1.8	7	tr	—
1	33	51	1.1	156	81	36	.10	.13	1.5	5	tr	—

Food	Measure	Weight (g)	Water (%)	Energy (Kcal)	Protein (g)	Carbohydrate (g)	Fat (g)	SFA (g)
Cake, home recipe, yellow layer, no icing	1/16 23 CM	54	24	196	2	31	7	2
Cheesecake	1/12 23 DM	92	46	278	5	26	18	10

Bread, Cereals, Related Products — Cookies

Food	Measure	Weight (g)	Water (%)	Energy (Kcal)	Protein (g)	Carbohydrate (g)	Fat (g)	SFA (g)
Cookies, brownies with nuts, home recipe	1 brownie	20	10	97	1	10	6	1
Cookies, chocolate chip, commercial	2 6 cm DM	22	3	104	1	15	5	1
Cookies, chocolate chip, home recipe	2 6 cm DM	20	3	103	1	12	6	2
Cookies, chocolate marshmallow (mallows)	1 biscuit	17	10	70	tr	12	2	1
Cookies, fig bars	2 bars	28	14	100	1	21	2	tr
Cookies, oatmeal with raisins	2 cookies	26	3	117	2	19	4	1
Cookies, peanut butter home recipe	2 cookies	24	3	123	2	14	7	2
Cookies, sandwich, chocolate/vanilla, commercial	2 round	20	2	99	tr	14	5	1
Cookies, shortbread, commercial	2 large	28	3	139	2	18	6	2
Cookies, shortbread, home recipe (margarine)	2 large	28	3	145	2	17	8	1
Cookies, social tea or arrowroot	2 biscuits	13	6	57	tr	9	2	tr
Cookies, sugar, from refigerated dough	2 cookies	24	4	118	1	16	6	1
Cookies, vanilla wafers	5 cookies	20	4	93	1	15	4	tr

Bread, Cereals, Related Products — Flours and Grains

Food	Measure	Weight (g)	Water (%)	Energy (Kcal)	Protein (g)	Carbohydrate (g)	Fat (g)	SFA (g)
Barley, pearled, light uncooked	125 mL	106	11	370	9	84	1	tr
Bulgur	250 mL	185	10	655	21	140	3	1
Carob, flour	250 mL	148	11	266	7	119	2	tr
Cornmeal, degermed, dry form	125 mL	73	12	266	6	57	tr	tr
Cornstarch	125 mL	68	12	246	tr	60	0	0
Potato flour	250 mL	38	8	133	3	30	tr	tr
Rice, brown, cooked	250 mL	180	70	214	5	46	1	tr

PUFA (g)	Cholesterol (mg)	Calcium (mg)	Iron (mg)	Sodium (mg)	Potassium (mg)	Vitamin A (RE)	Thiamin (mg)	Riboflavin (mg)	Niacin (NE)	Folate (mcg)	Vitamin C (mg)	Dietary Fibre (g)
1	29	38	.9	139	42	24	.09	.10	1.3	5	tr	—
—	170	52	.4	204	90	69	.03	.12	1.3	—	5	—
1	17	8	.4	50	38	12	.04	.03	.4	2	0	—
1	9	9	.6	88	29	8	.04	.04	.5	2	0	—
1	10	7	.5	70	23	7	.03	.03	.5	2	0	—
tr	13	4	.3	36	15	13	.02	.02	.3	2	tr	—
tr	11	22	.6	71	55	9	.05	.05	.6	3	0	—
tr	10	5	.8	42	96	4	.07	.05	.8	5	tr	—
1	11	11	.6	71	55	3	.04	.04	1.3	—	0	—
tr	8	5	.4	97	8	0	.05	.03	.6	1	0	—
1	11	20	.8	17	18	7	.13	.08	1.2	2	0	—
3	0	6	.6	125	18	89	.08	.06	1.1	—	0	—
tr	tr	4	.4	48	20	0	.07	.06	.7	1	tr	—
2	15	25	.5	131	17	6	.05	.03	.7	—	0	—
tr	13	8	.4	75	25	7	.04	.05	.7	—	0	—
tr	0	17	2.1	3	170	0	.13	.05	4.9	21	0	—
1	0	54	6.8	7	424	0	.52	.26	12.1	78	0	—
tr	0	521	6.0	25	1348	tr	.07	.07	2.4	—	0	—
tr	0	4	.8	tr	88	96	.10	.04	1.8	16	0	—
0	0	0	.0	0	0	0	.00	.00	.0	—	0	—
tr	0	13	6.5	13	603	0	.16	.05	2.1	19	7	—
tr	0	22	.9	508	126	0	.16	.04	3.3	17	0	2.2

Food	Measure	Weight (g)	Water (%)	Energy (Kcal)	Protein (g)	Carbohydrate (g)	Fat (g)	SFA (g)
Rice, white unenriched short grain, cooked	250 mL	185	73	202	4	45	tr	tr
Rice, white unenriched short grain, raw	250 mL	211	12	766	14	170	tr	tr
Rice, white, enriched, instant, ready-to-serve, hot	250 mL	174	73	190	4	42	tr	tr
Rice, white, enriched, long-grain, parboiled, cooked	250 mL	169	73	179	4	39	tr	tr
Rye, flour, light	250 mL	100	11	357	9	78	1	tr
Soybean, flour, defatted	250 mL	106	8	346	50	40	tr	0
Wheat Bran	15 mL	3	12	6	tr	2	tr	tr
Wheat Germ	15 mL	7	12	25	2	3	tr	tr
Wheat, flour, all purpose	250 mL	133	12	484	14	101	1	tr
Wheat, flour, all purpose, calcium carbonate added	250 mL	133	12	484	14	101	1	tr
Wheat, flour, cake	250 mL	114	12	415	9	91	1	tr
Wheat, flour, whole	250 mL	127	12	423	17	90	3	tr

Bread, Cereals, Related Products — Muffins

Food	Measure	Weight (g)	Water (%)	Energy (Kcal)	Protein (g)	Carbohydrate (g)	Fat (g)	SFA (g)
Muffins, blueberry, home recipe	6DMX5DMX4	40	39	112	3	17	4	1
Muffins, bran, home recipe	6DMX5DMX4	40	35	104	3	17	4	1
Muffins, corn, made from mix + milk + eggs	6DMX5DMX4	40	30	130	3	20	4	1
Muffins, plain, home recipe	8DMX5DMX4	40	38	118	3	17	4	1

Bread, Cereals, Related Products — Pancakes and Waffles

Food	Measure	Weight (g)	Water (%)	Energy (Kcal)	Protein (g)	Carbohydrate (g)	Fat (g)	SFA (g)
Pancakes, buckwheat, made from mix + eggs + milk	1 10.2DM	27	58	54	2	6	2	tr
Pancakes, plain, made from mix + eggs + milk	1 10.2 DM	27	51	61	2	9	2	tr
Waffles, made from mix + eggs + milk	1 round	75	42	206	7	27	8	3

Bread, Cereals, Related Products — Pasta

Food	Measure	Weight (g)	Water (%)	Energy (Kcal)	Protein (g)	Carbohydrate (g)	Fat (g)	SFA (g)
Macaroni, enriched, cooked	250 mL	148	72	164	5	34	1	tr

PUFA (g)	Cholesterol (mg)	Calcium (mg)	Iron (mg)	Sodium (mg)	Potassium (mg)	Vitamin A (RE)	Thiamin (mg)	Riboflavin (mg)	Niacin (NE)	Folate (mcg)	Vitamin C (mg)	Dietary Fibre (g)
tr	0	19	.4	692	52	0	.04	.02	1.4	16	0	.6
tr	0	51	1.7	11	194	0	.15	.06	6.0	61	0	—
tr	0	5	1.4	0	0	0	.22	.02	2.6	—	0	.5
tr	0	32	1.4	605	73	0	.19	.02	2.7	14	0	.5
tr	0	22	1.1	1	156	0	.15	.07	2.3	78	0	4.5
0	0	281	11.8	1	1929	4	1.16	.36	11.9	403	0	—
tr	0	4	.4	tr	34	0	.02	.01	.7	4	0	1.2
tr	0	5	.7	tr	58	0	.14	.05	.6	15	0	—
r	0	21	3.9	3	126	0	.85	.53	9.6	28	0	3.9
r	0	166	3.9	3	126	0	.85	.53	9.6	28	0	3.9
r	0	19	3.0	2	108	0	.69	.43	7.4	24	0	3.3
1	0	52	4.2	4	470	0	.70	.15	8.6	54	0	11.3
r	33	34	.8	253	46	26	.09	.10	1.3	4	tr	—
tr	41	57	1.6	179	172	28	.07	.10	2.3	3	tr	—
tr	23	96	.8	192	44	29	.08	.09	1.2	3	tr	—
tr	21	42	.9	176	50	12	.09	.12	1.5	3	tr	—
tr	18	59	.4	125	66	19	.04	.05	.6	3	tr	—
tr	20	58	.3	152	42	20	.04	.07	.6	3	tr	—
1	45	179	1.2	515	146	52	.14	.23	2.1	9	tr	—
tr	0	12	2.2	1	90	0	.21	.38	2.6	5	0	1.2

Food	Measure	Weight (g)	Water (%)	Energy (Kcal)	Protein (g)	Carbohydrate (g)	Fat (g)	SFA (g)
Noodles, chow mein, canned	250 mL	47	11	230	6	27	11	2
Noodles, egg, enriched cooked	250 mL	169	70	211	7	39	2	tr
Spaghetti, enriched, cooked	250 mL	148	73	164	5	34	1	tr
Bread, Cereals, Related Products — Pies								
Pie, apple, 2 crust	1/6 23 DM	158	48	404	3	60	18	5
Pie, blueberry, 2 crust	1/6 23 DM	158	51	382	4	55	17	4
Pie, cherry, 2 crust	1/6 23 DM	158	47	412	4	61	18	5
Pie, custard, 1 crust	1/6 23 DM	152	58	331	9	36	17	6
Pie, lemon meringue, 1 crust	1/6 23 DM	140	47	357	5	53	14	4
Pie, mincemeat, 2 crust	1/6 23 DM	158	43	428	4	65	18	5
Pie, peach, 2 crust	1/6 23 DM	158	48	403	4	60	17	4
Pie, pumpkin, 1 crust	1/6 23 DM	152	59	321	6	37	17	6
Pie, raisin, 2 crust	1/6 23 DM	158	43	427	4	68	17	4
Piecrust, baked shell	1 23 cm DM	180	15	900	11	79	60	15
Pies, fried, fast food apple	1 pie	85	43	255	2	31	14	6
Pies, fried, fast food cherry	1 pie	85	42	250	2	32	14	6
Bread, Cereals, Related Products — Snack Foods								
Cone for Ice Cream	1 cone	4	9	15	tr	3	tr	tr
Popcorn, air popped, plain	250 mL	8	4	31	1	6	tr	tr
Popcorn, popped with oil and salt	250 mL	12	3	55	1	7	3	2
Popcorn, sugar coated	250 mL	37	4	142	2	32	1	tr
Potato chips	10 chips	20	3	105	1	10	7	2
Pretzels, bread stick	5 pretzels	15	5	59	1	11	tr	tr
Pretzels, 3 ring	1	3	5	12	tr	2	tr	tr
Bread, Cereals, Related Products — Sweet Baked Goods								
Danish Pastry, plain, round	1 11X2.5	65	22	274	5	30	15	5
Date Squares	1	90	—	226	2	45	5	—
Doughnuts, cake type	1	43	24	168	2	22	8	2
Doughnuts, yeast-leavened	1	42	28	174	3	16	11	3

PUFA (g)	Cholesterol (mg)	Calcium (mg)	Iron (mg)	Sodium (mg)	Potassium (mg)	Vitamin A (RE)	Thiamin (mg)	Riboflavin (mg)	Niacin (NE)	Folate (mcg)	Vitamin C (mg)	Dietary Fibre (g)
	5	15	.4	470	34	0	.05	.03	1.8	—	0	—
	52	17	2.5	3	74	35	.24	.43	3.3	7	0	—
	0	12	2.2	1	90	0	.21	.38	2.6	6	0	1.2
	0	13	1.6	476	126	5	.17	.13	2.2	10	2	—
	0	17	2.1	423	103	5	.17	.14	2.4	11	5	—
	0	22	1.6	480	166	70	.19	.14	2.3	12	0	—
	160	146	1.5	436	208	105	.14	.32	2.6	11	0	—
	130	20	1.4	395	70	71	.10	.14	1.8	8	4	—
	2	44	2.7	708	281	tr	.16	.14	2.3	7	2	—
	0	16	1.9	423	235	115	.17	.16	3.1	9	5	—
	93	78	1.4	325	243	375	.14	.21	2.3	13	0	—
	0	28	2.5	450	303	tr	.17	.14	2.5	7	2	—
	0	25	4.5	1100	90	0	.54	.40	7.1	21	0	—
	14	12	.9	326	42	3	.09	.06	1.4	—	1	—
	13	11	.7	371	61	19	.06	.06	1.0	—	1	—
	0	6	tr	9	10	0	tr	tr	tr	—	0	—
	0	tr	.2	tr	20	0	.03	.01	.4	—	0	—
	0	tr	.3	233	31	0	.04	.01	.4	—	0	—
	0	2	.5	tr	95	0	.14	.02	.8	—	0	—
	0	5	.2	94	260	0	.03	tr	1.1	9	8	—
	0	3	.2	252	20	0	tr	tr	.4	—	0	—
	0	tr	tr	50	4	0	tr	tr	tr	—	0	—
	42	33	1.2	238	73	60	.18	.20	2.5	23	0	—
	—	24	1.3	135	270	3	.07	.05	tr	14	—	—
	26	17	.9	215	39	10	.09	.09	1.1	4	0	—
	11	16	.9	98	34	8	.10	.09	1.3	9	0	—

Food	Measure	Weight (g)	Water (%)	Energy (Kcal)	Protein (g)	Carbohydrate (g)	Fat (g)	SFA (g)
Eclairs, chocolate, custard filled	1	100	56	239	6	23	14	4
Combination Dishes								
Beans and wieners, canned	250 mL	269	71	387	20	34	19	8
Beans with tomato sauce and pork, canned	250 mL	269	71	328	16	51	7	3
Beef and vegetable stew, canned	250 mL	259	83	205	15	18	8	5
Beef pot pie, baked	1/3 pie	210	55	517	21	39	30	8
Cheeseburger, regular	1	112	46	300	15	28	15	7
Cheeseburger, 4 oz patty	1	194	46	525	30	40	31	15
Chicken a la king, home recipe	250 mL	259	68	495	29	13	36	13
Chicken and noodles, home recipe	250 mL	254	71	389	24	27	20	6
Chicken pot pie, baked	1/3 pie	232	57	545	23	42	31	11
Chili con carne without beans, canned	250 mL	269	67	538	28	16	40	19
Chili con carne with beans, canned	250 mL	269	72	358	20	33	16	8
Chop suey with meat or chicken	250 mL	264	75	317	27	13	18	9
Chow mein, chicken, canned, without noodles	250 mL	264	89	100	7	19	tr	0
Chow mein, chicken, home recipe, without noodles	250 mL	264	78	269	33	11	11	3
English muffin, egg, cheese and bacon	1	138	49	360	18	31	18	8
Fish cakes, fried	1 6.5DMX2	60	66	103	9	6	5	2
Fish sandwich, large, without cheese, fast food	1	170	48	470	18	41	27	6
Fish sandwich, regular with cheese, fast food	1	140	43	420	16	39	23	6
Hamburger, regular	1	98	46	245	12	28	11	4
Hamburger, 4 oz patty	1	174	50	445	25	38	21	7
Luncheon meat, canned	SL 8X5X1 cm	45	52	150	6	tr	14	5
Macaroni and cheese, canned	250 mL	254	80	241	10	27	10	4

PUFA (g)	Cholesterol (mg)	Calcium (mg)	Iron (mg)	Sodium (mg)	Potassium (mg)	Vitamin A (RE)	Thiamin (mg)	Riboflavin (mg)	Niacin (NE)	Folate (mcg)	Vitamin C (mg)	Dietary Fibre (g)
2	136	80	.7	82	122	102	.04	.16	1.2	9	0	—
8	35	100	5.1	1450	705	35	.19	.16	7.2	64	0	—
tr	11	145	4.8	1245	565	35	.22	.08	4.6	64	5	19.6
tr	36	31	2.3	1064	451	754	.08	.13	5.3	35	8	—
6	44	29	3.8	596	334	517	.29	.29	8.7	17	6	—
1	44	135	2.3	672	219	65	.26	.24	6.5	—	1	—
2	104	236	4.5	1224	407	128	.33	.48	12.9	—	3	—
4	197	135	2.6	803	427	357	.10	.44	11.0	23	13	—
4	102	28	2.3	635	157	137	.05	.18	8.9	13	0	—
5	72	70	3.0	594	343	926	.33	.33	9.0	21	5	—
0	70	102	3.8	1428	627	40	.05	.32	11.0	22	0	—
tr	46	86	4.6	1428	627	16	.08	.19	7.2	96	0	—
tr	106	63	5.0	1111	449	63	.29	.40	10.3	30	34	—
0	8	48	1.3	766	441	16	.05	.11	2.3	21	13	—
3	82	61	2.6	758	499	29	.08	.24	10.5	21	11	—
tr	213	197	3.1	832	201	160	.46	.50	7.0	—	1	—
1	25	7	.2	106	209	0	.02	.04	2.6	7	0	—
10	91	61	2.2	621	375	15	.35	.23	6.8	—	1	—
8	56	132	1.8	667	274	25	.32	.26	6.2	—	2	—
tr	32	56	2.2	463	202	14	.23	.24	6.0	—	1	—
tr	71	75	4.8	763	404	28	.38	.38	12.4	—	1	—
2	28	3	.3	580	97	0	.17	.09	2.3	3	tr	—
2	25	211	1.0	772	147	84	.13	.25	2.8	21	tr	—

Food	Measure	Weight (g)	Water (%)	Energy (Kcal)	Protein (g)	Carbohydrate (g)	Fat (g)	SFA (g)
Macaroni and cheese, home recipe	250 mL	211	58	454	18	42	23	13
Meat loaf, homemade	SL 10X8X1	73	64	117	12	3	6	—
Pizza, cheese	1/8 35 DM	65	48	153	8	18	5	2
Pizza, sausage	1/8 35 DM	65	43	183	8	18	9	2
Quiche lorraine	1/8 20 DM	176	47	600	13	29	48	23
Roast beef sandwich, fast food	1	150	52	345	22	34	13	4
Spaghetti, with meat balls and tomato sauce, homemade	250 mL	262	70	351	20	41	12	4
Spaghetti, with tomato sauce and cheese, canned	250 mL	264	80	201	6	41	2	tr
Taco, fast food	1 taco	81	55	195	9	15	11	4
Tourtiere (pork pie)	1/6 23 DM	139	37	482	21	32	30	8
Fats and Oils — Butter								
Butter	250 mL	240	16	1720	2	tr	195	121
Butter	15 mL	14	16	100	tr	tr	11	7
Butter	1 pat	5	16	36	tr	tr	4	3
Fats and Oils — Cooking Fats								
Lard	250 mL	217	0	1957	0	0	217	89
Lard	15 mL	13	0	117	0	0	13	5
Shortening, vegetable oils	250 mL	217	0	1953	0	0	217	67
Shortening, vegetable oils	15 mL	13	0	117	0	0	13	4
Fats and Oils — Margarine								
Margarine, tub, vegetable oils, no declaration	250 mL	240	16	1719	2	1	193	31
Margarine, tub, vegetable oils, no declaration	15 mL	14	16	100	tr	tr	11	2
Margarine, tub, vegetable oils, with declaration	250 mL	240	16	1719	2	1	193	35
Margarine, tub, vegetable oils, with declaration	15 mL	14	16	100	tr	tr	11	2
Fats and Oils — Oils								
Canola (rapeseed, colza) oil	250 mL	230	0	2033	0	0	230	17

PUFA (g)	Cholesterol (mg)	Calcium (mg)	Iron (mg)	Sodium (mg)	Potassium (mg)	Vitamin A (RE)	Thiamin (mg)	Riboflavin (mg)	Niacin (NE)	Folate (mcg)	Vitamin C (mg)	Dietary Fibre (g)
1	72	382	1.9	1146	253	272	.21	.42	5.1	18	tr	—
—	67	28	1.7	477	273	—	.05	.14	8.1	—	1	—
tr	12	144	1.4	456	85	123	.14	.20	2.9	10	5	—
tr	19	122	.9	434	127	109	.05	.12	2.4	10	6	—
4	285	211	1.0	653	283	454	.11	.32	2.5	—	0	—
2	55	60	4.0	757	338	32	.40	.33	10.0	—	2	—
tr	79	131	3.9	1066	702	503	.26	.31	7.8	21	24	—
tr	8	42	2.9	1008	319	293	.37	.29	5.8	14	11	—
tr	21	109	1.2	456	263	57	.09	.07	3.1	—	1	—
5	53	27	3.9	707	235	3	.56	.32	8.2	15	tr	—
7	525	56	.4	1984	62	1810	.01	.08	.6	7	0	—
tr	31	3	tr	116	4	106	tr	tr	tr	tr	0	—
tr	11	1	tr	41	1	38	.00	tr	tr	tr	0	—
24	206	tr	.0	tr	tr	0	.00	.00	.0	0	0	—
1	12	tr	.0	tr	tr	0	.00	.00	.0	0	0	—
—	0	0	.0	tr	tr	0	.00	.00	.0	—	0	—
—	0	0	.0	0	0	0	.00	.00	.0	—	0	—
36	0	64	.0	2589	90	2541	.02	.08	.5	3	tr	—
2	0	4	.0	151	5	148	tr	tr	tr	tr	tr	—
81	0	64	.0	2589	90	2541	.02	.08	.5	3	tr	—
5	0	4	.0	151	5	148	tr	tr	tr	tr	tr	—
77	0	0	.0	0	0	0	.00	.00	.0	0	0	—

Food	Measure	Weight (g)	Water (%)	Energy (Kcal)	Protein (g)	Carbohydrate (g)	Fat (g)	SFA (g)
Canola (rapeseed, colza) oil	15 mL	14	0	124	0	0	14	1
Corn oil	250 mL	230	0	2033	0	0	230	29
Corn oil	15 mL	14	0	124	0	0	14	2
Olive oil	250 mL	230	0	2033	0	0	230	31
Olive oil	15 mL	14	0	124	0	0	14	2
Peanut oil	250 mL	228	0	2016	0	0	228	39
Peanut oil	15 mL	14	0	124	0	0	14	2
Soybean oil	250 mL	230	0	2033	0	0	230	33
Soybean oil	15 mL	14	0	124	0	0	14	2
Sunflower oil	250 mL	230	0	2033	0	0	230	24
Sunflower oil	15 mL	14	0	124	0	0	14	1

Fats and Oils — Salad Dressings

Food	Measure	Weight (g)	Water (%)	Energy (Kcal)	Protein (g)	Carbohydrate (g)	Fat (g)	SFA (g)
Mayonnaise, >65% oil	15 mL	14	16	102	tr	tr	11	1
Salad dressing, mayonnaise type, >35% oil	15 mL	15	40	58	tr	4	5	2
Salad dressing, thousand island, commercial	15 mL	16	46	64	tr	3	6	tr
Salad dressing, blue cheese	15 mL	16	32	77	tr	2	8	tr
Salad dressing, french calorie reduced, commercial	15 mL	16	69	24	tr	2	2	tr
Salad dressing, french regular, commercial	15 mL	16	38	64	tr	2	6	tr
Salad dressing, home cooked, boiled	15 mL	16	69	25	tr	2	2	tr

Sugars and Sweets — Candy

Food	Measure	Weight (g)	Water (%)	Energy (Kcal)	Protein (g)	Carbohydrate (g)	Fat (g)	SFA (g)
Candy, caramels, plain or chocolate	3	30	8	120	1	23	3	2
Candy, chocolate coated peanuts	15 pieces	30	1	168	5	12	12	3
Candy, chocolate fudge	1 3X3X2.5	29	8	116	tr	22	4	1
Candy, gum drops	5 drops	30	12	104	tr	26	tr	0
Candy, hard	6	30	1	116	0	29	tr	0
Candy, jelly beans	10 beans	30	6	110	0	28	tr	0

UFA (g)	Cholesterol (mg)	Calcium (mg)	Iron (mg)	Sodium (mg)	Potassium (mg)	Vitamin A (RE)	Thiamin (mg)	Riboflavin (mg)	Niacin (NE)	Folate (mcg)	Vitamin C (mg)	Dietary Fibre (g)
0	0	.0	0	0	0	.00	.00	.0	0	0	—	
0	0	.0	0	0	0	.00	.00	.0	0	0	—	
0	0	.0	0	0	0	.00	.00	.0	0	0	—	
0	tr	.9	tr	0	0	.00	.00	.0	0	0	—	
0	tr	tr	tr	0	0	.00	.00	.0	0	0	—	
0	tr	tr	tr	tr	0	.00	.00	.0	0	0	—	
0	tr	tr	tr	tr	0	.00	.00	.0	0	0	—	
0	tr	tr	0	0	0	.00	.00	.0	0	0	—	
0	tr	tr	0	0	0	.00	.00	.0	0	0	—	
0	0	.0	0	0	0	.00	.00	.0	0	0	—	
0	0	.0	0	0	0	.00	.00	.0	0	0	—	
8	1	tr	73	2	4	tr	tr	tr	tr	tr	—	
4	2	tr	107	1	13	tr	tr	tr	tr	0	—	
4	2	tr	112	17	15	tr	tr	tr	1	0	—	
3	13	tr	188	4	11	tr	.02	.2	1	tr	—	
tr	2	tr	310	6	0	.00	.00	tr	0	0	—	
9	2	tr	255	tr	3	tr	tr	tr	tr	0	—	
9	13	tr	117	19	20	.01	.02	.5	0	tr	—	
tr	44	.4	68	58	tr	tr	.05	.3	—	0	—	
tr	35	.5	18	151	0	.11	.05	3.1	17	0	—	
tr	22	.3	55	43	0	tr	.03	.2	—	0	—	
0	2	.2	11	2	0	.00	.00	.0	0	0	—	
0	6	.6	10	1	0	.00	.00	.0	0	0	—	
0	4	.3	4	tr	0	.00	.00	.0	0	0	—	

Food	Measure	Weight (g)	Water (%)	Energy (Kcal)	Protein (g)	Carbohydrate (g)	Fat (g)	SFA (
Candy, licorice	3 sticks	33	7	104	1	24	tr	0
Candy, marshmallows	4	28	17	89	tr	23	0	0
Candy, mints or fondant		30	8	109	tr	27	tr	tr
Chocolate, baking, bitter	1 square	28	2	141	3	8	15	8
Chocolate, baking sweet	1 square	28	tr	148	1	16	10	5
Gum, chewing	1 stick	4	4	13	0	4	0	0
Sugars and Sweets — Chocolate Bars								
Chocolate bars, "Caravan/ Caramilk" type		30	8	125	1	23	4	1
Chocolate bars, "Oh Henry" type with nuts		30	7	138	3	18	7	2
Chocolate bars, all varieties		30	4	141	2	19	7	3
Chocolate bars, milk, plain		30	tr	156	2	17	10	5
Sugars and Sweets — Chocolate Flavoured Beverage Powder								
Chocolate flavoured powder + skim milk, made with water	250 mL	270	86	131	4	29	1	tr
Chocolate flavoured powder, no milk, made with whole milk	250 mL	264	81	224	9	30	9	5
Sugars and Sweets — Chocolate Flavoured Syrup								
Chocolate syrup, fudge type	15 mL	19	25	63	tr	10	3	1
Chocolate syrup, thin type	15 mL	19	32	47	tr	12	tr	tr
Sugars and Sweets — Icings								
Icing, chocolate, made with milk and fat	250 mL	291	14	1094	9	196	40	23
Icing, creamy fudge, from mix made with water	250 mL	259	15	878	7	193	17	5
Icing, white, boiled	250 mL	99	18	313	1	79	0	0
Sugars and Sweets — Other								
Popsicle	1	85	80	61	0	16	0	0
Sugars and Sweets — Spreads								
Honey, strained, liquid	15 mL	21	17	64	tr	17	0	0
Jams and preserves	15 mL	20	29	54	tr	14	tr	0
Jellies	15 mL	19	29	52	tr	13	tr	0

PUFA (g)	Cholesterol (mg)	Calcium (mg)	Iron (mg)	Sodium (mg)	Potassium (mg)	Vitamin A (RE)	Thiamin (mg)	Riboflavin (mg)	Niacin (NE)	Folate (mcg)	Vitamin C (mg)	Dietary Fibre (g)
0	21	2.6	25	71	0	.00	.00	.2	0	0	—	
tr	5	.4	11	2	0	.00	.00	.0	0	0	—	
0	4	.3	64	2	0	.00	.00	.0	—	0	—	
0	22	1.9	1	232	5	.01	.07	1.0	3	0	—	
tr	26	.4	9	75	tr	tr	.04	.3	3	0	—	
0	0	.0	0	0	0	.00	.00	.0	0	0	—	
2	38	.5	52	63	4	.02	.05	.3	2	0	—	
tr	38	.3	38	67	0	.08	.05	1.6	9	0	—	
1	35	.5	39	87	—	.02	.05	.3	6	0	—	
6	68	.3	28	115	24	.02	.10	.5	2	0	—	
1	118	.4	182	292	tr	.04	.22	1.0	—	tr	—	
33	297	.9	175	506	76	.10	.43	1.9	—	3	—	
0	24	.2	17	54	9	tr	.04	.3	—	0	—	
0	3	.3	10	54	0	tr	.01	.2	—	0	—	
47	175	3.5	178	567	183	.06	.29	2.3	8	tr	—	
0	101	2.8	601	251	—	.05	.21	2.1	3	0	—	
0	2	.0	142	18	0	.00	.03	.0	tr	0	—	
0	0	tr	9	4	0	.00	.00	.0	0	0	—	
0	1	.1	1	11	0	tr	tr	tr	tr	tr	—	
0	4	.2	2	18	tr	tr	tr	tr	2	tr	—	
0	4	.3	3	14	tr	tr	tr	tr	—	tr	—	

Food	Measure	Weight (g)	Water (%)	Energy (Kcal)	Protein (g)	Carbohydrate (g)	Fat (g)	SFA (
Molasses, blackstrap or cooking	15 mL	21	24	45	0	12	0	0
Molasses, fancy, (usually consumed)	15 mL	21	24	53	0	14	0	0
Sugars and Sweets — Sugars								
Sugar, brown	250 mL · pk	232	2	865	0	224	0	0
Sugar, brown	15 mL	9	2	34	0	9	0	0
Sugar, white, granulated	250 mL	211	tr	812	0	210	0	0
Sugar, white, granulated	15 mL	13	tr	50	0	13	0	0
Sugar, white, powdered	250 mL · pkd	127	tr	489	0	126	0	0
Sugars and Sweets — Syrups								
Maple syrup	15 mL	20	33	50	0	13	0	0
Table syrup (blends)	15 mL	21	24	61	0	16	0	0
Miscellaneous Items — Beverages, Alcoholic								
Beer	341 mL	346	92	145	1	13	0	0
Liquor, gin, rum, vodka, whiskey	50 mL	48	67	111	0	0	0	0
Wine, dessert	100 mL	100	77	137	tr	8	0	0
Wine, red table	100 mL	98	88	72	0	3	0	0
Wine, white table	100 mL	98	87	77	0	3	0	0
Miscellaneous Items — Beverages, Non-Alcoholic								
Coffee, beverage	250 mL	254	99	5	tr	1	0	0
Postum, beverage, made with water	250 mL	252	—	17	tr	4	0	0
Soft drinks, club soda (soda water)	280 mL	280	99	0	0	0	0	0
Soft drinks, cola type beverage	280 mL	291	89	119	0	29	0	0
Soft drinks, cola type beverage with aspartame	280 mL	280	0	0	0	24	0	0
Soft drinks, gingerale	280 mL	289	91	90	0	23	0	0
Soft drinks, tonic water	280 mL	289	91	98	0	25	0	0
Tea, beverage	250 mL	254	3	0	0	tr	0	0
Tea, beverage, made from sweetened instant powder	250 mL	277	91	94	tr	24	tr	tr

PUFA (g)	Cholesterol (mg)	Calcium (mg)	Iron (mg)	Sodium (mg)	Potassium (mg)	Vitamin A (RE)	Thiamin (mg)	Riboflavin (mg)	Niacin (NE)	Folate (mcg)	Vitamin C (mg)	Dietary Fibre (g)
0	0	144	3.4	20	615	0	.02	.04	.4	—	0	—
0	0	35	.9	3	193	0	.02	.01	tr	—	0	—
0	0	197	7.9	70	798	0	.02	.07	.5	—	0	—
0	0	8	.3	3	31	0	tr	tr	tr	—	0	—
0	0	0	.2	2	6	0	.00	.00	.0	—	0	—
0	0	0	tr	tr	tr	0	.00	.00	.0	—	0	—
—	0	0	.1	1	4	0	.00	.00	.0	—	0	—
0	0	21	.2	2	35	0	.03	.01	.0	—	0	—
0	0	10	.9	14	tr	0	.00	.00	.0	—	0	—
0	0	17	.0	24	87	0	.00	.10	2.3	21	0	—
0	0	0	.0	tr	tr	0	.00	.00	.0	—	0	—
0	0	8	.0	4	75	0	.01	.02	.2	—	0	—
0	0	8	.4	5	109	—	.00	.03	tr	—	0	—
0	0	9	.3	5	80	—	.00	.01	tr	—	0	—
0	0	5	1.0	5	137	0	.00	.00	.6	tr	0	—
0	0	7	.7	7	131	—	.05	.00	—	—	0	—
0	0	14	.0	59	6	0	.00	.00	.0	0	0	—
0	0	9	.0	12	3	0	.00	.00	.0	0	0	—
0	0	8	.5	20	3	0	.00	.00	.0	0	0	—
—	0	0	.0	0	0	0	.00	.00	.0	—	0	—
0	0	3	.0	12	0	0	.00	.00	.0	0	0	—
0	0	0	tr	8	94	0	.00	.04	.0	13	0	—
tr	0	6	tr	tr	52	0	.00	.04	.2	10	0	—

Food	Measure	Weight (g)	Water (%)	Energy (Kcal)	Protein (g)	Carbohydrate (g)	Fat (g)	SFA (g)
Miscellaneous Items — Condiments								
Bouillon cubes	1 cube	6	3	10	1	tr	tr	tr
Ketchup	15 mL	17	69	18	tr	4	tr	0
Mustard, prepared, yellow	15 mL	16	80	12	tr	1	tr	tr
Salt, table	5 mL	6	tr	0	0	0	0	0
Shake and Bake, dry	15 mL	6	5	24	tr	4	tr	tr
Vinegar, white	15 mL	15	95	2	0	tr	0	0
Miscellaneous Items — Gelatin								
Gelatin dessert powder "Jello"	1 package	85	2	315	8	75	0	0
Gelatin dessert, dietetic	125 mL	127	99	10	3	tr	tr	0
Gelatin dessert, prepared with water, "Jello"	125 mL	127	84	75	2	18	0	0
Gelatin, dry powder	1 envelope	7	13	23	6	0	tr	0
Miscellaneous Items — Sauces and Gravy								
Barbecue sauce	250 mL	264	81	198	5	34	5	tr
Gravy, brown, canned	15 mL	15	87	8	tr	tr	tr	tr
White sauce, medium	250 mL	264	73	428	10	23	33	18
Miscellaneous Items — Soups								
Soup, bean with bacon, canned, + water	250 mL	267	84	182	8	24	6	2
Soup, beef broth, bouillon/consomme, canned + water	250 mL	255	96	31	6	2	0	0
Soup, beef noodle, canned + water	250 mL	258	92	88	5	9	3	1
Soup, clam chowder, manhattan with tomato, + water	250 mL	258	90	83	4	13	2	tr
Soup, clam chowder, without tomato, + whole milk	250 mL	262	85	173	10	18	7	3
Soup, cream of mushroom, canned, + water	250 mL	258	90	137	2	10	9	3
Soup, cream of mushroom, canned, + whole milk	250 mL	262	85	215	6	16	14	5

PUFA (g)	Cholesterol (mg)	Calcium (mg)	Iron (mg)	Sodium (mg)	Potassium (mg)	Vitamin A (RE)	Thiamin (mg)	Riboflavin (mg)	Niacin (NE)	Folate (mcg)	Vitamin C (mg)	Dietary Fibre (g)
tr	tr	4	.1	1440	24	tr	.01	.01	.4	2	0	—
0	0	4	.1	177	62	24	.02	.01	.3	3	3	—
tr	0	13	.3	200	21	0	.00	.00	.0	—	0	—
0	0	15	tr	2325	tr	0	.00	.00	.0	0	0	—
tr	0	4	.2	210	12	0	.01	.00	.2	2	0	—
0	0	0	.0	tr	2	0	.00	.00	.0	0	0	—
0	0	0	.0	270	179	0	.00	.00	.0	0	0	—
tr	0	0	.0	9	47	0	.00	.00	.0	0	0	—
0	0	0	.0	65	2	0	.00	.00	.0	0	0	—
0	0	tr	.0	6	2	0	.00	.00	tr	0	0	—
2	0	50	2.4	2152	459	230	.08	.05	3.2	11	18	—
tr	tr	tr	.1	8	12	0	tr	tr	tr	tr	0	—
1	108	304	.5	1001	367	364	.13	.45	2.7	12	2	—
2	3	85	2.2	1004	425	93	.09	.04	2.1	34	2	—
0	0	10	.6	673	163	0	.02	.03	.8	3	1	—
tr	5	15	1.2	1006	106	67	.07	.06	1.9	5	tr	—
4	3	36	2.0	1912	276	98	.07	.05	1.0	10	3	—
4	24	197	1.6	1048	317	42	.07	.25	3.1	10	4	—
4	3	49	.5	1091	106	0	.05	.10	1.4	5	1	—
5	21	189	.6	1137	286	39	.08	.30	2.4	10	2	—

Food	Measure	Weight (g)	Water (%)	Energy (Kcal)	Protein (g)	Carbohydrate (g)	Fat (g)	SFA (g)
Soup, cream of chicken canned, + water	250 mL	258	91	124	4	10	8	2
Soup, cream of chicken canned, + whole milk	250 mL	262	85	202	8	16	12	5
Soup, minestrone, canned, + water	250 mL	255	91	87	5	12	3	tr
Soup, split pea with ham, canned, + water	250 mL	267	82	200	11	30	5	2
Soup, tomato, canned, + water	250 mL	258	90	90	2	18	2	tr
Soup, tomato, canned, + whole milk	250 mL	262	85	170	6	24	6	3
Soup, vegetable beef, canned, + water	250 mL	258	92	83	6	11	2	tr
Soup, vegetable, vegetarian, canned, + water	250 mL	255	92	77	2	13	2	tr
Soup, chicken noodle, dehydrated, + water	250 mL	267	94	56	3	8	1	tr
Soup, onion, dehydrated, + water	250 mL	260	96	29	1	5	tr	tr
Soup, tomato vegetable dehydrated, + water	250 mL	267	94	59	2	11	tr	tr

Miscellaneous Items — Leavening Agents

Food	Measure	Weight (g)	Water (%)	Energy (Kcal)	Protein (g)	Carbohydrate (g)	Fat (g)	SFA (g)
Baking powder, continuous action	15 mL	13	1	18	0	4	0	0
Yeast, baker's, dry, granulated	1 envelope	8	5	23	3	3	tr	0
Yeast, brewer's, dry	15 mL	8	5	23	3	3	tr	0

UFA (g)	Cholesterol (mg)	Calcium (mg)	Iron (mg)	Sodium (mg)	Potassium (mg)	Vitamin A (RE)	Thiamin (mg)	Riboflavin (mg)	Niacin (NE)	Folate (mcg)	Vitamin C (mg)	Dietary Fibre (g)
10	36	.6	1042	93	59	.03	.07	1.6	2	tr	—
29	191	.7	1106	288	100	.08	.27	2.7	8	1	—
3	36	1.0	964	332	247	.06	.05	1.5	17	1	—
8	24	2.4	1063	422	48	.16	.08	3.3	3	2	—
0	13	1.9	921	279	72	.09	.05	1.8	15	70	—
18	168	1.9	985	474	115	.14	.26	3.0	22	72	—
5	18	1.2	1011	183	201	.04	.05	2.0	11	3	—
0	23	1.1	870	222	319	.06	.05	1.2	11	2	—
3	35	.5	1359	32	5	.08	.06	.5	2	tr	—
0	13	.2	897	68	0	.03	.06	.5	2	tr	—
0	8	.7	1210	109	21	.06	.05	.5	11	6	—
0	379	.6	855	28	0	.00	.00	.0	0	0	—
0	4	1.3	4	160	0	.19	.43	3.5	—	0	—
0	17	1.4	10	152	0	1.25	.34	3.6	—	0	—

SUMMARY EXAMPLES OF RECOMMENDED NUTRIENT INTAKES

Age	Sex	Weight kg	Protein g	Vitamin A REa	Vitamin D μg	Vitamin E mg	Vitamin C mg	Folate μg	Vitamin B12 μg
Months									
0–4	Both	6.0	12b	400	10	3	20	25	0.3
5–12	Both	9.0	12	400	10	3	20	40	0.4
Years									
1	Both	11	13	400	10	3	20	40	0.5
2–3	Both	14	16	400	5	4	20	50	0.6
4–6	Both	18	19	500	5	5	25	70	0.8
7–9	M	25	26	700	2.5	7	25	90	1.0
	F	25	26	700	2.5	6	25	90	1.0
10–12	M	34	34	800	2.5	8	25	120	1.0
	F	36	36	800	2.5	7	25	130	1.0
13–15	M	50	49	900	2.5	9	30e	175	1.0
	F	48	46	800	2.5	7	30e	170	1.0
16–18	M	62	58	1000	2.5	10	40e	220	1.0
	F	53	47	800	2.5	7	30e	190	1.0
19–24	M	71	61	1000	2.5	10	40e	220	1.0
	F	58	50	800	2.5	7	30e	180	1.0
25–49	M	74	64	1000	2.5	9	40e	230	1.0
	F	59	51	800	2.5	6	30e	185	1.0
50–74	M	73	63	1000	5	7	40e	230	1.0
	F	63	54	800	5	6	30e	195	1.0
75+	M	69	59	1000	5	6	40e	215	1.0
	F	64	55	800	5	5	30e	200	1.0
Pregnancy (additional)									
1st Trimester			3	0	2.5	2	0	200	0.2
2nd Trimester			15	0	2.5	2	10	200	0.2
3rd Trimester			24	0	2.5	2	10	200	0.2
Lactation (additional)			22	400	2.5	3	25	100	0.2

a   Retinol Equivalents
b   Protein is assumed to be from breast milk and must be adjusted for infant formula.
c   Infant formula with high phosphorus should contain 375 mg calcium.
d   Breast milk is assumed to be the source of the mineral.
e   Smokers should increase vitamin C by 50%.
f   Niacin Equivalents
g   Level below which intake should not fall.

Calcium mg	Phosphorous mg	Magnesium mg	Iron mg	Iodine µg	Zinc mg	Energy kcal	Thiamin mg	Riboflavin mg	Niacin NE[f]
250[c]	150	20	0.3[d]	30	2[d]	600	0.3	0.3	4
400	200	32	7	40	2	900	0.4	0.5	7
500	300	40	6	55	4	1100	0.5	0.6	8
550	350	50	6	65	4	1300	0.6	0.7	9
600	400	65	8	85	5	1800	0.7	0.9	13
700	500	100	8	110	7	2200	0.9	1.1	16
700	500	100	8	95	7	1900	0.8	1.0	14
900	700	130	8	125	9	2500	1.0	1.3	18
1100	800	135	8	110	9	2200	0.9	1.1	16
1100	900	185	10	160	12	2800	1.1	1.4	20
1000	850	180	13	160	9	2200	0.9	1.1	16
900	1000	230	10	160	12	3200	1.3	1.6	23
700	850	200	12	160	9	2100	0.8	1.1	15
800	1000	240	9	160	12	3000	1.2	1.5	22
700	850	200	13	160	9	2100	0.8	1.1	15
800	1000	250	9	160	12	2700	1.1	1.4	19
700	850	200	13	160	9	1900	0.8[g]	1.0[g]	14[g]
800	1000	250	9	160	12	2300	0.9	1.2	16
800	850	210	8	160	9	1800	0.8[g]	1.0[g]	14[g]
800	1000	230	9	160	12	2000	0.8	1.0	14
800	850	210	8	160	9	1700	0.8[g]	1.0[g]	14[g]
500	200	15	0	25	6	100	0.1	0.1	1
500	200	45	5	25	6	300	0.1	0.3	2
500	200	45	10	25	6	300	0.1	0.3	2
500	200	60	0	50	6	450	0.2	0.4	3

Designed for the Maintenance of Good Nutrition of Practically All Healthy People in the U.S.A.

	Age (years)	Weight (kg)	Weight (lbs)	Height (cm)	Height (in)	Protein (g)	Fat-Soluble Vitamins			Water-Soluble Vitamins						
							Vitamin A (µg)[b]	Vitamin D (µg)[c]	Vitamin E (mg α)[d]	Vitamin C (mg)	Thiamin (mg)	Riboflavin (mg)	Niacin (mg NE)[e]	Vitamin B6 (mg)	Folacin[f] (µg)	Vitamin B12
Infants	0.0–0.5	6	13	60	24	kg × 2.2	420	10	3	35	0.3	0.4	6	0.3	30	0.5[g]
	0.5–1.0	9	20	71	28	kg × 2.0	400	10	4	35	0.5	0.6	8	0.6	45	1.5
Children	1–3	13	29	90	35	23	400	10	5	45	0.7	0.8	9	0.9	100	2.0
	4–6	20	44	112	44	30	500	10	6	45	0.9	1.0	11	1.3	200	2.5
	7–10	28	62	132	52	34	700	10	7	45	1.2	1.4	16	1.6	300	3.0
Males	11–14	45	99	157	62	45	1000	10	8	50	1.4	1.6	18	1.8	400	3.0
	15–18	66	145	176	69	56	1000	10	10	60	1.4	1.7	18	2.0	400	3.0
	19–22	70	154	177	70	56	1000	7.5	10	60	1.5	1.7	19	2.2	400	3.0
	23–50	70	154	178	70	56	1000	5	10	60	1.4	1.6	18	2.2	400	3.0
	51+	70	154	178	70	56	1000	5	10	60	1.2	1.4	16	2.2	400	3.0
Females	11–14	46	101	157	62	46	800	10	8	50	1.1	1.3	15	1.8	400	3.0
	15–18	55	120	163	64	46	800	10	8	60	1.1	1.3	14	2.0	400	3.0
	19–22	55	120	163	64	44	800	7.5	8	60	1.1	1.3	14	2.0	400	3.0
	23–50	55	120	163	64	44	800	5	8	60	1.0	1.2	13	2.0	400	3.0
	51+	55	120	163	64	44	800	5	8	60	1.0	1.2	13	2.0	400	3.0
Pregnant						+30	+200	+5	+2	+20	+0.4	+0.3	+2	+0.6	+400	+1.0
Lactating						+20	+400	+5	+3	+40	+0.5	+0.5	+5	+0.5	+100	+1.0

Minerals

Calcium (mg)	Phosphorus (mg)	Magnesium (mg)	Iron (mg)	Zinc (mg)	Iodine (μg)
360	240	50	10	3	40
540	360	70	15	5	50
800	800	150	15	10	70
800	800	200	10	10	90
800	800	250	10	10	120
1200	1200	350	18	15	150
1200	1200	400	18	15	150
800	800	350	10	15	150
800	800	350	10	15	150
800	800	350	10	15	150
1200	1200	300	18	15	150
1200	1200	300	18	15	150
800	800	300	18	15	150
800	800	300	18	15	150
800	800	300	10	15	150
+400	+400	+150	h	+5	+25
+400	+400	+150	h	+10	+50

[a] The allowances are intended to provide for individual variations among most normal persons as they live in the United States under usual environmental stresses. Diets should be based on a variety of common foods in order to provide other nutrients for which human requirements have been less well defined.

[b] Retinol equivalents. 1 retinol equivalent = 1 μg retinol or 6 μg β-carotene.

[c] As cholecalciferol. 10 μg cholecalciferol = 400 IU vitamin D.

[d] α-tocopherol equivalents.
1 mg d-α-tocopherol = 1 α TE.

[e] 1 NE (niacin equivalent) is equal to 1 mg of niacin or 60 mg of dietary tryptophan.

[f] The folacin allowances refer to dietary sources as determined by *Lactobacillus casei* assay after treatment with enzymes (conjugases) to make polyglutamyl forms of the vitamin available to the test organism.

[g] The RDA for Vitamin B_{12} in infants is based on average concentration of the vitamin in human milk. The allowances after weaning are based on energy intake (as recommended by the American Academy of Pediatrics) and consideration of other factors such as intestinal absorption.

[h] The increased requirement during pregnancy cannot be met by the iron content of habitual American diets nor by the existing iron stores of many women; therefore, the use of 30–60 mg of supplemental iron is recommended. Iron needs during lactation are not substantially different from those of non-pregnant women, but continued supplementation of the mother for 2–3 months after parturition is advisable in order to replenish stores depleted by pregnancy.

Source: Reprinted, with permission, from "Recommended Dietary Allowances," 9th ed. (Washington, D.C.: National Academy Press, 1980).

Bibliography

Adlercreutz, H. "Western Diet and Western Diseases: Some Hormonal and Biochemical Mechanisms and Associations." *Scandinavian Journal Clin Lab* 201 (May 1990): 3-23.

American Heart Association. "Rationale of the Diet-Heart Statement of the American Heart Association." *Circulation* 65 (1982): 839A-854A.

Anderson, J., L. Story, et al. "Hypocholesterolemic Effects of Oat Bran or Bean Intake for Hypercholesterolemic Men." *American Journal of Clinical Nutrition* 40 (1984): 1146.

Arts, C.J., et al. "In Vitro Binding of Estrogens by Dietary Fiber and the In Vivo Apparent Digestibility Tested in Pigs." *Journal Steroid Biochemistry Molecular Biology* 38 (May 1991): 621-628.

Bain, R.J. "Accidental Digitalis Poisoning due to Drinking Herbal Tea." *British Medical Journal* 290 (1985): 1624.

Beaudette, T. "Caffeine: Clinical Implications." *Seminars in Nutrition* 4 (1984): 1.

Black, M.R., D.M. Madeiros, et al. "Zinc Supplements and Serum Lipids in Young Adult White Males." *American Journal of Clinical Nutrition* 47 (1988): 970–75.

Burkitt, D., A. Walker, et al. "Dietary Fiber and Disease." *Journal of the American Medical Association* 229 (1974): 1068.

Canada. Department of Consumer and Corporate Affairs. "Guide for Food Manufacturers and Advertisers." Ottawa, 1984.

Canada. Department of National Health and Welfare. "Action Towards Healthy Eating. Technical Report." Ottawa, 1990.

Canada. Department of National Health and Welfare. "Canada's Food Guide For Healthy Eating." Ottawa, 1992.

Canada. Department of National Health and Welfare. "Canada's Food Guide Handbook (Revised)." Ottawa, 1985.

Canada. Department of National Health and Welfare. "Feeding Babies." Ottawa, 1986.

Canada. Department of National Health and Welfare. "Nutrients in Canadian Foods." Rev. ed. Ottawa, 1986.

Canada. Department of National Health and Welfare. "Nutrition Recommendations. The Report of the Scientific Review Committee." Ottawa, 1990.

Canada. Department of National Health and Welfare. "Promoting Healthy Weights." Ottawa, 1988.

Canada. Department of National Health and Welfare. "Recommended Nutrient Intakes for Canadians." Ottawa, 1983.

Canada. Department of National Health and Welfare. "Report of the Expert Advisory Committee on Dietary Fibre." Ottawa, 1985.

Canada. Department of National Health and Welfare. "Report of the Expert Advisory Committee on Herbs and Botanical Preparations." Ottawa, 1986.

Canada. Department of National Health and Welfare. "Sorting out Sulphites." Ottawa, 1986.

Canadian Atherosclerosis Society. "Canadian Consensus Conference on Cholesterol." Ottawa, 1988.

Canadian Paediatric Society. Nutrition Committee. "Infant Feeding." *Canadian Journal of Public Health* 70 (1979): 376.

Consensus Development Conference. "Lowering Blood Cholesterol to Prevent Heart Disease." *Journal of the American Medical Association* 253 (1985): 2080–86.

Dalton, K. "Pyridoxine Overdose in Pre-Menstrual Syndrome." *Lancet* 1 (1985): 1168.

DeBakey, M.E., A.M. Gotto, et al. "Diet, Nutrition and Heart Disease." *Journal of the American Dietetic Association* 86 (1986): 729–31.

Eastwood, M.A., and R. Passmore. "Nutrition: The Changing Scene—Dietary Fibre." *Lancet* (July 1983): 202–206.

Franz, M. "Nutrition Update." *The Diabetes Educator* 11 (1986): 3.

Garland, C.F., et al. "Can Colon-Cancer Incidence and Death Rates Be Reduced with Calcium and Vitamin D?" *American Journal of Clinical Nutrition* 54 (1991): 193S-201S.

Glomset, J.A. "Fish, Fatty Acids and Human Health." *New England Journal of Medicine* 319 (1985): 1253–54.

Hamet, P., et al. "Interactions among Calcium, Sodium, and Alcohol Intake as Determinants of Blood Pressure." *Hypertension* 17 (1991): 150–154.

Hilton, E., et al. "Ingestion of Yogurt Containing *Lactobacillus acidophilus* as Prophylaxis for Candidal Vaginitis." *Annals of Internal Medicine* 116 (1992): 353-57.

Isolauri, E., et al. "A Human *Lactobacillus* strain (*Lactobacillus casei* sp Strain GG) Promotes Recovery from Acute Diarrhea in Children." *Pediatrics* 88 (1991): 90-97.

Jenkins, D.J., et al. "Nibbling versus Gorging: Metabolic Advantages of Increased Meal Frequency." *New England Journal of Medicine* 321 (October 1989): 929–934.

Kaila, M., et al. "Enhancement of the Circulating Antibody Secreting Cell Response in Human Diarrhea by a Human *Lactobacillus* Strain." *Pediatric Research* 32 (1992): 141-44.

Kirkley, B.G. "Bulimia: Clinical Characteristics, Development and Etiology." *Journal of the American Dietetic Association* 86 (1986): 468–72.

Kremer, J.M. "Clinical Studies of Omega-3 Fatty Acid Supplementation in Patients Who Have Rheumatoid Arthritis." *Rheum Dis Clin North America* 17 (May 1991): 391-402.

Kromhout, D., E.B. Bosschieter, et al. "The Inverse Relation between Fish Consumption and 20-Year Mortality from Coronary Heart Disease." *New England Journal of Medicine* 312 (1985): 1205-1209.

Lanza, E., and R.R. Butrum. "A Critical Review of Food Fiber Analysis and Data." *Journal of the American Dietetic Association* 86 (1986): 732-40.

Lieber, C.S. "To Drink (Moderately) or Not to Drink?" *New England Journal of Medicine* 310 (1984): 846.

Lipid Research Clinics Program. "The Lipid Research Clinics Coronary Primary Prevention Trial Results, I: Reduction in Incidence of Coronary Heart Disease." *Journal of the American Medical Association* 251 (1984): 351-64.

"The Lipid Research Clinics Coronary Primary Prevention Trial Results, II: The Relationship of Reduction in Incidence of Coronary Heart Disease to Cholesterol Lowering." *Journal of the American Medical Association* 251 (1984): 365-74.

Mirkin, G., and M. Shangold. "Sports Medicine." *Journal of the American Medical Association* 254 (1985): 2340.

North York. Department of Health. Nutrition Services. "Nutrition Matters." North York, Ont., 1982.

Ontario. Milk Marketing Board. "Calcium Absorption and Utilization from Food." *Spotlight on Nutrition Issues* (June 1986).

Ontario. Ministry of Health. "Healthy Beginnings—A Teacher's Kit." Toronto, 1983.

Ontario. Ministry of Health. "Infant Nutrition: A Guide for Professionals." Toronto, 1985.

Pennington, J.A., and H.N. Church. *Bowes and Church's Food Values of Portions Commonly Used.* J.B. Lippincott Company, 1985.

Phillipson, B.E., D.W. Rothrock, et al. "Reduction of Plasma Lipids, Lipoproteins, and Apoproteins by Dietary Fish Oils in Patients with Hypertriglyceridemia." *New England Journal of Medicine* 312 (1985): 1210-16.

Pusateri, D.J., et al. "Dietary and Hormonal Evaluation of Men at Different Risks for Prostate Cancer: Plasma and Fecal Hormone-Nutrient Interrelationships" *American Journal of Clinical Nutrition* 51. (March 1990): 371-377.

Ross, J.K., C. English, et al. "Dietary Fiber Constituents of Selected Fruits and Vegetables." *Journal of the American Dietetic Association* 85 (1985): 1111-16.

Rossignal, A.M. "Caffeine-Containing Beverages and Pre-Menstrual Syndrome in Young Women." *American Journal of Public Health* 75 (1985): 1335.

Siegel, R.K., M.A. Eisohly, et al. "Cocaine in Herbal Tea." *Journal of the American Medical Association* 255 (1986): 40.

Simopoulos, A.P., and T.B. Van Itallie. "Body Weight, Health, and Longevity." *Annals of Internal Medicine* 100 (1984): 285-94.

Slattery, M.L. "Dietary Calcium Intake as a Mitigating Factor in Colon Cancer." *American Journal of Epidemiology* 128 (March 1988): 504-514.

Spencer, H. "Minerals and Mineral Interactions in Human Beings." *Journal of the American Medical Association* 86 (1986): 864-67.

Spencer, H., and L. Kramer. "NIH Consensus Conference: Osteoporosis: Factors Contributing to Osteoporosis." *Journal of Nutrition* 116 (1986): 316-19.

Superko, H.R., et al. "Caffeinated and Decaffeinated Coffee Effects on Plasma Lipoprotein Cholesterol, Apolipoproteins and Lipase Activity: a Controlled Randomized Trial." *American Journal Clinical Nutrition* 54. (September 1991): 599-605.

Swiatlo, N., et al. "Relative Folate Bioavailability from Diets Containing Human, Bovine and Goat Milk." *Journal of Nutrition* 120. (February 1990): 172-177.

Thys-Jacobs, S., et al. "Calcium Supplementation in Premenstrual Syndrome: A Randomized Crossover Trial." *Journal General Internal Medicine* 4. (March 1989): 183-189.

United States. Department of Agriculture and Department of Health, Education and Welfare. "Nutrition and Your Health: Dietary Guidelines for Americans." 2d ed. Washington, D.C., 1985.

United States. National Academy of Sciences—National Research Council. Food and Nutrition Board. "Diet, Nutrition and Cancer." Washington, D.C., 1985.

United States. National Academy of Sciences—National Research Council. Food and Nutrition Board. "Recommended Dietary Allowances." 9th rev. ed. Washington, D.C. 1980.

Van Horn, L.V., K. Liu, et al. "Serum Lipid Response to Oat Product Intake with a Fat-Modified Diet." *Journal of the American Dietetic Association* 86 (1986): 759-64.

Van Dusseldorp, M., et al. "Effect of Decaffeinated versus Regular Coffee on Serum Lipoproteins: a 12-Week Double-blind Trial." *American Journal Epidemiology* 132. (July 1990): 33-40.

Watson, R.R., and T.K. Leonard. "Selenium and Vitamins A, E, and C: Nutrients with Cancer Prevention Properties." *Journal of the American Dietetic Association* 86 (1986): 505-510.

Wood, P.D. "The Science of Successful Weight Loss." *Medical and Health Annual* (1984).

Recipe Index

Subject Index

Additives, 42, 297, 298
Adolescents
    eating habits of, 253–55
    iron deficiency in, 14
    and vegetarian diet, 215
Aerobic exercise, 202–3, 210; see also
    Exercise
Aging, 255–58; see also Older adults
Alcohol, 177, 182–85
    and blood pressure, 13
    and breast-feeding, 248
    and exercise, 207
    and pregnancy, 183, 244
Alcohol and Caloric Content of Various
    Alcoholic Beverages, 184
Allergies, 294
    and breast-feeding, 246
    and infants, 249, 250
    and milk, 164–65
Amino acids, 36, 37, 214
Amphetamines, 295–96
Anemia, pernicious, 8
Anorexia nervosa, 254–55, 272
Arthritis, 273
Atherosclerosis, 22; see also Heart
    disease
Athletes and diet, 290–91; see also
    Exercise

Babies; see Infants
Barbecued foods, 300
Barley, 92
Beans, 44–45
Bee pollen, 290, 291
Beef, 39–40
Beta-carotene, 9, 126, 127–29
    Fruits and Vegetables Rich in Beta-
    Carotene, 128
Beverages, 126, 176–85, 207, 244,
    248; see also Alcohol, Caffeine,
    Milk, Water
Biotin, 7
Blood cholesterol; see Cholesterol
Blood pressure, 13, 16, 19, 162, 183
Blood sugar, 38–39, 179, 183, 187–89,
    206–7, 301
Body Mass Index (BMI), 272–73
    How to Find Your BMI, 273–75

Bones, 11, 19; see also Osteoporosis
Botulism, 42, 251, 289
Bran; see oats, oatbran; wheat, wheat
    bran
Bread, 84–85, 190, 191, 213
Breakfast, 39, 186–91
    and adolescents, 254
    and fast foods, 226
    and pregnancy, 245
Breast-feeding, 215–16, 245–49
Brunch, 191
Buckwheat, 92
Bulgur wheat, 89
Bulimia, 254–55, 272
Butter vs. margarine, 27

Caffeine, 179–82, 188–89, 294
    and athletic competitions, 291
    and breast-feeding, 248
    and pregnancy, 244
Caffeine Content of Various Foods and
    Medications, 180
Calcium, 38, 39, 162, 181
    and adolescents, 253, 255
    and blood pressure, 13
    deposits, 9
    described, 11–14, 162
    and exercise, 211
    and pregnancy, 244
    supplements, 14, 163, 300
    and vegetarian diet, 215–16
    see also Osteoporosis
Calcium Content of Various Foods, 12
Calories, 2
    in alcohol, 2, 183
    daily requirements, 244
    Energy Cost of Various Activities, 206
    Energy Requirements of Individuals,
    279
Canada's Food Guide For Healthy
    Eating, 1
Canadian Guidelines for Healthy
    Weights, 275
Cancer, 21, 30, 42, 43, 128–29, 162,
    182, 273
Carbohydrates, 2–3, 43, 83, 207; see
    also Grains, Starch, Sugar
Carcinogens, 21

Garlic, 130
Glucose, 3, 83, 295
Grains, 83–95, 213
Granola, 85–86
Grapefruit, 299

Hair analysis, 293
Heart disease, 7, 21–22, 30, 41, 128,
    162, 273
    and body weight, 273
    and exercise, 203
Hemoglobin, 14; *see also* Iron
Herbs, herbal teas, 185, 294
High-colonic enemas, 293–94
Honey, 3, 85, 289
    and botulism in infants, 251, 289
Hydrogenation, 28
Hypertension, 13, 16, 19, 162, 273
Hypoglycemia, 183, 301

Ice cream, 156, 168–70
Immune system, 246
Infants
    and allergies, 249
    and formula, 249
    and solid food, 250–51
    and vegetarian diet, 205
    see also Breast-feeding, Pregnancy
Iodine, 20
Iron, 14–15, 86, 89, 90, 244, 247
    and athletes, 211, 291–92
    and protein, 38, 39
    and older adults, 257
    and vegetarian diet, 215
Iron Content of Various Foods, 15

Kidney stones, 8, 14

Labels of products, 27, 84, 86, 164,
    258, 292, 297, 298, 300, 301
Lactose, 3, 43, 165
Lactose intolerance, 13, 165
Lead poisoning, 178–79, 185, 299
Lecithin, 289–90
Legumes, 30, 43–46
Lentils, 43, 45
"Light foods," 300
Linoleic acid, 6, 27
Lipoproteins (HDL, LDL, VLDL), 23, 26,
    28, 129–30, 183, 203

Magnesium, 19–20, 38, 89, 90, 300
Malnutrition, 182–83
Manganese, 20, 84, 89
Margarine vs. butter, 27

Meat, red, 38–39, 190, 213
Meats, luncheon, 42–43
Medication
    caffeine content of, 180
    and older adults, 257
Menopause, 2, 11, 211, 255–56
Milk, milk products, 9, 162–70,
    212–13
    and breakfast, 190
    maximum benefits from, 166–67
    nutrients in, 162–63
    storing, 212–13
    see also Dairy products, Lactose
        intolerance
Minerals, 6, 10–20, 215, 291
Moulds, 47, 296–97
Muffins, 94

"Natural foods," 298
Niacin, 7
Nitrates, nitrites, 42
Noodles, 92–93
Nutrients
    described, 1–20
    Nutrients in Canadian Foods,
        306–63
    Recommended Nutrient Intakes
        (RNI), 1
    *Recommended Nutrient Intakes for
        Canadians* (summary), 364–65
Nuts, 46–47

Oats, oat bran, 30, 31, 43, 79, 90–91,
    292
Obesity, 30–31, 253
Older adults, 256–58
    shopping tips for, 258
Omega-3 fatty acids, 27, 41–42, 193
Onions, and blood cholesterol, 129–30
Osteoporosis, 11, 162, 183, 253, 256, 257, 275

Palm oil, 26
Pantothenic acid, 7
Pasta, 92–93
Pasteurization, 166
Pastry, 94
Peanut butter, 47
Phosphorus, 14, 38, 89
Pollution, 42, 178–79
Popcorn, 90, 292–93
Potassium, 19
Poultry, 40, 190
Pregnancy
    and alcohol, 183, 244
    and caffeine, 181, 244

and diet, 8, 10, 16, 215–16, 243–45
and smoking, 244
see also Breast-feeding
Pre-Menstrual Syndrome, 7, 181
Preservatives, 85
Protein, 3, 36–48, 89, 90
Complementary Proteins, 37
excess, 39
for older adults, 257
sources of, 36–48, 84
and vegetarian diet, 36–37, 214–15
Pyridoxine (vitamin B$_6$), 7

Raw milk, 166
Restaurant food, 39, 190–92, 216–25, 297
Restaurant food, 39, 190–92, 216–25, 297
Riboflavin (vitamin B$_2$), 6–7, 44, 89, 90, 91
Rice, 91
Rye, 92

Salad bars, 132, 297
Salads, 166; *see also* Vegetables
Salt; *see* Sodium
Scurvy, 8
Seeds, 46–47
Selenium, 20, 42, 183
Seniors; *see* Older Adults
Singles, 212–13
Smoking
and breast-feeding, 248–49
and calcium balance, 13–14
effect on cholesterol, 23
and pregnancy, 244
Snack ideas, 252–53
Sodium, 13, 16–19, 42–43, 166, and blood pressure, 13
in cereals, 86
and exercise, 207
and pregnancy, 245
Sodium Content of Various Foods, 17–18
Soybeans, 45–46, 249
Starch, 83; *see also* Carbohydrates, Fibre, Grains
Stearic acid, 293
Stress, 23, 203–4
Sucrose, 43, 295
Sugar, 3, 43, 168
and cereals, 85–86
and exercise, 205, 207
vs. honey, 289

in snacks, 252
sources of, 3, 295
and weight control, 3
see also Blood sugar
Sugar Content of Popular Cereals, 87–88
sulphites, 297

Tea, 180
Teenagers; *see* Adolescents
Teeth, 13, 19, 163, 257
Thiamin (vitamin B$_1$), 6, 44, 89, 90, 91, 183
Tofu, 45–46
Trans fatty acids, 28, 301
Triglycerides, 23, 25, 183

Vegetables, 126–32, 213, 244
and beta-carotene, 128
and breakfast, 193
cruciferous, 128
and fibre, 126–27, 129
Fruits and Vegetables Rich in Beta-Carotene, 128
Fruits and Vegetables Rich in Vitamin C, 129
and hidden fats, 132
and cancer prevention, 128–29
storing and cooking, 130–32
and vitamin C, 129, 130–31
Vegetarian diet, 36–37, 38, 45, 164, 213–16
Vitamins, 6–10, 38
supplements, 291
Vitamin A, 9, 14, 90, 126, 128, 163
Vitamin B$_1$ (thiamin), 6, 44, 89, 90, 91, 183
Vitamin B$_2$ (riboflavin), 6–7, 44, 89, 90, 91
Vitamin B6 (pyridoxine), 7
Vitamin B12, 8, 215
Vitamin C, 8, 16, 43, 126, 127–29, 130–31, 215
Fruits and Vegetables Rich in Vitamin C, 129
Vitamin D, 9, 14, 163, 216
Vitamin E, 9–10, 20, 84, 127
Vitamin K, 10

Walking, 205
Water, 19, 127, 176–78, 207, 244, 248; *see also* Beverages